Longevity and Life Preservation in Eastern Medicine

Longevity and Life Preservation in Eastern Medicine

Written by Lee Je-ma
Translated by Choi Seung-hoon

Kyung Hee University Press

Longevity and Life Preservation in Eastern Medicine

Written by Lee Je-ma, Translated by Choi Seung-hoon

Published by Kyung Hee University Press,
1 Hoegi-dong Dongdaemun-gu, Seoul 130-701, Republic of Korea
http://www.khupress.com

First edition published in 1996
Revised edition published in 2009

ISBN 978-89-8222-319-8 93510

Dedicated to my wife, Sung-hye,
and our children, Su-on and Kyu-ha,
and to all those who share Lee Je-ma's dreams.

On the Revised Edition of "Longevity and Life Preservation in Eastern Medicine"

More than ten years has passed since "Longevity and Life Preservation in Oriental Medicine" was published at the end of 1996. There is a traditional proverb mentioning "ten years can change even nature (rivers and hills, originally)."

Without exception, in the field of traditional medicine, there have been a number of innovations over the last ten years. Above all accomplishments, the development of 『*WHO International Standard Terminologies on Traditional Medicine in the Western Pacific Region* (*WHO-IST*)』, which was published in 2007 by the Western Pacific Regional Office for the WHO, could be listed as the most profound progress in the traditional medicine world.

Fortunately, I had a chance to be in the center of the project as the Regional Adviser in traditional medicine, working for the Western Pacific Regional Office of the WHO. As I was driving the project, I felt a strong demand to revise the "Longevity and Life Preservation in Oriental Medicine" personally. I could confess that my experience involved in the translation of "Longevity and Life Preservation in Oriental Medicine" twelve years ago was an undeniable cause to promote the development of *WHO-IST*.

Then I decided to change even the title of the book to "Longevity and Life Preservation in Eastern Medicine." In addition, I made some corrections and modifications based upon *WHO-IST*. Through such endeavours, I hope Sasang Constitutional Medicine will become more globalized as Lee Je-ma

(李濟馬) dreamed more than one hundred years ago.

2009. 7. 10

Choi Seung-hoon

Preface

Over a hundred years ago, Philosopher Lee Je-ma left his will as follows; "The Sasang Constitutional Medicine will hold sway over the world a century hence." Now is the time Philosopher Lee predicted.

Born in the social turmoil of the latter part of the Joseon dynasty, Philosopher Lee Je-ma experienced the difficulties of the times. He diligently studied the liberal and martial arts, and especially medical science. Throughout his thoroughgoing life, he grafted an Oriental Medicine based on the traditions of Taoism to Confucianism, and established new guidelines in the field of philosophy and medical science. Philosopher Lee is the great genius in the history of science of Korea.

"The Sasang Constitutional Medicine" initiated by Philosopher Lee is not a universal theory applicable to everybody, but a philanthropic philosophy respecting the diversity of individuals. Philosopher Lee refuted totalitarian reasoning, and instead espoused a liberal and democratic approach to the field of medicine.

It was in 1965 that I first encountered the philosophy of Lee Je-ma. Not having then a profound knowledge of Oriental Medicine, I read the 『*Dongui Suse Bowon*』 at the prodding of my colleagues. After reading the book, I was deeply touched by the philosophical profundity of Lee Je-ma. I also resolved to transform the Dongyang Medical College, which was experiencing financial difficulties, into present day Kyung Hee University's College of Oriental

Medicine. It is remarkable that his philosophy, fully elaborated over a hundred years, offers such brilliant insights, though it is not perfect for our times. Most notable is his categorization of the physical constitution into four types, and his development of therapeutics for the respective types; both contributions reaffirmed the eminence of Korean Oriental Medicine.

Since the national liberation of Korea, Oriental Medicine has enjoyed the full interest and love from the Korean people, thanks to the noble efforts of the Oriental Medicine societies centered on Kyung Hee University. With such great public interest and support, Sasang Constitutional Medicine can finally be disseminated nationwide, and Lee Je-ma's prediction realized.

We have a historical mission of developing our traditional medicine by following Lee Je-ma's philosophy and of creating a "Third Medicine" through the ideal combination of Oriental and Western medical traditions. In order to accomplish this, we have to do our best in globalizing Philosopher Lee Je-ma's Sasang Constitutional Medicine. In this regard, Dr. Choi Seung-hoon's publication of the English version of the 『*Dongui Suse Bowon*』 is a very meaningful and important event. I would like to take this opportunity to express my wholehearted congratulations and best wishes to Dr. Choi Seung-hoon, who is now playing a critical role in creating a Third Medicine with his noble devotion to the globalization of Sasang Constitutional Medicine.

1996. 12. 5

Choue Young-seek

Chancellor of Kyung Hee University System

Translator's Note

The『*Dongui Suse Bowon*』consists of two parts: basic theory and clinical studies. Lee Je-ma opens his basic theory by defining the environments that surround man and the body itself using a quarternary paradigm. This paradigm is an extension of the Confucian tradition in employing the number four.

The terminology, which Lee Je-ma employs, is quite hard to understand as his philosophical ideas are of his own development based on Neo-Confucianism (新儒學). Even widely experienced Oriental medical doctors find it hard to comprehend, which has resulted in many doctors exhibiting interest only in the clinical aspects. However, understanding his philosophical attitude is required prior to studying his Sasang Constitutional Medicine. Additionally, a thorough understanding of the『*Shanghanlun*』(傷寒論: "Treatise on Cold-induced Diseases") written by Zhang Zhongjing (張仲景) is a prerequisite to understanding Lee Je-ma's clinical studies.

As a translator, I have tried to translate the terminology literally and avoided including my own interpretations, so as to allow the readers to understand Lee Je-ma's original words.

The terminology used in the translation, such as stomach and blood, which can be translated into English without much difficulty, does not necessarily denote the stomach and blood as understood in western medicine. Those words having no equivalents in English have been inscribed phonetically in italic letters. Some of the terms newly employed in this translation are provided with explanations or footnotes in brackets; this also applies to the names of prescriptions. To pervent confusion, all titles of books are written in italic letters inside the punctuation marks 『』.

The following table of the pinyin phonetic alphabet shows pronunciations with approximate English equivalents. In parentheses are the corresponding letters in the Wade-Giles system.

Pronunciation Guide

a	(a) as in *father*
b	(b) as in *book*
c	(ts', tz') like *ts* in *its*
ch	(ch) as in *church*, strongly aspirated
d	(t) as in *door*
e	(e) as in *her*
f	(f) as in *finger*
g	(k) as in *go*
h	(h) as in *her*, strongly aspirated
i	(i) like the vowel sound in *eat* or the *i* in *sir*
j	(ch) as in *jeep*
k	(k') as in *kite*, strongly aspirated
l	(l) as in *love*
m	(m) as in *me*
n	(n) as in *no*
o	(o) like the vowel sound in *law*
p	(p') as in *park*, strongly aspirated
q	(ch') like the *ch* in *cheese*

r	(r) as in *red of*
s	(s, ss, sz) as in *sister*
sh	(sh) as in *show*
t	(t') as in *tough*, strongly aspirated
u	(u) as in *too*; also in the French *tu*
w	(w) semi-vowel in syllables begin ning with *u* when not preceded by' conso nants, pronounced as in *want*
x	(hs) like *sh* in *sheety*
y	semi-vowel in syllables beginning with *i* or *u* when not preceded by consonants, pronounced as in *yes*
z	(ts, tz) as in *zone*
zh	(ch) like the first consonant in *jump*
ai	like *ie* in *pie*
ao	like *ow* in *how*
ei	like *ay* in *day*
ie	like *ie* in *experience*
ou	like *oe* in *toe*

Acknowledgements

In 1989, I was fortunate to be the first visiting professor from Korea to teach at China Medical College, currently China Medical University in Taiwan. There, I had an opportunity to teach a graduate course in English about the『*Dongui Suse Bowon*』(東醫壽世保元). That opportunity laid the foundation, which inspired me to further my study of Lee Je-ma and to launch this task, one of the most meaningful endeavors in my life. I wish to express my gratitude to China Medical College and its graduate students.

This work is a product of the many people who volunteered their time, energies and talents in countless ways.

Professor Moon Joon-jeon, who showed me the joys of scholastic pursuit, and Professor Kim Young-oak, who taught me how to be a true scholar. Chancellor Choue Young-seek, the founder of Kyung Hee University, who, early on, suggested the birth of a third medicine through the development of an East-West Cooperative Medicine, and who gave both financial and moral support to this task. And the patrons organized by Chancellor Choue, Professor Song Il-byung, Professor Goh Byung-hee of Kyung Hee University, and other scholars of the Sasang Medical Society whose input during our group discussions was truly invaluable.

My assistants and students: Dr. Shim Bum-sang, Dr. Park Gyeong-mo, Dr. Lee Neung-ki, Dr. Lee Hang-jae, Dr. Kim Sung-woo, and Dr. Jang Hwan-sun and Sun- woo in Los Angeles. Their energies and efforts in all the tasks–big and small–I assigned, kept the project alive. Professor Fred J. Seligson of Hankuk University of Foreign Studies, who since my college days has been my big brother in heart and spirit; to Professor Kim Nam-hee of Chung-ang Sangha College, Andy Douglas of Iowa State University, and especially my student, David Rhee from the University of Chicago, all of whom helped the project to take shape.

There were many others who were truly unsparing with their assistances to the completion of this task. I regret I could not name them all.

Finally, I thank the Lord, who sent the great man, Lee Je-ma, to our nation, Korea, and who also allowed me to bring Lee Je-ma's dream to fruition by opening the doors of Sasang Constitutional Medicine to the world.

1996. 12. 5

CONTENTS

PART Ⅲ

PART Ⅳ

PART V

PART VI

Introduction

Traditional Chinese medicine (TCM) regards the human body as a black box, and diagnoses the condition of the internal organs by their external manifestations. Every individual's face, shape and temperament are different. TCM understands that each human being has a different internal structure, as do the main organs. TCM also recognizes that those differences can be categorized as certain types. For example, in the『*Lingshu*』(靈樞: "Miraculous Pivot"), the bible of TCM, the discourses of the 'Tongtian' (通天: "Communication with Heaven") and the 'Yinyang Ershewuren'(陰陽二十五人: "Yin - yang with Twenty Five Types of People") present very sophisticated theories using yin-yang and five phases ideas as categorizing guidelines.

Confucianism (儒家) and Taoism (道家) have traditionally dominated Chinese thought. While Confucianism has become the root and trunk of the philosophy applied to political, social and moral problems, Taoism represents Chinese natural science. This includes TCM, which, from the beginning, has been totally rooted in Taoist thought. In ancient times, the natural environment directly affected living conditions, but as human science and civilization developed, the relationship between man and nature became less important than the relationship between man and his social environment. The incidence of mental or psychological problems from social relationships increased relative to that of physical diseases from the natural environment.

TCM doctors, who had been mostly concerned with the physical universe (the Taoist mind), gradually realized the importance of our mental and moral natures, which are the main objects of Confucian philosophy. Consequently, Confucianism and Taoism became unified under the auspices of Sasang (four types) Constitutional Medicine (SCM).

The influence of TCM had made human beings passive by putting more emphasis on the natural environment rather than on themselves. However, the theories of SCM tell us that men can control both their physical and mental condition through their own efforts. In this way, we are presented with a method of treating people that does more than just eliminate the pathogenic factors (邪氣) as in TCM focusing on man's relationship with natural influences. This new medicine can do that and also transforms what we are at our core. Even though SCM is an encounter between Taoist and Confucian thought, it essentially adopts a TCM view of pathogenesis. This includes the concept that healthy qi (正氣) is the first consideration in promoting health and treating disease. TCM states that disease occurs when the pathogen is stronger than the healthy qi. Therefore, the primary treatment principle is the cultivation and preservation of healthy qi. However, the compositions of quantity and quality of healthy qi are different in each individual. There are some people with more yang qi, while others have more yin blood. While the 『*Huangdi Neijing*』(黃帝內經: "Huangdi's Internal Classic") and Chinese medical doctors had a vague concept of constitution and only touched upon constitutional problems superficially, SCM has extensively and systematically resolved this issue. SCM focuses on the different constitutional manifestations of the individual's nature and emotions. A person's nature and emotions drive the ascending and descending of qi in the body, and this dynamic of the qi's ascent and descent shapes the different types of structures, functions and temperaments.

The ideas of the『*Huangdi Neijing*』,『*Shanghanlun*』and Confucianism have existed for a long time, but each took a different path. The prototypes of the four constitutional types (greater yang, lesser yang, greater yin and lesser yin) were brought forth in the discourses of the 'Tongtian' in the『*Huangdi Neijing*』, and the treatment principle of each constitutional type is rooted in the『*Shanghanlun*』. For the Confucianist element, the『*Zhongyong*』(中庸 : The

"Doctrine of the Mean") discusses in depth the four emotions: sorrow, anger, joy and pleasure.

Taoism and Confucianism finally meet in SCM. This has allowed the physical and mental planes of human beings to actually meet and become one. At the same time, it is also a successful unification of philosophy and science. Herein lies the greatness of SCM.

It is an interesting question as to how SCM bore fruit in Korea, and not in China where Confucianism, Taoism and TCM originated. Since the two countries have the same Taoist tradition, we cannot find any further clues in the Taoistic field. Therefore, we need to compare the two countries' Confucianist history. During the Song dynasty (宋代), through the neo-Confucianist Zhu Xi (朱熹: 1130-1200), Confucianism underwent a huge revival and spread throughout large areas of Asia, including the Joseon (朝鮮) kingdom. At that time, China and Joseon held a common Confucian tradition. However, after that period, China passed on to the metaphysics of the Ming (明) and Qing (淸) dynasties and continued changing and evolving with the doctrines of Wang Yangming (王陽明) and the bibliographical study of Chinese classics. This trend did not take hold in Joseon. During the Joseon dynasty, the country was absolutely controlled by the neo-Confucianist philosophy for hundreds of years. The rigidness and absoluteness of authority favored by neo-Confucianism brought much hardship to the people and stifled the gradual development of new ideas. However, towards the end of Joseon, centuries of repressed creativity and suffering led to an explosion. In contrast, China did not experience such a revolution, but rather underwent a gradual change from one new system to another. As modern western science sprang out from the long, dark Middle Ages, the new revolutionary Confucianist mind, which gave birth to SCM was able to spring out of these difficult times at the end of the Joseon dynasty. This was the climate into which SCM's founder Lee Je-ma – a Confucianist doctor – was born.

Just before his death, Lee Je-ma predicted that SCM would become a universal medicine in one hundred years. In recent decades, TCM has disclosed its long-held medical secrets and made significant inroads in the West. As an advanced type of TCM, still following the essence of TCM and its techniques, SCM, now presented in English, can move on to worldwide renown and application.

Life Story of Lee Je-ma

Lee Je-ma was born in 1836, during the reign of King Heonjong (憲宗), in the Joseon dynasty. His birthplace was Cheonseo Township (川西面), Hamheung County (咸興郡), Hamgyeong Province (咸鏡道), in northern Korea. He lived for 64 years and died in 1900. The period in which he lived was chaotic, with extreme political confusion mainly caused by party strife. There were serious economic difficulties, and the people were dissatisfied with the seemingly endless internal and external problems. The Joseon dynasty finally collapsed in 1910.

The founder of the Joseon dynasty was King Taejo (太祖), who was born in Yeongheung County (永興郡) in Hamgyeong Province. He did not like the temperament of the northern people and began a tradition that lasted for more than 500 years: no one fr:m the north, not even a man of talent, would be appointed to a high-ranking official post. Because of this, none of Lee Je-ma's family in the past 20 generations had been given a government post. Finally, his father, Lee Ban-o (李攀五), passed the civil -and military-service exams, and became a noble in the northern part of the nation.

There is an interesting story about the birth of Lee Je-ma. One day, Je-ma's father was coming home from the school where he was studying Confucian philosophy. On the road he ran into some of his friends, who were drinking at a tavern.

An older barmaid lived there with her daughter, still single but made unmarriageable by age. The daughter was not very attractive, being gifted with neither beauty nor intelligence. Because of this, the barmaid realized that it would be difficult to find a husband for her daughter.

Ban-o was not accustomed to drinking, but on that evening, his friends persuaded him to join them. He soon lost consciousness and remained in the tavern sleeping. At twilight, his friends left, asking the barmaid to take care of him. The barmaid thought that this was a good opportunity to try to bring her daughter and the young nobleman together, so she made a bed for him and sent her daughter in to warm it.

One day, ten months later at dawn, Ban-o's father was asleep and having a marvelous dream. He was given a charming colt by a mysterious person and told, "This colt is from Jeju (濟州) Island. No one claims it. I am giving it to you. Please feed it and take good care of it." The person tied the colt to a stake and disappeared. Ban-o's father looked at the colt and found it lovely and attractive. He was patting the colt on its back when he woke up.

Ban-o's father was pondering his wonderful dream when he heard someone calling from the gate. His servant opened the gate and brought the guests to him. The lady said, "This is your son's baby. Please accept him."

Ban-o's father called his son and asked him how this could have happened. Even though the younger Lee had been drunk, he was able to remember everything and told his father the truth. On any other day, the new grandfather might have been angry, but recalling his special dream, he decided that it was a good omen. The baby and the mother were taken in. Grandfather Lee named the baby Je-ma, after his dream's Jeju Island and Ma (meaning 'horse'). The elder Lee thus had always expected his grandson to become a great man, and showered the child with love.

Since Ban-o had not as yet sired any children, he was able to enter Je-ma's name into the family register as legitimate offspring. However, the feudalistic society did not accept Je-ma. His birth from unmarried parents left him with physical and mental barriers to overcome.

By nature, Je-ma was a very cheerful and brave boy. Moreover, his grandfather's heartfelt love nourished and supported him. Because of this, in later years, Je-ma left a will to his descendants, which declared that his grandfather was to be considered the founder of their line.

When Je-ma turned seven, he was sent to be taught by his uncle. He studied one to ten pages every day. There was, at first, concern that he seldom reviewed his lessons; but the next morning, Je-ma would always recite what he had learned the previous day.

During childhood, Je-ma was more fond of the military arts than of reading or writing. When young Je-ma played outside, he always chose a sword or a bow and arrow. Je-ma wanted to be a military commander when he grew up.

One day, while studying the『*Tongshi*』(通史: "Introduction to History"), young Je-ma came upon a sentence, which read, "··· Warrior Xiang Yu (項羽) committed suicide at Niao River (烏江) ···." He closed the book. The legendary hero Xiang Yu had incredible strength and was strong enough to move a mountain, but life had been harsh, and he suffered a miserable fate. Je-ma sighed, "Alas! It is so sad" and cried. His family and teachers were astonished at how a seven-year-old boy could experience such mature insight.

When Je-ma was thirteen years old, his uncle gave a poetry examination to all the young scholars. While all of the scholars were concentrating on their exam, Je-ma came in and got a piece of paper. He quickly wrote something on it and left. When Je-ma's writing won first place, all the scholars were surprised, and they began to admire Je-ma.

Because of Je-ma's illegitimate birth, he was discriminated against by many of the townspeople. This affected his temperament, and he found that he could not control his anger. It was during this same time that Joseon society was experiencing instability. Je-ma could not bear these burdens in his hometown, so he left home at the age of thirteen.

For many long years, between the ages of fourteen and forty, Je-ma led a wandering life. Many of the details of this period, including those of his whereabouts, are unknown, but it is clear that this period had a great influence on his knowledge and writing. What is known is that this period was spent seeking the ultimate truth.

According to various scholars' research, at thirty, Lee Je-ma had the rare opportunity to read the 『*Myeongseonlok*』(明善錄: "Book of Illuminating Goodness") written by Han Seok-ji (韓錫地). This book criticized the metaphysics of the Joseon dynasty, overburdened with academic discussion. The 『*Myeongseonlok*』 made brave assertions for that era and contained very original thinking. Joseon Confucianists who followed the government's philosophy would have deemed this book politically harmful. For this reason, Han Seok-ji had requested that his descendants withhold the book from the public. Je-ma stayed at the home of Han's descendants for a while during the time of his search for the truth. This is how he had the opportunity to read this book, which was unpublished at the time. Later, the 『*Myeongseonlok*』 was to become an important book in Korean academic society. Je-ma was inspired to systematize Han's thoughts. Je-ma acknowledged Han's work from then on, and wrote books to spread Han's thoughts to the world. As a result, he became the target of criticism.

Je-ma studied for three years with Gi Jeong-jin (奇正鎭), who developed a creative type of metaphysics. Je-ma suffered from *jieyi* (generalized fatigue and lassitude) disease, which inspired Gi Jeong-jin to tell him that he was a genius, but one who needed to learn humility and control his quick temper. Je-ma followed Gi's directions and his health improved.

Je-ma's thought was influenced by the ideas of Han Seok-ji and Gi Jeong-jin. At the end of the 19th century, in eastern Asia, in the small town of Joseon, the foundation of Sasang Constitutional Medicine came to maturity through the insightful teachings of his talented mentors.

Je-ma was ill for a long period of time. This illness enabled him to discover SCM. Je-ma suffered from generalized fatigue and lassitude, *yege* (dysphagia) and *fanwei* (regurgitation of food from stomach). He knew that these diseases tend to affect a greater yang person. Generalized fatigue and lassitude results in restriction of movement to the upper body, preventing the lower limbs from functioning properly, but it is neither a paralysis nor is it accompanied by swelling or pain. According to the 『*Neijing*』(內經: "Canon of Internal Medicine"), generalized fatigue and lassitude appears as weakness, but in reality is not. Moreover, the symptoms resemble those of sthenia. It is also mistaken for a coldness disease or a febrile disease. It was, in a word, very hard to identify.

Je-ma's Liver and Kidney channels were depleted; the *chi* (cubit) pulse was slow and choppy. Heat stagnating in the middle-*jiao* caused the slow pulse. The choppy pulse was caused by collapse of the blood. These symptoms rarely happen to the greater yin type or the lesser yin type. When they do, it is as a complication of another disease.

Lumbar vertebral disease affecting the greater yang type causes the lower limbs to be too weak to walk. The kidney is located in the lumbar region. These symptoms occur when someone is in deep sorrow. Symptoms of dysphagia and regurgitation of food from the stomach are different, but the causes are identical. The small intestine qi is blocked. Dysphagia creates difficulty in swallowing (gagging), or results in vomiting soon after the food is swallowed. Regurgitation of food from the stomach is milder than dysphagia, with the person vomiting in the evening whatever he ate in the morning, and vice versa. A person with this disease should not eat greasy food. He should also avoid anger and sorrow. According to the 『*Neijing*』, at certain times, yin qi should predominate, but does not; at other times, yang qi should predominate, but does not.

Je-ma suffered from the above-mentioned diseases. He had been treated with traditional medicine, but never had been cured. Je-ma became aware that each individual's constitution is different, and that the symptoms and treatment of disease depend on the individual's constitution. At this point, Je-ma devoted his life to research the constitutional types. After a long period, he was finally cured, but people were frightened of him because he acted like an insane man trying to refine his theories on SCM.

For example, one day, a lady came in with a severe illness. Je-ma had a difficult time defining which constitutional type she belonged to. The lady was shy and did not express any emotion, which he needed to observe in order to make a proper diagnosis. Je-ma decided to use a trick and asked the other people to leave the room. When he was alone with the lady, he asked her to take off her clothes one piece at a time. She could not disobey him, because in those days, one always did as the doctor asked, but she felt ashamed. When the patient was left wearing only her undergarments, Je-ma asked her to take off everything. She was about to stand up, when Je-ma tugged on her underwear. The lady was astonished at his dishonorable attitude and she screamed, thinking that he was trying to rape her. In this display of emotion, he was able to figure out her original nature. She was then asked to put her clothes back on. He decided that her constitution was of the lesser yang type, and he used the proper medication to cure her. This sort of medical subterfuge was resorted to many times during the process of his research.

Choi Lin (崔麟) wrote in his autobiography, "When I was ill, I went to see Je-ma to be treated by him. In order for him to know my constitutional type, he analyzed my handwriting and palpated my arms and legs. Later, he took me to a detached room, reserved for men only, and asked me to carry firewood, which I did three times. This was to see my movements and complete the diagnosis. He figured out that I was of the lesser yin type and prescribed medication that cured me." This type of diagnostic method was common with Lee Je-ma.

Je-ma was a philosopher as well as a doctor, writing several books, including the『*Cheonyucho*』(闡幽抄: "Writings of Elucidations"),『*Jejung Sinpyeon*』(濟衆新編: "New Compilation for Relieving People"),『*Gwangjeseol*』(廣濟說: "Discourse on General Health Maintenance"),『*Gyeokchigo*』(格致藁: "Draft on an Inquiry into the Properties of Things") and『*Dongui Suse Bowon*』(東醫壽世保元: "Longevity and Life Preservation in Eastern Medicine"). The『*Cheonyucho*』was only two or three pages long, but its denotation is so profound that it is difficult to comprehend the contents. The purpose of these works was to provide lessons to his disciples; he did not intend them to be handed down to posterity.

The『*Gwangjeseol*』teaches about the care of the health and states: "Therefore, being jealous of the wise and able is the most prevalent disease in the world. Respecting the wise and practicing virtue is the greatest medicine in the world." In order for us to live a long and healthy life, we should distinguish right from wrong and be ethical in all our actions. The『*Gwangjeseol*』was added while the『*Dongui Suse Bowon*』was in the process of being edited. The『*Jejung Sinpyeon*』was written on ethics and attached to the『*Gyeokchigo*』as an appendix.

Je-ma began writing the『*Gyeokchigo*』at the age of forty four. It took him thirteen years to complete the book. It progressed intermittently, showing us the development of his thoughts. The ideas of this book are a completion of Confucianism and, at the same time, helped open up a new path for Joseon philosophy.

While Je-ma was writing the 『*Jejung Sinpyeon*』, he passed the special military service examination and was appointed head of the Jinhae District (鎭海縣). He was fifty years old at the time and interested in medical research. He completed the 『*Gyeokchigo*』 seven years later in 1893, and began work on the 『*Dongui Suse Bowon*』. This book is a continuation of the 『*Gyeokchigo*』's philosophy, and is an achievement of Joseon Confucianism. It opened up new academic possibilities during the Joseon dynasty.

Neither in the East nor in the West did most of the medical world recognize the specific characteristics of an individual's constitution, as human beings and specific diseases were all considered to have the same nature. This thinking has been an obstacle in preventing effective treatment, and also had led to less than desirable results. The internal organs are different because of the individual's constitution; if recovery from disease depends on the patient's reaction to the medicine, then prevention, treatment principles and prescriptions ought to be different for each different type. In the 『*Dongui Suse Bowon*』, Je-ma classified the constitutional types of human beings into greater yang type, lesser yang type, greater yin type and lesser yin type, thus introducing SCM as a new accomplishment presenting constitutional physiology, pathology and its treatment.

After he finished writing the 『*Dongui Suse Bowon*』, Je-ma returned to his hometown. He quelled a rebellion, which occurred in Gangwon Province (江原道), and was appointed to be the acting provincial governor of Hamheung for his meritorious deed. He retired from his government position at the age of 62 in 1898. Later, he opened a private clinic, named Bowon-guk (保元局: Clinic for Life Preservation) in the city of Hamheung.

Je-ma again devoted himself to medical research and revised the 『*Dongui Suse Bowon*』. He revised the discourses from the 'Origin of Eastern Medicine' to the 'Lesser Yin Person's Disease', although the discourse on the 'Greater Yang Person's Disease' was never touched and has remained in its original form.

In Je-ma's later years, he offered treatment to the poor. When he was recompensed, he only accepted a small amount of hulled millet. He did not want to exchange money for treatment, and was not preoccupied with worldly gain. His second son, Yong-su (龍水), took over Je-ma's clinic after he died.

One day, Je-ma went to his hometown with his disciples to choose his own grave. He selected a place, which looked wonderful. However, when the disciples took a good look, they saw that, in *fengshui* (風水) terms, there was a white tiger on the right side, but no blue dragon on the left. The disciples pointed this out to him. Then Je-ma responded, "It is only temporary; the water dragon will come by and by," and decided on that place. The disciples were doubtful as to the auspiciousness of this location, but in the year he died, a reservoir was built, creating the missing water dragon. The disciples were astonished at his foresight.

Lee Je-ma died at the age of 64 in 1900. He left a will that states as follows: "One hundred years after I die, Sasang Constitutional Medicine will dominate the world."

Chronological Table of Lee Je-ma's Life

Age	Year	Historical Events	Personal History	Academic Works	Medical Works
1	1837		Born in Hamheung City (Mar. 9)		
7	1843		Began to study under his uncle		
13	1849		Took first place in regional exam., left home		
14 - 29	1850 - 1865		Details of his where-abouts are unknown		
30	1866	The invasion of Kangwha Island by a French Fleet		Read 「*Myeongseonlok*」	
39	1875				Administered *Liuwei Dihuang Tang* to a *mangyin* patient
44	1880			Began to write 「*Gyeokchigo*」	
46	1882	The Military Revolt			
50	1886		Passed the special military exam., appointed in charge of the Jinhae District and its army		
57	1893			Finished writing 「*Gyeokchigo*」	Began to write 「*Dongui Suse Bowon*」 (Jul. 13)
58	1894	Donghak Revolution			Finished writing 「*Dongui Suse Bowon*」 (Apr. 13)
59	1895		Returned to his home-town	Began to write 「*Jejung Sinpyeon*」 (Nov. 24)	
60	1896	Choi Moon-hwan's Revolution	Supressed Choi Moon-hwan's Revolution and appointed in charge of Gowon County		
61	1897	Korean Empire began		Finished writing 「*Jejung Sinpyeon*」	
62	1898		Resigned from public life and opened his private clinic		Administered *Jingfang Dihuanang Tang* to a *mangyin* patient. Revised and modified 「*Dongui Suse Bowon*」
64	1900	Opening of the Kyungin Railway	Died (Sep. 21)		

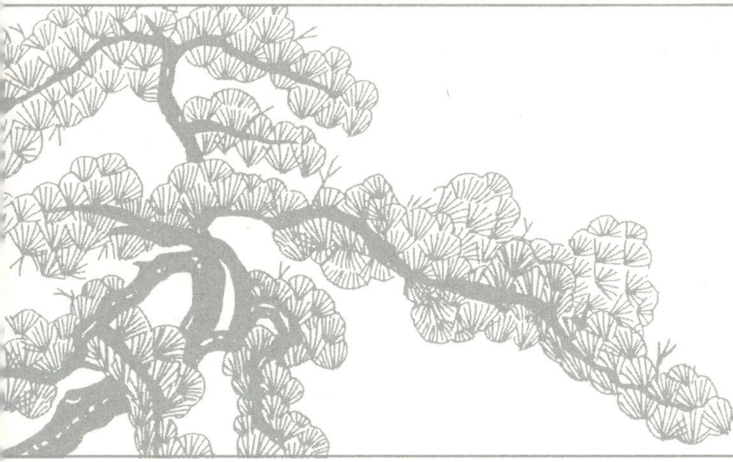

PART I

1

Discourse on Nature and Order*

1 There are four environmental frames: locality, human relationships, social relationships, and times of heaven.

2 There are four human affairs: living quarters, clanships, social acquaintances and appointed roles.

3 The ears are capable of hearing times of heaven. The eyes are capable of seeing social relationships. The nose is capable of smelling human relationships. The mouth is capable of tasting locality.

4 Times of heaven are extremely variable. Social relationships are extremely extensive. Human relationships are extremely wide. Locality is extremely diverse.

5 The Lung executes appointed roles well. The Spleen harmonizes social acquaintances. The Liver establishes clanships. The Kidney determines living quarters.

6 Appointed roles should be well developed. Social acquaintances should be well arranged. Clanships should be well organized. Living quarters should be well managed.

---

* 性命論

7 There is cleverness in the jaw. There is administration in the chest. There is moderation in the navel. There is generosity in the abdomen.

8 Cleverness should not be arrogant. Administration should not be overconfident. Moderation should not be too domineering. Generosity should not be excessive.

9 There is discernment in the head. There is nobility in the shoulders. There is resourcefulness in the waist. There is method in the hips.

10 Discernment should not be deprived. Nobility should not be extravagant. Resourcefulness should not be idle. Method should not include pilfering.

11 The ears, eyes, nose and mouth perceive the environment. The Lung, Spleen, Liver and Kidney are established among human affairs. The jaw, chest, navel and abdomen actualize wisdom. The head, shoulders, waist and hips add conduct to action.

Environmental frames (Sensory organ)	Times of heaven	Social relationships	Human relationships	Locality
	Ears	Eyes	Nose	Mouth
Human affairs (Organ)	Appointed roles	Social acquaintances	Clanships	Living quarters
	Lung	Spleen	Liver	Kidney
Wisdom (Body)	Cleverness	Administration	Moderation	Generosity
	Jaw	Chest	Navel	Abdomen
Action (Body)	Discernment	Nobility	Resourcefulness	Method
	Head	Shoulders	Waist	Hips

12 Times of heaven are universal. Appointed roles are established individually. Social relationships are universal. Social acquaintances are established individually. Human relationships are universal. Clanships are established individually. Localities are universal. Living quarters are established individually.

13 Cleverness is universally accepted. Discernment is undertaken individually. Administration is universally accepted. Nobility is undertaken individually. Moderation is universally accepted. Resourcefulness is expressed

individually. Generosity is universally accepted. Method is carried out individually.

14 The universally renowned is heaven. The individually established is human. The generally accepted is nature. The individually generated is order.

15 The ears are fond of pleasant sounds. The eyes are fond of beautiful colors. The nose is fond of sweet smells. The mouth is fond of good tastes.

16 Pleasant sounds please the ears. Beautiful colors please the eyes. Sweet smells please the nose. Good tastes please the mouth.

17 The Lung dislikes unpleasant sounds. The Spleen dislikes ugly colors. The Liver dislikes unpleasant odors. The Kidney dislikes bad-tasting foods.

18 Unpleasant sounds displease the Lung. Ugly colors displease the Spleen. Unpleasant odors displease the Liver. Bad tastes displease the Kidney.

19 There can be an arrogant mind in the jaw. There can be an overconfident mind in the chest. There can be a domineering mind in the navel. There can be a boastful mind in the abdomen.

20 The arrogant mind is arrogant intention. The overconfident mind is confident thinking. The domineering mind is domineering resolution. The boastful mind is boastful will.

21 There is covetousness in the head. There is extravagance in the shoulders. There is idleness in the waist. There is greed in the hips.

22 Covetousness has a tendency to deprive others of their share. Extravagance is prone to self-glorification. Idleness is inclined towards self-loathing. Greed is disposed to steal.

23 There is nothing comparable to the fondness that human ears, eyes, nose and mouth have for the good, and the dislike that the Lung, Spleen, Liver and Kidney have for the bad. There is nothing comparable to the wickedness of the human jaw, chest, navel and abdomen, and the idleness of the human head, shoulders, waist and hips.

24 King Yao[1] and King Shun[2] reigned with perfect virtue 5,000 years ago, and to this day, people mention their names when it comes to virtue. This demonstrates that there is nothing comparable to the people's love for virtue. King Chieh[3] and King Chou[4] governed with tyranny 4,000 years ago, and everyone mentions their names when it comes to vice. This demonstrates that there is nothing comparable to the people's hatred for vice. Three thousand disciples studied under Confucius[5], but only Yen Hui did not stray from perfect virtue for three months. Among the rest, only 72 disciples did the same for only a few days to a month, but no longer were their hearts filled with joy in following Confucius. This demonstrates that there is nothing comparable to the people's wickedness. There was a king, Wen[6], to whom all virtue belonged, the virtue which prevailed for a hundred years. King Wu[7] and the Duke of Zhou succeeded Wen's achievements until virtue widely prevailed. Nevertheless, Kwan Shu and Chai Shu promoted a rebellion against their brother, the Duke of Zhou, so this demonstrates that there is nothing comparable to the people's idleness.

25 Therefore, through the ears, eyes, nose and mouth, everyone can become like King Yao and King Shun; but through the jaw, chest, navel and abdomen, not everyone can spontaneously become like Yao and Shun. Through the Lung, Spleen, Liver and Kidney, everyone can become Yao and Shun; but through the head, shoulders, waist and hips, not everyone can spontaneously be Yao and Shun.

26 When people's ears, eyes, nose and mouth love goodness, their minds are not inferior to Yao's and Shun's mind. When people's Lung, Spleen, Liver and Kidney detest vice, their minds are not inferior to Yao's and Shun's. So it follows that everyone can become like Yao and Shun. In the jaw, chest, waist and abdomen, frequently the tendencies to deceive others are hidden. They cannot become as wise as Yao and Shun, unless they preserve their minds and nourish their natures. In the head, shoulders, waist and hips, occasionally the tendencies to deceive others are covered in darkness. They cannot become like Yao and Shun, unless they cultivate their personal characters and establish their orders. The above-mentioned

explain why not everyone can spontaneously become like Yao and Shun.

27 The people on the street all agree upon righteousness, so the sentiment of ears, eyes, nose and mouth loves benevolence. Therefore, it is very natural and fair. Being fair means being unselfish. Even though people are together in the same room, they still stay selfish and only think about their own benefit, so the sentiment of the Lung, Spleen, Liver and Kidney detests evil. It is extremely unselfish. Unselfishness means extreme fairness. There is wisdom, ceaseless and like polished ivory, in the jaw, chest, navel and abdomen. If arrogance, overconfidence and a domineering or boastful mind suddenly appear, wisdom will spontaneously disappear and cannot be generally accepted. There is ceaseless glowing conduct in the head, shoulders, waist and hips; but if a covetous mind, extravagance, idleness or greed suddenly appear, consequently, conduct will be resigned and unable to act righteously.

28 All people's ears, eyes, nose, and mouth are extremely clever, while their jaw, chest, navel and abdomen are stupid. All people's Lung, Spleen, Liver and Kidney are wise, while their head, shoulders, waist and hips are unwise.

29 The ears, eyes, noses and mouths of human beings are connected to heaven, and heaven is perceptive. The Lung, Spleen, Liver and Kidney of human beings are related to man, and man is reflective. Our jaws, chests, navels and abdomens constitute our minds, but they are not free from stupidity. Being free from stupidity depends upon us. Our head, shoulders, waist and hips constitute our body, but they are not free from a lack of wisdom. Having wisdom depends upon us.

30 Heaven created human beings and bestowed on to us good sense as a part of our nature. Good sense is necessary in order to live. Without it, one may die. Virtue originates from good sense.

31 Heaven created human beings and bestowed on to us the means of livelihood that originates from heaven's order. The means of livelihood are necessary in order to live. Without it, one may die. The Tao originates from the means of livelihood.

32 Every virtue–benevolence, righteousness, propriety, wisdom, loyalty, filial piety, friendship and fraternal love–originates from good sense. Every function–the scholar, the farmer, the craftsman, the merchant, fields, houses, countries and states–originates from the means of livelihood.

33 If one's good sense is used for service, then one can teach others. If one's means of livelihood is honest, one can receive merit. Despite an excellent nature, if one's good sense is selfish and trivial, and one is cunning like Cao Cao[8)], one cannot teach others. Though a man is heroic, if his lifestyle is selfishly willful, and he is violent and ill tempered like the first Emperor of Chin[9)], he can receive no merit.

34 If one appreciates the virtues of others and at the same time practices virtue, this is the ultimate nature of virtue. If one hates the vices of others and at the same time never has any vices himself, then this is the way of right order. If knowledge and deeds are accumulated, then this is the way and the virtuous. If the way and the virtuous are performed, this is the state of benevolence and sacredness. The way and the virtuous are just as good as the knowledge and the deeds, and the nature and the order are also just as good as the knowledge and the deeds.

35 Someone asked, "If it is possible to discourse on nature by referring to knowledge, then what is the meaning of the discourse on order by referring to deeds?" Order is a kind of destiny. If someone does good deeds, then his destiny will surely be glorious; but if he does bad deeds, his destiny will be surely ruined. We can understand this situation without divination. This has the same meaning as the verse "Always be studious in order to be in harmony with the ordinances of Heaven, and you will obtain much happiness," in the 『*Shijing*』[10)] (詩經 : "Classic of Poetry").

36 Someone asked, "You said that the ears are capable of hearing times of heaven, the eyes are capable of seeing social relationships, the nose is capable of smelling human relationships, and the mouth is capable of tasting localities. That the ears are capable of hearing times of heaven, and the eyes are capable of seeing social relationships is acceptable, but how is it possible that the nose is capable of smelling human relationships, and the

mouth is capable of tasting localities?" "Participating in human relationships–observing the outer appearances of others and trying to evaluate whether each individual's ability and conduct are wise or not–is what is meant by smelling. Living in a certain place–broadly experiencing the interests of human life–is what is meant by tasting."

37 To preserve one's mind, one must rebuke one's mind. It may seem that the mind is naturally clear. Actually, however, one must rebuke one's mind to make it clear; if not, the mind will be cloudy. The awakening mind of a horse is far quicker than that of a cow, because the mind of a horse is more self-rebuking and thus quicker than that of a cow. The mental vitality of the hawk is braver than that of the kite, because the self-rebuking mind of a hawk is far braver than that of the kite. From the above-mentioned, we can understand the clarity of mind and strength of mental vitality of animals. The same may be said of human beings. In human beings, the degrees of differences among individuals range from two to ten thousand fold. Then how can we say that the highest capacity is attainable without any efforts?

2

Discourse on the Four Principles*

1 There are four types of human beings based upon the congenital formation of the organs. Those who have a large Lung and a small Liver are greater yang persons. Those who have a large Liver and a small Lung are greater yin persons. Those who have a large Spleen and a small Kidney are lesser yang persons. Those who have a large Kidney and a small Spleen are lesser yin persons.

2 There are four kinds of inclinations in the human mind. Those who neglect propriety and who are self-indulgent are called the mean. Those who neglect righteousness and who are idle are called the weak. Those who neglect wisdom and who use flattery are called the sycophantic. Those who neglect benevolence and who are very greedy are called the avaricious.

3 Among the five organs, the Heart is the Taichi (太極), the Great Absolute, located in the center. Among the five organs, the Lung, the Spleen, the Liver and the Kidney are the four symbols related to the four corners. The Great Absolute in the center, the Heart, of the sage is higher than that of the ordinary person. The four symbols related to the four corners of the

* 四端論

sage are similar to those of the ordinary person.

4 There are four different categories based upon the formation of the organs, but there is one thing that is common to all, the transformation according to the principles of nature. The sage and the ordinary person are the same. There are four different classes of the mind, and in each class, there are 10,000 different levels, because of the varieties of selfish desires. For this reason, the sage and the ordinary person are different in 10,000 ways.

5 The changes of yin and yang are based on one principle and have four different aspects. This is the reason why the sage admires heaven. The degree of chasteness and generosity, among the four inclinations of the mind–the mean, the weak, the sycophantic and the avaricious–varies in 10,000 ways. Among this variety, there is one thing in common. This is the reason why the ordinary person admires the sage.

6 There are four types of organ formation in the sage, and there are four types of organ formation in ordinary people, too. When one sage dwells among 10,000 ordinary people, the ordinary people are delighted by his presence. The sage is not avaricious, but the ordinary people are avaricious. When one sage dwells among 10,000 ordinary people, the sage is concerned about the ordinary people.

7 The organs of the ordinary person are the same as those of the sage. Their abilities are the same as that of the sage. Since ordinary people have the same Lung, Spleen, Liver and Kidney ability as that of the sage, claiming that they have no ability is the fault not of the ability, but of the Heart.

8 The vast flowing qi issues forth from the Lung, the Spleen, the Liver and the Kidney. The vast flowing principle issues forth from the observing mind. When the qi of the four organs, which are benevolence, righteousness, propriety and wisdom, is amplified, the vast flowing qi issues forth from those four organs. When the desires of the four types of people, which are the mean, the weak, the sycophantic and the avaricious, are identified, the vast flowing principle issues forth from the Heart.

9 They say that the sage has no desire, but having no desire is not the same as the nothingness of Taoism or the nirvana of Buddhism. This means that the sage is so deeply concerned that the world is not well ordered, that he has no desire about himself, and that, moreover, he has no time to think about it. That the sage is deeply concerned that the world is not ordered, and thus has no time to think about his own desires, certainly means that he learns without satiety, and teaches without being tired. Learning without satiety and teaching without being tired is nothing less than the desirelessness of the sage. If there was even a little desire, it is not the mind of Yao and Shun. If there was no concern even momentarily for the world, it is not the mind of Confucius and Mencius[1)].

10 For the greater yang person, the nature of his sorrow is distantly dispersed, and the emotion of his anger is quick. Since his sorrow is distantly dispersed, the qi flows into the Lung, and the Lung qi becomes excessive. Since his anger is quick, the qi stimulates the Liver, and the Liver qi becomes depleted. This is why the greater yang's organ formation is "a large Lung and a small Liver." For the lesser yang person, the nature of his anger is widely encompassing, and the emotion of his sorrow is quick. Since his anger is widely encompassing, the qi flows into the Spleen, and the Spleen qi becomes excessive. Since his sorrow is quick, the qi stimulates the Kidney, and the Kidney qi becomes depleted. This is why the lesser yang's organ formation is "a large Spleen and a small Kidney." For the greater yin person, the nature of his joy is broadly extended, and the emotion of his pleasure is quick. Since his joy is broadly extended, the qi flows into the Liver, and the Liver qi becomes excessive. Since his pleasure is quick, the qi stimulates the Lung, and the Lung qi becomes depleted. This is why the greater yin's organ formation is "a large Liver and a small Lung." For the lesser yin person, the nature of his pleasure is firm in depth, and the emotion of his joy is quick. Since his pleasure is firm in depth, the qi flows into the Kidney, and the Kidney qi becomes excessive. Since his joy is quick, the qi stimulates the Spleen, and the Spleen qi becomes depleted. This is why the lesser yin's organ formation is "a large Kidney and a small Spleen."

Type	Greater Yang (Tai-yang)	Lesser Yang (So-yang)	Greater Yin (Tai-eum)	Lesser Yin (So-eum)
Congenital formation of their organs	a large Lung a small Liver	a large Spleen a small Kidney	a large Liver a small Lung	a large Kidney a small Spleen
Nature	Sorrow	Anger	Joy	Pleasure
Emotion	Anger	Sorrow	Pleasure	Joy

11 The Lung qi extends straight up. The Spleen qi embraces like the shell of the chestnut. The Liver qi is generous and relaxed. The Kidney qi slowly accumulates.

12 Becauser the Lung exhales and the Liver inhales, the Liver and the Lung are the gates of respiration for air and fluids. Because the Spleen draws in and the Kidney sends out, the Kidney and the Spleen are the storerooms that control the drawing in and sending out of foodstuffs.

13 Sorrow qi ascends straight up. Anger qi ascends obliquely. Joy qi descends obliquely. Pleasure qi drops straight down.

	Lung	Spleen	Liver	Kidney
Qi	Extend straight up	Embrace like the shell of the chestnut	Generous and relaxed	Softly accumulated
	Ascend straight up	Ascend obliquely	Descend obliquely	Drop down
Nature	Distantly disperse	Widely encompassing	Broadly extend	Firm in depth
	Sorrow	Anger	Joy	Pleasure

14 Sorrow qi and anger qi ascend, and joy qi and pleasure qi descend. If ascending qi is excessive, the lower part of the body will be damaged. If descending qi is excessive, the upper part of the body will be damaged.

15 If sorrow qi and anger qi move in an orderly way, they will ascend gently. If joy qi and pleasure qi move in an orderly way, they will descend in a relaxed way. Sorrow qi and anger qi are yang, and this is the reason why if they move smoothly, they will ascend gently. Joy qi and pleasure qi are yin, and this is the reason why if they move smoothly, they will descend gently.

16 If sorrow qi and anger qi move in a disorderly manner, they will ascend explosively and amass in the upper part of the body. If joy qi and pleasure qi move in a disorderly manner, they will descend violently and accumulate in the lower part of the body. When the ascending qi moves in a disorderly manner, accumulating in the upper part of the body, the Liver and Kidney will be damaged. When the descending qi moves in a disorderly manner, accumulating in the lower part of the body, the Spleen and Lung will be damaged.

17 Due to frequent anger, the waist constricts frequently. The waist is the dwelling place of the Liver, therefore, if the waist becomes constricted irregularly, the Liver will be damaged. Due to sudden fluctuations of joy, the chest will expand and contract. The chest is the dwelling place of the Spleen, so that if the chest expands and contracts irregularly, the Spleen will be damaged. Due to sudden fluctuations of sorrow, the lumbar vertebrae will flex and straighten suddenly. The lumbar vertebrae are the dwelling place of the Kidney, so that if the lumbar vertebrae flex and straighten suddenly, the Kidney will be damaged. Due to repeated fluctuations of pleasure, the upper back will be pushed up and thrust down. The upper back is the dwelling place of the Lung, so that if the upper back is pushed up and thrust down irregularly, the Lung will be damaged.

18 The greater yang person is prone to explosive anger and deep sorrow, so he must be cautious about this. The lesser yang person is prone to sudden sorrow and deep anger, so he must be cautious about this. The greater yin person is prone to fluctuating pleasure and deep joy, so he must be cautious about this. The lesser yin person is prone to fluctuating joy and deep pleasure, so he must be cautious about this.

19 Kao Yao said, "Everything lies in knowing others and allowing them to live peacefully." Yu[2)] said, "This is so. Yet even King Yao felt this to be difficult. To know others is wisdom. One who knows others can properly award a government post to the right person. To allow people to live peacefully is merciful. People will follow and respect such a merciful leader. If the king is wise and merciful, why should he worry about Huan

Dou, and the exile You Miao, or be afraid of the flattery of Kong Ren?"

20 Repeating the above story of King Yu three times and saying admiringly, "Since knowing others is very difficult, King Yao controlled pleasure, anger, sorrow and joy, so that they acted in their due degree. Since he dared not disregard knowing others, King Yu controlled pleasure, anger, sorrow and joy, so that they acted in this due degree. The sudden fluctuation of pleasure, anger, sorrow, and joy in the world comes from insincere deeds and not knowing others well enough. Knowing others was difficult even for King Yao and King Yu lamented over this matter; so what person can easily be satisfied that he know others? One should reflect more on one's own sincerity and never make light of the selection of the right people."

21 Though one has a good and loving mind, if he expresses it in a disorderly way, his virtuous mind will not be clear. Though one has a hatred of the bad mind, if he does so in a disorderly way, his hatred of the bad will not be widely recognized. It is advisable that public affairs be engaged in by good men. If not, joy and pleasure will certainly be disturbed. It is not advisable that public affairs be engaged in by bad men. If so, sorrow and anger will increase.

22 Sorrow and anger feed off each other, and joy and pleasure complement each other. If sorrow becomes extreme, anger will be generated. If anger becomes extreme, sorrow will be generated. If pleasure becomes extreme, joy will be generated. If joy becomes extreme, pleasure will be generated. If the greater yang person's sorrow cannot be controlled, in the end, anger will spring forth. If the lesser yang person's anger cannot be controlled, in the end, sorrow will stir deeply within. If the lesser yin person's pleasure cannot be controlled, in the end, joy becomes unstable. If the greater yin person's joy cannot be controlled, in the end, pleasure becomes unrestrained. Such stirring of the emotions is comparable to cutting one's intestines with a sharp knife. Once the emotions are seriously stirred, it may take more than 10 years to recover. This is the key to longevity, so we must be aware of this.

23 The various formations of the four types are due to the changes of yin and

yang. We need not mention those congenital formations. In addition, there are incomplete manifestations of the above formations. Such people's destiny is dependent upon their cultivation of human affairs, so we must be cautious.

24 Just one greater yang person's anger can trigger the anger of a thousand, or tens of thousands of other people; but if his anger cannot handle those people, he will certainly not be equal to the task of dealing with them. Just one lesser yin person's joy can trigger the joy of a thousand, or tens of thousands of other people; but if his joy cannot handle those people, he will certainly not be equal to the task of dealing with them. Just one lesser yang person's sorrow can trigger the sorrow of a thousand, or tens of thousands of other people; but if his sorrow cannot handle those people, he will certainly not be equal to the task of dealing with them. Just one greater yin person's pleasure can trigger the pleasure of a thousand, or tens of thousands of other people; but if his pleasure cannot handle those people, he will certainly not be equal to the task of dealing with them.

25 The greater yang and lesser yang persons should always be cautious about having too much sorrow and anger; pretending to have joy and pleasure would be useless. If they try to pretend, their joy and pleasure will not be from the bottom of their hearts, and their sorrow and anger will become distorted. The greater yin and lesser yin persons should always be cautious about having too much joy and pleasure; pretending to have sorrow and anger would be useless. If they try to pretend, their sorrow and anger will not be from the bottom of their hearts, and their joy and pleasure will become distorted.

26 When there are no stirrings of pleasure, anger, sorrow or joy, the mind may be said to be in a state of equilibrium. When those feelings have been stirred, and they act in their due degree, what ensues may be called the state of harmony. When there are no stirrings of pleasure, anger, sorrow or joy, and the mind is always cautious, isn't such a person gradually becoming closer to the state of equilibrium? When pleasure, anger, sorrow, or joy has already been stirred, and one reflects upon them, isn't such a person gradually becoming closer to the state of harmony?

3

Discourse on the Establishment and Supplement*

1 The greater yang person's sorrow is distantly dispersed, and his anger is quick. "Sorrow is distantly dispersed" means that the ears of the greater yang person perceive the times of heaven, and he feels sorrow that people deceive each other. Sorrow is nothing other than "listening." "Anger is quick" means that the Spleen of the greater yang person enters into social acquaintances, and he becomes angry when others disregard him. This anger is nothing other than becoming angry. The lesser yang person's anger is widely encompassing, and his sorrow is quick. "Anger is widely encompassing," means that the eyes of the lesser yang person can see social relationships, and he feels angry that people mutually disregard each other. Anger is nothing other than "observing." "Sorrow is quick" means that the Lung of the lesser yang person engages in appointed roles, and he becomes sorrowful when others deceive him. This sorrow is nothing other than becoming sorrowful. The greater yin person's joy is broadly extended, and his pleasure is quick. "Joy is broadly extended" means that the nose of the greater yin person perceives human relationships, and he feels joy that people help each other. Joy is nothing other than "smelling." "Pleasure is quick" means that the Kidney of the greater yin person engages in living quarters, and he feels pleasure when others pro-

---

* 擴充論

tect him. This pleasure is nothing other than becoming pleased. The lesser yin person's pleasure is firm in depth, and his joy is quick. "Pleasure is firm in depth," means that the mouth of the lesser yin person perceives localities, and he feels pleasure when people protect each other. Pleasure is nothing other than "tasting." "Joy is quick" means that the Liver of the lesser yin person engages in clanships, and he becomes joyful when others help him. This joy is nothing other than becoming joyful.

2 The ears of the greater yang person are able to extensively comprehend the times of heaven, but his nose is unable to extensively comprehend human relationships. The nose of the greater yin person is able to extensively comprehend human relationships, but his ears are unable to extensively comprehend the times of heaven. The eyes of the lesser yang person are able to extensively comprehend social relationships, but his mouth is unable to extensively comprehend localities. The mouth of the lesser yin person is able to extensively comprehend localities, but his eyes are unable to extensively comprehend social relationships.

3 The Spleen of the greater yang person is well integrated with social acquaintance, but his Liver cannot get along with clanships. The Liver of the lesser yin person can get along with clanships, but his Spleen cannot be well integrated with social acquaintances. The Lung of the lesser yang person smartly handles appointed roles, but his Kidney cannot maintain constant stability within living quarters. The Kidney of the greater yin person can maintain constant stability within living quarters, but his Lung cannot smartly handle appointed roles.

4 Since the listening of the greater yang person is able to extensively comprehend the times of heaven, his *shen* (mental vitality) is sufficient to fill the brain, and a large amount of it gathers in the Lung. Since the smelling of the greater yang person is unable to extensively comprehend human relationships, his blood is insufficient to fill the lumbar vertebrae, and a small amount of it gathers in the Liver. Since the smelling of the greater yin person is able to extensively comprehend human relationships, his blood is sufficient to fill the lumbar vertebrae, and a large amount of it gathers in the Liver. Since the listening of the greater yin person is unable

to extensively comprehend the times of heaven, his mental vitality is insufficient to fill the brain, and a small amount of it gathers in the Lung. Since the sight of the lesser yang person is able to extensively comprehend social relationships, his qi is sufficient to fill the mid-back area, and a large amount of it gathers in the Spleen. Since the tasting of the lesser yang person is unable to extensively comprehend localities, his essence is insufficient to fill the bladders, and a small amount of it gathers in the Kidney. Since the tasting of the lesser yin person is able to extensively comprehend localities, his esssence is sufficient to fill the bladders, and a large amount of it gathers in the Kidney. Since the sight of the lesser yin person is unable to extensively comprehend social relationships, his qi is insufficient to fill the mid-back area, and a small amount of it gathers in the Spleen.

5 Since the anger of the greater yang person is well integrated with social acquaintances, he is not disregarded within these acquaintances. Since the joy of the greater yang person cannot keep its standing within clanships, he is disregarded by clanships. The exploding anger of the greater yang person is not caused by social acquaintances, but certainly caused by clanships. Since the joy of the lesser yin person can keep its standing with clanships, he is helped by these clanships. Since the anger of the lesser yin person cannot be well integrated within social acquaintances, he cannot be helped by these acquaintances. The joy experienced by a lesser yin person is not caused by clanships, but certainly caused by social acquaintances. Since the sorrow of the lesser yang person can smartly handle appointed roles, he is not deceived by these appointed roles. Since the pleasure of the lesser yang person is not able to maintain stability within living quarters, he is deceived by living quarters. His overflowing sorrow is not caused by appointed roles, but to these living quarters. Since the pleasure of the greater yin person always maintains stability within living quarters, he is protected by living quarters. Since the sorrow of the greater yin person is not able to smartly handle appointed roles, he cannot be protected by appointed roles. The outpour of pleasure from a greater yin person is not caused by living quarters, but caused by appointed roles.

6 The social acquaintances of the greater yang person are governed by

anger, but his involvement in clanships should not be constrained by anger. If his anger is directed against clanships, nothing beneficial for these groups can come out of it, and it may even damage his Liver. The involvement in clanships of the lesser yin person is governed by joy, but his social acquaintances should not be constrained by joy. If his joy is directed towards social acquaintances, nothing beneficial for these acquaintances can come out of it, and it may even damage his Spleen. The appointed roles of the lesser yang person are governed by sorrow, but his living quarters should not be constrained by sorrow. If his sorrow is directed towards living quarters, nothing beneficial for living quarters can come out of it, and it may even damage his Kidney. The living quarters of the greater yin person are governed by pleasure, but his appointed role should not be constrained by pleasure. If his pleasure is directed towards appointed roles, nothing beneficial for appointed roles can come out of it, and it may even damage his Lung.

7 Due to his temperament, the greater yang person always tends to move forward, not backward. Due to his temperament, the lesser yang person always tends to be active, without finishing what he begins. Due to his temperament, the greater yin person always tends towards stillness, and does not move. Due to his temperament, the lesser yin person always tends to remain in one place, and does not go out.

8 The greater yang person always tends to move forward according to his capacity. However, he realizes that his capacities are meager, and when he reflects upon it, he will not be able to move forward. The lesser yang person always tends to be active according to his ability. However, he realizes that his power is not so firm, and when he reflects upon it, he will not be able to be so active. The greater yin person always tends towards stillness according to his comprehension. However, he realizes that his knowledge is not so thorough, and when he reflects upon it, he will not be able to be still. The lesser yin person always tends to remain in one place according to his plans. However, he realizes that his plans are not so far-reaching, and when he reflects upon it, he will not be able to remain in one place.

9 The emotional character of the greater yang person tends to be masculine, not feminine. The emotional character of the lesser yin person tends to be feminine, not masculine. The emotional character of the lesser yang person tends towards achievements in the outside world and not towards attending to his domestic affairs. The emotional character of the greater yin person tends towards attending to his domestic affairs, but not towards achievement in the outside world.

10 Though the greater yang person tends to be masculine, it is advisable for him to be feminine to some extent. If he tries to be totally masculine, he will become overly self-indulgent. Though the lesser yin person tends to be feminine, it is advisable for him to be masculine to some extent. If he tries to be totally feminine, he will become idle. Though the lesser yang person tends towards achievements in the outside world, it is advisable for him to attend to his domestic affairs to some extent. If he pursues achievements in the outside world totally, he will become overly attached to his own urgencies. Though the greater yin person tends towards attending to his domestic affairs, it is advisable for him to pursue achievements in the outside world to some extent. If he attends but to his domestic affairs, he will become overly avaricious.

11 No matter how stupid the greater yang person is, he can easily comprehend others. Even though he may be very unworthy, he can distinguish between the good and evil in others. No matter how stupid the lesser yang person is, he is highly respectful to others. Even though he may be very unworthy, he can distinguish between cleverness and foolishness in others. No matter how stupid the greater yin person is, he can guide others confidently. Even though he may be very unworthy, he can distinguish between diligence and idleness in others. No matter how stupid the lesser yin person is, he can easily pacify others. Even though he may be very unworthy, he can distinguish between ability and inability in others.

12 Since the greater yang person is good at social acquaintances, he always has anger generated by his anxiety when encountering strangers. This anger comes from a fair and respectful mind, so it is very virtuous. Since

he neglects clanships, his acquaintances in clanships always create pitfalls for him. Thus, he gets angry, and this damages his organs. The reason is that he is not very sociable.

13 Since the lesser yin person is good at clanships, he always has joy coming from acquaintances with familiar company. This joy comes from a fair and respectful mind, so it is very virtuous. Since he neglects social acquaintances, unfamiliar people could always deceive him. Thus, he becomes excessively joyful, and this damages his organs. The reason is that his anxiety is not very comprehensive.

14 Since the lesser yang person is cautious of appointed roles, he always has sorrow coming from his tendency to engage in outside business. This sorrow comes from a fair and respectful mind, so it is very virtuous. Since he is not cautious of living quarters, those who always tend to maintain stability within living quarters create pitfalls for him. Thus, he becomes sorrowful, and this damages his organs. The reason is that he cherishes the outside world and neglects his domestic affairs.

15 Since the greater yin person is cautious of living quarters, he always has pleasure coming from his maintaining stability within living quarters. This pleasure comes from a fair and respectful mind, so it is very virtuous. Since he is not good at appointed roles, he can be deceived by those who always tend to be active in outside affairs. Thus, he indulges in pleasure, and this damages his organs. The reason is that he but pays attention to his domestic affairs and neglects outside matters.

16 The jaw of the greater yin person has to be cautious about being arrogant. If his jaw has no arrogance, he will possess incomparable cleverness. The chest of the lesser yin person has to be cautious about being overconfident. If his chest has no overconfidence, he will become an incomparable administrator. The navel of the greater yang person has to be cautious about being domineering. If his navel shows no dominance, he will show incomparable moderation. The abdomen of the lesser yang person has to be cautious about being boastful. If his abdomen has no boastfulness, he will display incomparable generosity.

17 The head of the lesser yin person has to be cautious about being covetous. If his head has no covetousness, he will certainly possess the magnificent discernment of a great man. The shoulders of the greater yin person have to be cautious about being extravagant. If his shoulders have no extravagance, he will certainly display the magnificent nobility of a great man. The waist of the lesser yang person has to be cautious about being idle. If his waist has no idleness, he will certainly have the magnificent resourcefulness of a great man. The hips of the greater yang person have to be cautious about being greedy. If his hips do not have a greedy nature, he will certainly possess the magnificent method of a great man.

4

Discourse on Viscera and Bowels*

1 The area of the Lung corresponds to the neck/upper back region. The area of the epigastrium corresponds to the region between the jaw and the upper chest. Between the back and chest is the upper-*jiao*. The area of the Spleen corresponds to the mid-back area. The stomach corresponds to the region of the diaphragm. Between the mid-back area and the diaphragm is the upper-middle-*jiao*. The area of the Liver corresponds to the waist. The area of the small intestine corresponds to the navel level. Between the waist and the navel is the lower-middle-*jiao*. The area of the Kidney corresponds to the area below the lumbar. The area of the large intestine corresponds to the area of lower abdomen. Below the lumbar-navel region is the lower-*jiao*.

	Four *jiao*	Four region	Four viscera	Four bowels
Heart	upper-*jiao*	between the back and chest	Lung	Epigastrium
	upper-middle-*jiao*	between the mid-back region and the diaphragm	Spleen	Stomach
	lower-middle-*jiao*	between the waist and the navel	Liver	Small Intestine
	lower-*jiao*	between the lumbar-navel region	Kidney	Large Intestine

* 臟腑論

2 Ingested food moves from the epigastrium into the stomach, then to the small intestine, into the large intestine, and out from the anus. Most ingested food accumulates in the stomach and evaporates into hot qi or is digested in the small intestine and changes into cool qi. The lighter component of the hot qi rises to the epigastric region and becomes warm qi. The heavier component of cool qi descends into the large intestine and becomes cold qi.

3 The epigastric region is connected to the mouth and nose, so the qi of ingested food rises. The large intestine is connected to the anus, so the qi of ingested food descends. The stomach is very large and can contain a large amount of food, so that the qi of ingested food may accumulate there. The small intestine is narrow and convoluted, so that the qi of the ingested food can be digested there.

4 The warm qi of ingested food is transformed into *jin* (thin and clear body fluid) in the epigastric region, and then it rises up to the sublingual area to become the sea of thin and clear body fluid. The sea of thin and clear body fluid is the dwelling place of thin and clear body fluid. The clear qi of the sea of thin and clear body fluid flows out through the ear and becomes mental vitality, which then enters the brain and forms the sea of *ni* (greasy body fluid), which is the dwelling place of mental vitality. The clear fluid of the sea of greasy body fluid ultimately returns to the Lung internally, whereas the turbid substance exits through the skin. Therefore, the epigastric region, tongue, ears, brain and skin all are part of the Lung system.

5 The hot qi of ingested food transforms into *gao* (paste) in the stomach, and paste enters the area between the breasts to become the sea of paste. The sea of paste is the dwelling place of paste. The clear qi of the sea of paste goes out through the eyes and turns into qi, which then enters the mid-back area and forms the sea of *mo* (membrane), where the qi dwells. The clear fluid of the sea of membrane ultimately goes to the Spleen internally, whereas the turbid substance goes to the tendons externally. Therefore, the stomach, breasts, eyes, mid-back area and tendons all are part of the Spleen system.

6 The cool qi of ingested food transforms into *you* (oil) in the small

intestine, and then proceeds to the navel area to form the sea of *you*, where oil dwells. The clear qi of the sea of oil goes out through the nose, and turns into blood, and finally goes to the lumbar region to form the sea of blood, where blood dwells. The clear fluid of the sea of blood ultimately advances to the Liver internally, whereas the turbid substance enters the muscles externally. Therefore, the small intestine, navel, nose, lumbar region and muscles all are part of the Liver system.

7 The cold qi of ingested food transforms into *ye* (liquid) in the large intestine, and liquid goes to the upper margin of the pubic hair and becomes the sea of liquid, where liquid dwells. The clear qi of the sea of *zhi* (juice) leaves through the mouth and becomes *jing* (essence), and then it advances to the bladder to form the sea of essence, where essence dwells. The clear fluid of the sea of essence ultimately goes to the Kidney internally, whereas the turbid substance goes to the bones externally. Therefore, the large intestine, orifice of the urethra, mouth, bladder and bones all are part of the Kidney system.

8 The ears' capacity to listen to the times of heaven makes it possible to draw out the clear qi from the sea of thin and clear body fluid, which fills the upper-*jiao*. There, the clean qi turns into mental vitality, which then pours into the brain and becomes greasy body fluid. The greasy body fluid accumulates to form the sea of greasy body fluid. The eyes' capacity to see social relationships makes it possible to draw out the clear qi from the sea of paste, which fills the upper-middle-*jiao*. There, the clear qi pours into the mid-back area and becomes membrane. The membrane accumulates to form the sea of membrane. The nose's capacity to smell human relationships makes it possible to draw out the clear qi from the sea of oil, which fills the lower-middle-*jiao*. There, the clear qi turns into blood, which then pours into the lumbar region and becomes concentrated blood. The blood accumulates to form the sea of blood. The mouth's capacity to taste localities makes it possible to draw out the clear qi from the sea of liquid, which fills the lower-*jiao*. There, the clear qi turns into essence, which then pours into the bladder and becomes concentrated

essence. The essence accumulates to form the sea of essence.

9 The Lung's sorrowful power to master appointed roles makes it possible to suck out the clear juice from the sea of greasy body fluid, which enters the Lung. The clear juice nourishes the source of the Lung, supports the sea of thin and clear body fluid internally, stimulates the qi, and concentrates thin and clear body fluid. The Spleen's anger power to master social acquaintances makes it possible to suck out the clear juice from the sea of membrane, which enters the Spleen. The clear juice nourishes the source of the Spleen, supports the sea of paste internally, stimulates the qi, and concentrates paste. The Liver's joy power to master clanships makes it possible to suck out the clear juice from the sea of blood, which enters the Liver. The clear juice nourishes the source of the Liver, supports the sea of oil internally, stimulates the qi, and concentrates oil. The Kidney's pleasure power to master living quarters makes it possible to suck out the clear juice from the sea of essence, which enters the Kidney. The clear juice nourishes the source of the Kidney, supports the sea of liquid internally, stimulates the qi, and concentrates liquid.

10 The ascending power of the epigastrium to collect the turbid substance of the sea of thin and clear body fluid strengthens the epigastrium. The retaining power of the stomach to collect the turbid substance of the sea of paste strengthens the stomach. The removing and digesting power of the small intestine to collect the turbid substance of the sea of oil strengthens the small intestine. The descending power of the large intestine to collect the turbid substance of the sea of liquid strengthens the large intestine.

Four bowels	Four Qi	Four front seas	Power	Four back seas
Epigastrium	Warm Qi	Sea of *Jin*	The ascending power	Sea of *Ni*
Stomach	Hot Qi	Sea of *Gao*	The retaining power	Sea of *Mo*
Small Intestine	Cool Qi	Sea of *You*	The removing and digesting power	Sea of Blood
Large Intestine	Cold Qi	Sea of *Ye*	The descending power	Sea of *Jing*

11 The stretching capacity of the head refines and shapes the turbid substance of the sea of greasy body fluid into skin and hair. The grasping capacity of the hands refines and shapes the turbid substance of the sea of membrane into tendons. The dispersing capacity of the waist refines and shapes the turbid substance of the sea of blood into muscle. The flexing capacity of the feet refines and shapes the turbid substance of the sea of essence into bone.

12 Therefore, the ears must listen extensively, the eyes must see widely, the nose must smell broadly, and the mouth must taste deeply. The ears, eyes, nose and mouth should use their full capacities so that essence, mental vitality, qi and blood are well developed. If not, essence, mental vitality, qi and blood will be exhausted. The Lung must be good at learning. The Spleen must be good at inquiring. The Liver must be good at thinking. The Kidney must be good at differentiating. The Lung, Spleen, Liver and Kidney should use their capacities so that thin and clear body fluid, liquid, paste and oil are sufficient. If not, thin and clear body fluid, liquid, paste and oil will be consumed.

13 The sea of greasy body fluid stores mental vitality. The sea of membrane stores *ling* (soul). The sea of blood stores *hun* (ethereal soul). The sea of essence stores *po* (corporeal soul).

14 The sea of thin and clear body fluid stores intention. The sea of paste stores consideration. The sea of oil stores integrity. The sea of liquid stores will.

15 The sea of greasy body fluid in the head is the source of the Lung. The sea of membrane in the mid-back area is the source of the Spleen. The sea of blood in the lumbar region is the source of the Liver. The sea of essence in the bladders is the source of the Kidney.

16 The sea of thin and clear body fluid in the sublingual area is the source of the ears. The sea of paste in the breasts is the source of the eyes. The sea of oil in the navel is the source of the nose. The sea of liquid in the bladder is the source of the mouth.

17 The Heart is the supreme ruler of the whole body, located in the center of the chest, and is very bright and shiny. The ears, eyes, nose, and mouth observe all things. The Lung, Spleen, Liver and Kidney consider all things. The jaw, chest, navel and abdomen are sincere in all things. The head, hands, waist and feet respect all things.

5

Discourse on the Origin of Eastern Medicine*

1 In the 『*Shujing*[1]』 ("Classic of Document"), we read, "If the medicine does not cause a kind of dizziness, the illness cannot be cured." During the reign of Gaozong in the Shang dynasty, Gaozong experienced such dizziness after taking some medicine, and he greatly appreciated its effect. This tradition in medicine is very old, dating to before the era of Shennong[2] and Huangdi[3]. This is plausible, but most people believe that the 『*Bencao*[4]』 ("The Herbal") and 『*Suwen*[5]』 ("Plain Questions") were written by Shennong and Huangdi themselves. This is not possible. The reason is as follows. During the eras of Shennong and Huangdi, there were no written characters. Likewise, in the following era, the usage of written language was very approximate, so they could not have written those books. After the Zhou and during the Chin-Han dynasties, Bianque was the preeminent physician. Followed by him, Zhang Zhongjing[6] compiled the medical knowledge of that time. Soon afterwards, the practice of medicine began to flourish. After Zhang Zhongjing, following the Southern and Northern, Sui and Tang dynasties, and during the Song dynasty, Zhu Gong[7] also compiled the existing medical knowledge into the 『*Huorenshu*[8]』 ("Book for Saving Life"). After Zhu Gong, the Yuan

---

* 醫源論

dynasty's Li Gao[9)], Wang Haogu[10)], Zhu Zhenheng[11)] and Wei Yilin[12)] continued this tradition. Li Chan[13)] and Gong Xin[14)] inherited these medical teachings during the Ming dynasty, and later Heo Jun[15)]propagated them in the form of the『*Dongui Bogam*[16)]』("Treasure Mirror of Eastern Medicine"). This led to a renaissance in traditional medicine. Zhang Zhongjing propagated the medical and pharmacological theories dating back from the era of Shennong and Huangdi to the Chin-Han dynasties. Following this, Zhu Gong promoted similar medical and pharmacological theories from the era of the Wei and the Jin dynasties to the times of Sui and the Tang dynasties. Likewise, Li Chan and Gong Xin and Heo Jun spread the medical theories of the Song, Yuan and Ming dynasties. If we evaluate their contributions, Zhang Zhongjing, Zhu Gong and Heo Jun deserve the highest recognition, and Li Chan and Gong Xin follow just behind them.

2 As for the『Bencao』(本草經: Materia Medica), beginning with the days of Shennong and Huangdi, the knowledge of herbal medicine was used for several thousand years. In the era of Shennong, the『*Materia Medica*』already existed. The『*Tangye Bencao*[17)]』("Materia Medica of Decoction") came into being during the Yuan dynasty. During the Tang dynasty, the『*Shiliao Bencao*[18)]』("Dietetic Materia Medica") was written by Meng Xian[19)], and Chen Zangqi[20)] wrote the『*Bencao Shiyi*[21)]』("Supplement to Materia Medica"). During the Song dynasty, the『*Bencao Buyi*』("Reinforcing the Materia Medica") was written by Fang Anshang[22)], and the『*Rihuazi Bencao*[23)]』("Rihuazi Materia Medica") was published. During the Yuan dynasty, the『*Tangye Bencao*』was written by Wang Haogu.

3 The medical and pharmacological theories related to the lesser yin type were explained in detail by Zhang Zhongjing. However, it took the doctors of the Song, Yuan and Ming dynasties to develop these ideas to near completion. The medical and pharmacological theories related to the lesser yang type were partially explained by Zhang Zhongjing. Later, the doctors of the Song, Yuan and Ming dynasties also developed these ideas in detail. As for the medical and pharmacological ideas related to the greater yin type, Zhang Zhongjing only roughly sketched them out. The doctors

of the Song, Yuan and Ming dynasties imparted more details to those ideas. For the greater yang type, the medical and pharmacological theories were also only roughly sketched out by Zhu Zhenheng, and in the 『*Bencao*』, pharmacological theories were briefly mentioned, too.

4 Five to six thousand years after the development of this medical tradition, I perceived the principles of the four constitutional types by chance, and wrote a book titled the 『*Suse Bowon*[24]』 ("Longevity and Life Preservation"). The designations of greater yang disease, lesser yang disease, yang brightness disease, greater yin disease, lesser yin disease and reverting yin disease, mentioned by Zhang Zhongjing, were based on the terminology of symptoms. In my system, however, the designations of greater yang, lesser yang, greater yin and lesser yin types are based on the person's constitutions. We must not confuse these two viewpoints. First, we must perceive the roots and trunk, and afterward the branches and leaves. Taking the pulse is one of the methods for diagnosing symptoms and signs. When taking a pulse, we must remember that, fundamentally, there are but four main types of pulse, i. e. floating (superficial), deep, slow and fast. Aside from these, there is not much else of importance for diagnosis. The three yins and three yangs are differentiated according to their symptoms and the signs. Those principles originated from the symptoms and signs of the abdomen and back, and the outside and inside of the body, so there is no need to try to detect changes in the meridians.

5 In ancient times, doctors explained disease according to the theories of six meridians related to yin and yang, so when Zhang Zhongjing wrote his 『*Shanghanlun*[25]』, he also classified symptoms according to those assumptions. If the patient had a headache, aching of the body, fever, chills and a floating pulse, we can say that he has a greater yang disease. Bitterness in the mouth, parched throat, vertigo, deafness, fullness in the chest, chills and fever that come and go, headache, fever, and a tight-slender pulse indicate the lesser yang disease. Spontaneous perspiration, with an aversion to heat during fever, but no aversion to cold, and constipation indicate the yang brightness disease. Abdominal distention with occasional pain, without a thirst for water, or heartburn and diarrheas indicate the

greater yin disease. A feeble and weak pulse, constant drowsiness, thirst, heartburn, and diarrheas indicate the lesser yin disease. No abdominal pain and diarrheas at the onset, but appearing after the sixth or seventh day, feeble and loose pulse, cold limbs, curled tongue, and shrinkage of the scrotum indicate the reverting yin disease. Among the above six diseases, the three yin diseases are closely related to the lesser yin type. The lesser yang disease is closely related to the lesser yang type. The greater yang and yang brightness diseases may affect the lesser yang, lesser yin and greater yin types, but mostly they affect the lesser yin type. From ancient times, medical ideas and principles were widespread. Zhang Zhongjing compiled the prevalent ideas, as well as clinical experiences from ancient times, and wrote his 『*Shanghanlun*』. However, most ancient doctors did not understand that the propensities for love, hate, avarice, joy, anger, sorrow and pleasure in the mind were the causes of disease. Rather, they thought that an improper diet, wind, cold, summer heat and dampness were the causes of disease. If we analyze their ideas regarding disease and medicine, we can see that most of them were focused on the improper diet of the lesser yin type. Stomach-heat syndrome of the lesser yang type was described only a little, and those of the greater yin and the greater yang syndromes were not described at all.

6 Qibo[26)] answered, "On the first day, the febrile disease caused by cold is received by the greater yang meridian. Therefore, the head and the neck are in pain, and the waist and the back become rigid. On the second day, the yang brightness meridian contracts the disease. The yang brightness controls the flesh, its meridian supports the nose, and it is connected to the eyes. Thus the body is feverish, there is eyeball pain, the nose is dry and parched, and the patient finds it impossible to rest. On the third day, the lesser yang meridian contracts the disease. The region of the lesser yang controls the gall bladder. Its meridian follows the flanks and is connected to the ears. Thus, the ribs and chest are in pain, and the ears grow deaf. Now, the meridian of the three yangs have contracted the disease, but it has not yet entered the viscera; therefore, if one can produce perspiration, one can cure the disease. On the fourth day, the greater yin meridi-

an contracts the disease. The meridian of greater yin leads into the interior of the stomach and is connected to the throat. Thus, the stomach becomes replete (full), and the throat becomes dry and parched. On the fifth day, the lesser yin meridian contracts the disease. The meridian of lesser yin penetrates into the Kidney and is connected to the Lung; it is also connected to the root of the tongue. Thus, the mouth is dry, and the tongue is parched and dry. On the sixth day, the reverting yin meridian contracts the disease. The meridian of reverting yin passes through the sex organs and is connected to the Liver. The results are an affliction of fullness and shrinkage of the scrotum. Now, if the three yins, the three yangs, the five viscera and the six bowels have all contracted the disease, there is stagnation of the *ying* (nutrient) and the *wei* (defense), and no circulation of the five viscera. Death follows."

7 "If there is a patient in the simultaneous occurrence of syndromes of both the yang and yin meridians at the beginning of an exogenous febrile disease, he will die. When the syndromes of both the yang and yin meridians at the beginning of an exogenous febrile disease simultaneously occur, both the greater yang and lesser yin meridians are affected on the first day of illness. There will be a headache, a parched mouth, and discomfort in the chest. On the second day of illness, the yang brightness and greater yin meridians are both affected. The patient's abdomen feels full, and his body feverish. He does not want food and speaks deliriously. On the third day of illness, the lesser yang and reverting yin meridians are both affected. The ears grow deaf, and the scrotum shrinks and becomes deficient. Water and broth cannot be ingested, the patient cannot recognize other people, and on the sixth day, he will die. Their death always takes a period of six or seven days, their improvement ten days."

8 I have said, "The idea that the 『*Lingshu*[27)]』 and 『*Suwen*』 were attributed to Huangdi is nonsense and confuses the people. However, in those days, it was a common belief, so we need not criticize it. Since those books contain the medical experiences of ancient times concerning the theories of the five viscera, the six bowels, the meridians, acupuncture, disease and the cultivation of health, as well as many enlightening ideas, they are sov-

ereign in providing doctors with insightful knowledge of medical laws. Despite the fact that these books are not perfect, we must not criticize them or detract from their contributions. They recorded the wisdom and widespread knowledge of ancient times, including original ideas concerning the cultivation of health. We must take them into consideration, but should not accept them at face value."

9 "The greater yang, lesser yang and lesser yin meridian diseases mentioned by Qibo are actually diseases of the lesser yang person. The yang brightness and greater yin meridian diseases spoken of by Qibo are actually diseases of the greater yin person. The reverting yin meridian disease referred to by Qibo is actually a disease of the lesser yin person."

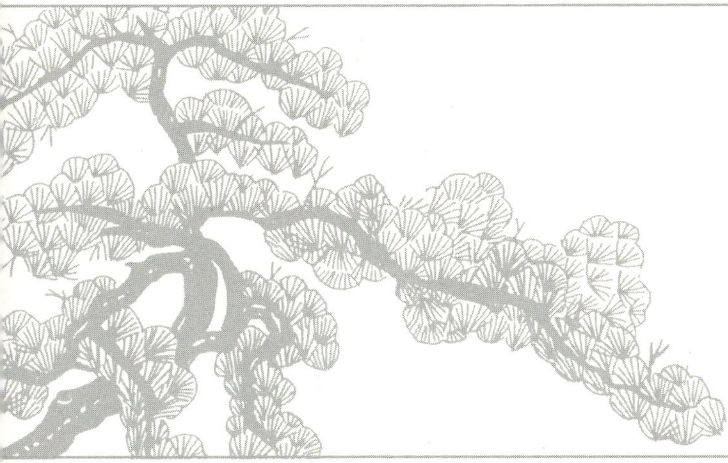

PART II

1

Discourse on the Soeum (Lesser Yin) Person's Exterior Febrile Disease Induced from the Kidney Affected by Heat*

1 In the 『*Shanghanlun*』, Zhang Zhongjing said, "Fever, chills and a floating pulse are the general symptoms and signs of the greater yang syndrome, which is in the exterior stage."

2 The pulse of the greater yang febrile disease caused by wind is floating when felt at the surface level and weak at the depth level. A pulse floating at the surface signifies spontaneous fever. A pulse weak in depth signifies spontaneous perspiration. *Guizhi Tang* (Decoction of Ramulus Cinnamomi) should be used when the patient feels chills and an aversion to wind, uneasy because of fever and nauseous with a tendency to snore.

3 In the 『*Dexiaofang*』[1] ("Effective Formulas"), Wei Yilin said, "The pestilences of the four seasons can be treated with *Xiangsu San* (Powder of Rhizoma Cyperi and Folium Perillae)."

4 In the 『*Yijian*』[2] ("Mirror of Medicine"), Gong Xin said, "The exogenous febrile disease with the symptoms of headache and aching of the body can be treated with *Huoxiang Zhengqi San* (Powder of Herba Agastachis for restoring healthy qi). It is difficult to determine whether this disease belongs to the exterior or interior syndrome."

---

* 少陰人腎受熱表熱病論

5 I have said, "The fever with chills in the greater yang febrile disease caused by wind mentioned by Zhang Zhongjing is the same as the lesser yin person's exterior febrile disease induced from the Kidney affected by heat. Fever and chills without perspiration should be treated with *Guizhi Tang, Cheongung Gyeji Tang* (Decoction of Rhizome Chuanxiong and Ramulus Cinnamomi), *Xiangsu San, Gunggui Hyangso San* (Powder of Rhizoma Cyperi and Folium Perillae with Rhizoma Chuanxiong and Radix Angelicae Sinensis) and *Gwakhyang Jeonggi San*. Fever and chills with perspiration is the start of *mangyang* (yang collapse), and should not be ignored. Begin treatment with *Hwanggi Gyeji Tang* (Decoction of Radix Astragali and Ramulus Cinnamomi), *Bojung Ikgi Tang* (Decoction for tonifying the middle and replenishing qi) and *Seungyang Ikgi Tang* (Decoction for ascending yang and replenishing qi) for three days. If sweating persists after the treatment, treat with *Guizhi Fuzi Tang* (Decoction of Ramulus Cinnamomi and Radix Aconiti Lateralis Praeparata), *Insam Gyeji Buja Tang* (Decoction of Radix Ginseng, Ramulus Cinnamomi and Radix Aconiti Lateralis Praeparata) and *Seungyang Ikgi Buja Tang* (Decoction of Radix Aconiti Lateralis Praeparata for lifting yang and replenishing qi)."

6 Zhang Zhongjing said, "If a patient suffering from greater yang disease has a fever, a floating and tense pulse and no perspiration, he will recover spontaneously after epistaxis."

7 In the case of the greater yang disease, after six to seven days, if the exterior syndrome still remains and the pulse is feeble and deep, the patient does not suffer from *jiexiong* (accumulation of pathogen in the chest), but behaves in a manic way. This is because the pathogenic heat has congealed in the lower-*jiao* and has formed a hard distension in the lower abdomen. If the patient's urination was normal, he can recover after discharging blood clots. *Didang Tang* (Decoction of *Didang*) is a curative.

8 In the greater yang syndrome, jaundiced skin, manic behavior, a hard distension in the lower abdomen and normal urination are the symptoms and signs of blood stasis. *Didang Tang* will be the curative. If a patient with an exogenous febrile disease caused by the cold has a distension of

the lower abdomen, there ought to be dysuria. However, if the patient's urination is normal, he has blood stasis.

9 Before the greater yang disease is gone, pathogenic heat congeals in the urinary bladder, and then the patient turns manic. The disease is gone when blood is passed. If the patient feels tightness and pain in the lower abdomen below the umbilicus, a purgative, *Taoren Chengqi Tang* (Decoction for purgation with Semen Persicae), can be used.

10 For the greater yang disease, there will be repeated diarrheas if purgatives are used several times before the exterior syndrome disperses. This shows that the exterior and interior syndromes still remain with hardness and stagnancy at the esophagus. *Renshen Guizhi Tang* (Decoction of Radix Ginseng and Ramulus Cinnamomi) can be adopted as a curative.

11 I have said, "The cause of the mania mentioned above is Kidney yang confronted by the heat. Meanwhile, the hardness and fullness in the lower abdomen indicates that his large intestine is averse to cold. When these two symptoms co-exist, we must treat the most urgent case first. If the former is urgent, the ascending supplement of *Cheongung Gyeji Tang, Hwanggi Gyeji Tang* and *Palmul Gunja Tang* (Decoction of eight noble ingredients) should be prescribed; if the latter is urgent, regulating with *Gwakhyang Jeonggi San* and *Hyangsa Yangwi Tang* (Decoction of Rhizoma Cyperi and Fructus Amomi for nourishing the stomach) should be adopted. If the exterior heat embraces the interior cold, then the poisonous qi gathers inside, becoming stronger as when one raises a tiger to know disaster later. If so, we must use *Padu Dan* (Pill of Semen Crotonis) to induce a bit of diarrheas, then give *Gwakhyang Jeonggi San* and *Palmul Gunja Tang,* which are regulating and strong tonifying drugs."

12 What Zhang Zhongjing referred to, as a blood disease of the lower-*jiao* is the same as the syndrome of the lesser yin patient whose Spleen yang qi is covered by cold and whose Kidney yang qi is obstructed by a pathogenic factor. Thus, the yang qi cannot go straight up to connect with the Spleen and is contracted in the bladder. "The manic behavior" means to speak in a confused state. "Having met a ghost," means emotional excitement and

delirium. "The exterior syndrome of the greater yang disease still remains" means that the patient sometimes has the symptoms of fever with uneasiness and chills. "The exterior syndrome of the greater yang disease is dispersed" means that the patient has no symptoms of fever with uneasiness and chills. The best way to treat this disease is to supplement the qi and to help the yang ascend, but to remove the blood stasis and to dispel the fever is not a good idea. Diarrhea caused by treatment with the purgative method described earlier indicates that treating the patients, who display the exterior symptoms of the greater yang disease, with *Chengqi Tang* (Decoction for purgation) is not suitable. Rather, one should replace it with *Didang Tang* or *Taoren Tang* (Decoction of Semen Persicae). While the exterior symptoms of the greater yang disease still remain, the yang qi is capable of fighting the pathogenic cold at the exterior level, although it is somewhat weakened. If the exterior symptoms have passed completely, then the yang qi is too weak to fight with the cold anymore. Finally, the yang qi is forced down by the cold. For this situation, how is it possible that purgative drugs are considered the ideal treatment? We do not have to wait until the yang qi reaches this stage to treat at with *Renshen Guizhi Tang*. By then, it is too late, is it not?

13 Zhang Zhongjing mentioned the febrile disease for women caused by the cold: At the onset of menstruation, the patient is feverish, delirious and insane at night, but returns to consciousness in the day. These are the symptoms of heat entering the blood chamber. Be careful not to disturb the stomach vital qi and the upper-middle-*jiao*. Self-healing will occur.

14 Yang brightness disease: Even though the patient has a parched throat with a thirst for water, if he can only hold the water in his mouth and can not swallow, then certainly he has epistaxis. Do not use a purgative.

15 Yang brightness disease: If the remedy of heat-elimination is adopted when anorexia is observed, hiccupping will occur. During the febrile disease caused by cold, if the patient has repeated nausea and vomiting, a purgative is prohibited, even though the yang brightness syndrome is observed. *Weijiashi* (Excess of the stomach and intestines) with constipa-

tion indicates that the exterior symptoms are not gone or the syndrome is half-exterior. A purgative will be applicable after regulation is achieved by taking Ramulus Cinnamomi and Radix Bupleuri.

16 I have said, "The syndrome mentioned above should be treated with *Gwakhyang Jeonggi San*, *Hyangsa Yangwi Tang* and *Palmul Gunja Tang*."

17 Zhang Zhongjing said, "The cause of the yang brightness disease is the excess of the stomach and intestines." One asked, "How does the yang brightness disease come into being?" Zhang Zhongjing answered, "When a diaphoretic, a purgative, or a diuretic is adopted for the greater yang disease, it will cause a loss of body fluid; and if the stomach is suffering from pathogenic dryness, then the disease transforms into the yang brightness. The patient suffering from interior excess will not change clothes (make stools) and experience constipation. What is described above is the so-called yang brightness disease."

18 If the exogenous febrile disease caused by cold changes into yang brightness, then a continuous light perspiration making the body wet will show itself; hence, the body becomes wet.

19 The exogenous febrile disease caused by cold: The syndrome is not gone after the adoption of an emetic or a purgative. There is no stool for five to six days, or even ten days, with tide fever in the afternoon, but no chills. The patient speaks to himself in an insane manner, as though he were observing ghosts. In a serious case, the patient unconsciously gropes at his clothes and bed in terror. He also has a slight dyspnea and stares out into nothingness. A tight pulse will indicate a curable case, while a hesitant pulse is the sign of a fatal case.

20 I have said, "When a doctor of the Chin-Han dynasties treated constipation, there was Radix et Rhizoma Rhei treatment, but no Semen Crotonis treatment. So Zhang Zhongjing also used *Da Chengqi Tang* (Drastic purgative decoction), which contains Radix et Rhizoma Rhei to treat a lesser yin patient who has the yang brightness disease transmitted from the greater yang disease. When a patient has continuous light perspiration, no stool

for five to six days, or for even longer than ten days, due to dryness, fidgetiness and excessiveness of the stomach, tide fever in the afternoon, but no chills, and speaks to himself in an insane manner, as though he were observing ghosts, the decoction will bring about a dramatic recovery. However, if the patient's condition is serious, he loses consciousness and gropes at his clothes and bed in terror, has a slight dyspnea and stares out into nothingness. After taking this decoction, if his pulse is tight, he will survive, while a hesitant pulse is the sign of a fatal case. This decoction can be applied to lesser yin patients who have had no stool for five to six days with tide fever in the afternoon as a result of the yang brightness disease transmitted from the greater yang disease. Zhang Zhongjing knew when to use this drug. Hence, he also knew that the symptoms and signs which show the transmission of the yang brightness disease from the greater yang disease in a lesser yin person. Zhang Zhongjing devoted his energy to determining the most suitable time to use *Da Chengqi Tang* in the treatment of this disease. Hence, he also knew when not to use this decoction. He found out that *Guizhi Tang* and *Renshen Guizhi Tang* are the only suitable drugs in the treatment of the greater yang and yang brightness diseases. To use this *Da Chengqi Tang* is like leaving the patient up to fate on the endless seaside (or the vast barren wasteland), waiting until the decoction can be used. In using *Da Chengqi Tang*, you must wait until the patient has had no stool for five to six days, with tide fever in the afternoon, and speaks to himself in an insane manner. How can it be said that this is an ideal treatment? Generally, if a lesser yin person has no spontaneous perspiration, his Spleen is not weak. Difficulties in defecating and dry stool indicate that his stomach is excess. That the lesser yin person with the greater yang and yang brightness diseases has no spontaneous perspiration means his Spleen is in fine condition. In this case, the illness is not so severe, even though the stools are very hard. There are drugs available to treat this condition easily. Radix et Rhizoma Rhei, Fructus Aurantii Immaturus, Cortex Magnoliae Officinalis and Natrii Sulfas are suitable for this case. In patients whose conditions are even more serious, there is only a fifty-percent chance of survival. When the condition is serious, we use *Palmul Gunja Tang and Seungyang Ikgi Tang with Padu Dan*. The result is dependent upon the following principles that in the case his pulse is tight, then he will survive, while a hesitant pulse is the sign of a fatal case. When the exterior symptoms of the greater yang disease remain, why do we not use the tonifying treatments to prevent and treat? For example, Semen Crotonis, a drug warm in nature and in vital function invigorating. Why should we wait till the occurrence of the yang brightness disease, which is accompanied by the tide fever in the afternoon, and the patient speaks to himself in an insane manner? If *Chengqi Tang* is used, there is only a fifty percent chance of survival."

21 In the 『*Benshifang*[3)]』 ("Effective Prescriptions"), Xu Shuwei[4)] said, "There was a patient suffering from the febrile disease caused by cold who had dyspnea, tachypnea, difficulty in defecation, tide fever recurring daily in the afternoon, and groping at his clothes, waving his hands in the air, looking straight ahead. Many doctors came to see him, but the patient's condition was very bad. Zhang Zhongjing wrote down these symptoms, but mentioned no effective treatment. He just said, 'The tight pulse indicates life, while the hesitant pulse indicates death.' At that time, I gave one pack of *Xiao Chengqi Tang* (Mild purgative decoction). Afterwards, he had a bowel movement, his symptoms began to disappear gradually, and his pulse also showed tauntness. In a fortnight, he had completely recovered."

22 In the 『*Haizangshu*[5)]』 ("Book of Haizang"), Wang Haogu said, "Once there was a patient suffering from the disease caused by cold who became insane enough with emotional excitement to run away, and had a weak, but rapid pulse. His condition worsened after he took *Chaihu Tang* (Decoction of Radix Bupleuri). Then he was treated with one pack of Radix Ginseng, Radix Astragali, Radix Angelicae Sinensis, Rhizoma Atractylodis Macrocephalae, Pericarpium Citri Reticulatae and Radix Glycyrrhizae decoction, his condition stabilized, and with one more dose, he slept soundly and was cured."

23 In the 『*Yixue Gangmu*[6)]』 ("Compendium of Medicine"), we read, "I have used qi invigorator and blood invigorator to cure some patients displaying symptoms of groping at their clothes and bed; only one of them

showed eyelid fasciculation and arrhythmia. I treated him with the same drugs, adding Ramulus Cinnamomi, after which the symptoms subsided."

24 In the 『*Minglilun*[7]』 ("Expounding on the Treatise"), Cheng Wuji said, "The tide fever is a symptom of yang brightness disease, but only the fever occurring in the afternoon can be called the tide fever. The yang brightness disease means the excess of the stomach and intestines. If there was the excess of the stomach and intestines, the patient shows symptoms of delirium and sticky perspiration on the hands and feet, accompanied by hard stool. If a patient displays the symptoms of delirious speech and tide fever, we may give him *Chengqi Tang*, but if the fever is not recurring tidal in the afternoon, the purgative must not be taken."

25 In the 『*Danxi Xinfa*[8]』 ("Danxi's Experiential Therapy"), Zhu Zhenheng said, "Whenever a deteriorated case of febrile disease caused by cold went into a coma, the nearly dying patient was made to drink 37.5g of Radix Ginseng boiled in water. Sweat then began to run down from the bridge of his nose."

26 I have said, "The discussions above indicate the difficulties in knowing when to use *Da Chengqi Tang*, so Zhang Zhongjing's *Da Chengqi Tang* cannot be relied upon. As shown already, there has been much confusion caused by his words. Zhang Zhongjing's *Da Chengqi Tang* might kill a person instead of curing him, so it should not be emphasized. The excess of the stomach and intestines, including difficulty in defecation and madness, should be treated with either whole Semen Crotonis or *Doksam Palmul Gunja Tang* (Decoction of eight noble ingredients with heavy dose of Radix Ginseng), or use Semen Crotonis first, then add *Palmul Gunja Tang*."

27 Zhang Zhongjing said, "The exterior symptoms of the yang brightness disease are fever, spontaneous perspiration with an aversion to heat during fever, but no chills."

28 Yang brightness disease caused by cold: If a patient has spontaneous perspiration and frequent urination, then the loss of body fluid will result in constipation and *piyue* (Spleen restriction). *Maren Wan* (Bolus of Fructus

Cannabis) will be a curative.

29 Yang brightness disease with spontaneous perspiration and normal urination will induce the exhaustion of the body fluid. Although there is constipation, no purgative should be adopted. Honey can be used as a constipation-dredging medication.

30 *Da Chengqi Tang* should be adopted immediately against yang brightness disease with fever and profuse sweating.

31 In the 『*Yixue Rumen*[9]』 ("Introduction to Medicine"), Li Chan said, "If the sweating can not be stopped, it is called yang collapse. If symptoms such as a feeling of stuffiness in the esophageal region, vexation in the chest, pale complexion, and twitching of muscles appear, the disease is difficult to treat. If the skin has a yellowish complexion and the limbs feel warm, the patient can be cured. When the sweating cannot be stopped, and genuine yang is lost, it is called yang collapse, and the body must be made cold. Numbness with coldness and contraction of the four limbs will appear, so *Guizhi Fuzi Tang* should be used."

32 Once, I treated an 11 year old lesser yin child who had yang collapse from too much sweating. He was always thinking seriously and suffered from diarrheas for a long time, and had heavy facial sweating at every meal. One day, headache, fever, spontaneous perspiration and constipation occurred suddenly. Since I was anxious about his frequent diarrheas, I didn't pay attention to the febrile symptoms such as headache, fever, constipation and perspiration, and just tried to dispel the exterior syndromes with Radix Astragali, Ramulus Cinnamomi and Radix Paeoniae Alba, etc. Four to five days after the treatment, the headache and fever had not disappeared. On the sixth day, I carefully observed his symptoms. The constipation lasted for four to five days. He urinated uncomfortably only two to three spoons of reddish urine two to three times a day. There were no chills with fever, and two to four times a day, he perspired over his face and whole body, and sometimes on the Renzhong (GV 26) point. The symptom was very serious, and I noticed that he got yang collapse from too much sweating. This syndrome was very serious, so I prescribed one

bean of Semen Crotonis and *Hwanggi Gyeji Buja Tang* (Decoction of Radix Astragali, Ramulus Cinnamomi and of Radix Aconiti Lateralis Praeparata), and he took two packs continuously. Later, at two o'clock in the afternoon, he had bowel movements and his urine became clean and slightly increased. The next day was the seventh day after the onset, and since I worried that he had taken too much Radix Aconiti Lateralis Praeparata, I prescribed one pack of *Hwanggi Gyeji Buja Tang* for two days. Two days later, yang collapse symptoms such as fever with no chills, profuse sweating, reddish and difficult urination, and constipation, a bluish face, and an intermittent tight cough appeared. His symptoms became more serious than before. It was around ten o'clock on the ninth day. Quickly, I gave him one bean of Semen Crotonis and two packs of *Insam Gyeji Buja Tang* containing 18.75g of Radix Ginseng and 7.5g of Radix Aconiti Lateralis Praeparata continuously. In the afternoon, bowel movement was possible, urination slightly increased, and the color of the urine was red, the same as before. Another pack of *Insam Gyeji Buja Tang* containing 18.75g of Radix Ginseng and 7.5g of Radix Aconiti Lateralis Praeparata was taken again. At midnight, the child was lying down laterally and could not raise his head. He vomited one or two spoonfuls of sputum, and consequently the tight coughing stopped. The next day, he took three packs of *Insam Gyeji Buja Tang* with 18.75g of Radix Ginseng and 7.5g of Radix Aconiti Lateralis Praeparata, and ate two or three spoonfuls of rice gruel. After each administration, he felt comfortable, stopped sweating, urinated a little more than before, and experienced no more constipation. The next day, he took another two packs, and could eat half a bowl of rice gruel. The next day, he took two more packs, and could eat more than half a bowl of rice gruel, felt comfortable without fever, and could move about in his house. It was the twelfth day after onset. During the last three days, the reason for his body experiencing no fever, no sweating, no constipation, and clean and fluent urine was due to taking 7.5g of Radix Aconiti Lateralis Praeparata two or three times a day. On the thirteenth day, he walked down to the garden, but he could not keep his head upright. Since I worried that he had taken too much Radix Aconiti Lateralis Praeparata, I gave him *Hwanggi Gyeji Buja Tang*, including 3.75g of Radix Aconiti

Lateralis Praeparata only twice a day. After seven to eight days, he could bring his head into a slightly upright position and his facial edema. was relieved. Thus, the same drug was used twice per day. After seven to eight days, he could put his head upright and his facial edema became milder than before. Afterwards, two packs of the drug were used every day. From the beginning, he took about 300g of Radix Aconiti Lateralis Praeparata for a month or more.

33 Zhang Zhongjing said, "There are three types of the yang brightness disease. *Piyue* (Spleen restriction) is called the yang brightness disease of the greater yang. The excess of the stomach and intestines is called the yang brightness disease of the yang brightness. The yang brightness disease of the lesser yang, which is caused by the adoption of a diaphoretic and a diuretic, manifests itself as dryness, fidgetiness and excessiveness of the stomach with constipation."

34 I have said, "Among the three types of yang brightness disease mentioned by Zhang Zhongjing, the first one is the Spleen restriction, which displays symptoms such as spontaneous sweating and smooth urination. The second one is the excess of the stomach and intestines, which contains symptoms such as the inability to change clothes and difficulty in defecation. The third one has symptoms such as dryness, fidgetiness and excessiveness of the stomach due to the adoption of a diaphoretic and a diuretic. This also belongs to the excess of the stomach and intestines, so there are not three, but only two types. Zhang Zhongjing regarded the Spleen restriction as the gradual decrease of body fluid, and the excess of the stomach and intestines as the dryness and excessiveness of the whole stomach region as the body fluid becomes exhausted. During the ancient middle ages, e.g. Warring States and Chin-Han dynasties, diaphoretic, emetic and purgative treatment began to be widely used after a long period of experiments using simpler drugs. For the exterior syndromes of the greater yang disease, one might use *Mahuang Tang* (Decoction of Herba Ephedrae) to induce sweating, or *Zhuling Tang* (Decoction of Polyporus) to induce smoother urination, or *Chengqi Tang* (Purgative decoction) to induce defecation.

Inducing defecation by *Chengqi Tang* may cause unceasing diarrheas. Taking *Mahuang Tang* and *Zhuling Tang*, which induce sweating and urination, will cause dryness, fidgetiness and excessiveness of the stomach with constipation. Zhang Zhongjing thought that the gradual restriction of Spleen fluid induced by the spontaneous sweating and the smooth urination of the Spleen restriction turned into dryness, fidgetiness and excessiveness of stomach. However, the Spleen restriction comes from the Spleen restriction, and the excess of the stomach and intestines comes from the excess of the stomach and intestines. It is unreasonable to assume that Spleen restriction should induce the excess of the stomach and intestines."

35 The excess of the stomach and intestines and the Spleen restriction are as different from each other as the deficient and excessive symptoms of greater yin and lesser yin disease, which belong to the yin syndrome. At the exterior syndrome of the greater yang disease, they have already separated into their own paths and cannot be remingled. When the exterior syndrome of the greater yang disease still remains and the patient behaves in a manic way, it is the initial stage symptoms of *yukuang* (oppressive mania). The inability to experience a bowel movement due to yang brightness disease with excess of the stomach and intestines belongs to the midstage symptoms of oppressive mania. Yang brightness disease with tide fever, manic speech, minor dyspnea, and staring straight are the terminal stage symptoms of oppressive mania. Greater yang disease with fever, chills, and spontaneous sweating is the initial stage of yang collapse. Yang brightness disease with no chills, but rather an aversion to heat, and spontaneous sweating are the midstage symptoms of yang collapse. Yang brightness disease with fever and profuse sweating are the terminal stage symptoms of yang collapse. Generally, most oppressive mania symptoms include fever with no sweating, while most yang collapse symptoms include fever with spontaneous sweating.

36 Among the yin syndromes, abdominal pain, diarrheas and the absence of abnormal sensation in the mouth are symptoms of the greater yin disease, while abnormal sensations in the mouth, abdominal pain and diarrheas are symptoms of the lesser yin disease. Among the yang syndromes, no

spontaneous sweating with headaches and fever are the oppressive maniac syndromes of the yang brightness disease of the greater yang, and spontaneous sweating, headaches and fever are the yang collapse syndromes of the yang brightness disease of the greater yang. Among the greater yin disease of yin syndrome and the oppressive maniac disease of yang syndrome, there are mild and severe symptoms. Among the lesser yin disease of yin syndrome and the yang collapse disease of yang syndrome, there are dangerous and critical symptoms, too. From the onset, yang collapse and the lesser yin disease already show a dangerous condition and which will grow increasingly critical.

37 Among the yang collapse symptoms, we should pay attention to the sweating, and, also, to the amount of urine. If there is clear and profuse urine flow and spontaneous sweating, it belongs to the Spleen restriction. They are dangerous symptoms. If there is yang collapse with reddish and difficult urination and spontaneous sweating, it belongs to the yang brightness disease with fever and profuse sweating. This too indicates a critical condition. However, there is also profuse sweating with reddish and difficult urination in the interior heat syndrome of the lesser yang person and the exterior heat syndrome of the greater yin person, so we should differentiate those diseases and avoid adopting the wrong drugs.

38 In the beginning of excess of the stomach and intestines, the symptoms are aversion to heat during fever, but no sweating or chills. When the condition becomes critical, there should be a little sticky sweating and tidal fever. A little sticky sweating and tidal fever indicate that the force dispersing and expelling the exterior cold evil is thoroughly exhausted. This is a sign of *weijie* (stomach exhaustion). In the beginning of the Spleen restriction, the symptoms are fever, spontaneous sweating, but no chills. When the condition becomes critical, the patient should display symptoms such as fever, profuse sweating and chills. Fever, profuse sweating and chills indicate that the force supporting the Interior Heat is already exhausted; this is also a sign of *pijue* (Spleen failure).

39 Zhang Zhongjing mentioned, "The reverting yin syndrome: *Danggui Sini*

Tang (Decoction for resuscitation with Radix Angelica Sinensis) is the curative for a case of cold limbs, lower abdominal pain, restlessness and fullness in the chest, constriction of the scrotum, and a slender pulse that is hardly detectable."

40 When the yin qi and yang qi cannot connect with each other, *jue* (syncope) will occur. The symptoms of syncope are a feeling of coldness on the hands and feet.

41 Six to seven days after the onset of exogenous febrile disease caused by cold, if the *chi* (inch) and *cun* (cubit) pulses are slightly moderate, it is the stage of reverting yin. When the symptoms of reverting yin include fullness in the lower abdomen and constriction of the scrotum, *Chengqi Tang* may be used.

42 Six to seven days after the onset of exogenous febrile disease caused by cold, if there is a big pulse, severe restlessness, stiffness of the mouth inducing an inability to speak and discomfor, he will certainly recover.

43 In the 『*Huorenshu*』, Zhu Gong said, "When one's limbs are cold, it is called syncope. When the tips of one's fingers and toes are slightly cold, it is called 'cool' and is a mild case. If one gets yin syncope, from the beginning, one will have cold limbs, a deep, weak, slow pulse pattern, and the feet may tremble."

44 Six to seven days after the onset of an exogenous febrile disease caused by cold, if there is restlessness and fullness in the chest, scrotum constriction and the inch and cubit pulses are moderate in nature; it means that the Liver meridian has been affected. If his pulse type is weak and floating, it indicates that he will recover; but if his pulse type is not floating, it indicates that his condition is difficult to cure. If his pulse type was floating and moderate, his scrotum is not constricted. If the patient had the exterior symptoms such as fever and chillness, his illness is about to be cured. *Guima Geban Tang* (Half and half combination of *Guizhi Tang* and *Mahuang Tang*) may be used. If his pulse type is deep and short on the inch and cubit, the scrotum constricts, and the toxic evil invades his abdomen, *Chengqi Tang* should be used. Emergency administration of *Chengqi Tang*

could save five in six patients. When a patient's pulse type becomes weak and floating on the sixth and seventh day, it means the condition is one of going up of water and going down of fire, according to the following principle: "If the *Pi* (䷋) goes to extremes, the *Tai* (䷊) will come." He will be fine after some chills and fever with profuse sweating.

45 A symptom such as cold limbs belongs to reverting yin, and we cannot adopt the diaphoretics and the purgative. However, the diaphoretics and the purgative can be used when the limbs of the patient get warm and the palms of the hands and feet feel warm from time to time. This is not *zhengjueni* (genuine cold limbs), so we must be careful.

46 Li Chan said, "If there are symptoms such as curled tongue, coldness over the elbow and the knee, and colic pain in the lower abdomen, *Sanwei Shenyu Tang* (Decoction of three drugs with Radix Ginseng and Fructus Evodiae) and *Sishun Tang* (Decoction of four drugs for a favorable condition) can be used. If there are symptoms such as constriction of the scrotum, alternating hot and cold limbs, and restlessness, *Da Chengqi Tang* may be used."

47 I have said, "The reverting yin disease, mentioned by Zhang Zhongjing, in which there is no abdominal pain or diarrhea at the onset, and sudden cold limbs on the sixth and seventh days, is not a case of yin syndrome. For a lesser yin person, the greater yang disease caused by wind has symptoms such as chills, fever and spontaneous sweating. These symptoms indicate a long-term conflict between the healthy qi and the pathogen. Eventually, this conflict brings about this syndrome, and this should be called the reverting yin syndrome of greater yang disease. It is not suitable to use *Danggui Sini Tang* or *Magui Geban Tang*, but *Shenyu Tang, Insam Osuyu Tang* or *Doksam Palmul Tang* could be used. *Da Chengqi Tang* is not suitable, but Semen Crotonis must be adopted."

48 A lesser yin person who gets an exogenous disease and cannot sweat for six to seven days will die from the reverting yin disease. After careful observation of his condition for four to five days, if the patient takes three to five packs of *Hwanggi Gyeji Tang* and *Palmul Gunja Tang,* death will be

prevented.

49 Zhu Gong said, "The reverting yin disease displays the following symptoms: great thirst with frequent urination, an uncomfortable feeling of ascending qi rushing up from below the esophagus, a hot and painful feeling in the chest (stomach), and hunger without being able to take in food. Once food is taken, ascarides will be regurgitated."

50 Gong Xin said, "Avoid adopting a purgative for a patient who, while suffering from the exogenous febrile disease caused by cold, regurgitated ascarides, even though he has a high fever. If the drug, which induces the body cold, was used, he will die. If there is coldness in the stomach, the ascarides will ascend to the esophagus, a very bad sign, indeed. In this situation, *Lizhong Tang* (Decoction for regulating the middle) should be quickly adopted."

51 I have said, "For the symptoms mentioned above, *Lizhong Tang* should be taken three to four times a day continuously, or Pericarpium Citri Reticulatae, Cortex Cinnamomi and Radix Polygoni Multiflori could be added."

52 For a serious illness and critical symptoms, unless the patient takes the medicine three to four times a day, he cannot benefit from the full effect of the medicine; and if he takes the medicine continuously, he may recover somewhat, but not completely. Continuous taking means taking the medicine once to three times a day, and two to three days or five to six days or several months continuously. The amount of doses per day and the number of days during which the patient takes the medicine will vary according to the illness's progress.

2

Discourse on the Lesser Yin Person's Interior Cold Disease Induced from the Stomach Affected by Cold*

1 Zhang Zhongjing said, "The symptoms of the greater yin disease are abdominal distension with vomiting, anorexia, and worsening diarrheas with occasional abdominal pain."

2 Abdominal distension, pain that appears time and again, vomiting and diarrheas without thirst are symptoms of the greater yin disease. *Sini Tang* (Decoction for warming cold limbs) or *Lizhong Tang* should be adopted. When abdominal distension is not reduced, or not significantly reduced, *Da Chengqi Tang* should be used.

3 Diarrhea without thirst in a febrile disease caused by cold is symptomatic of the greater yin disease. It is caused by coldness in the viscera. *Sini Tang* should be adopted to warm the viscera.

4 For the treatment of the greater yin syndrome, accompanied by abdominal pain and diarrheas without thirst, *Lizhong Tang*, *Lizhong Wan* or *Sishun Lizhong Tang* or *Wan* also can be adopted.

5 I have said, "For the symptoms mentioned above, *Lizhong Tang*, *Sishun Lizhong Tang* and *Sini Tang* may be used. Since they originated in the

* 少陰人胃受寒裏寒病論

early stage of ancient times by Zhang Zhongjing, they are not sufficiently effective. Thus, *Baikhao Ijung Tang* (Decoction for regulating the middle with Radix Polygoni Multiflori Alba) and *Baikhao Buja Ijung Tang* (Decoction for regulating the middle with Radix Polygoni Multiflori Alba and Radix Aconiti Lateralis Praeparata) should be used. The symptom of abdominal fullness, not reduced or significantly reduced, is due to an obstinate cold syndrome and indigestion. In this case, Semen Crotonis should be used, but not *Da Chengqi Tang*."

6 Zhang Zhongjing said, "If a purgative is given as a remedy for the syndrome originating from yin, *pi* (qi stagnancy) will take shape. If the patient has nausea and fever as a result of a febrile disease caused by cold, and the patient feels fullness at the esophagus, but no pain, it is qi stagnancy. *Banxia Xiexin Tang* (Decoction of Rhizoma Pinelliae for purging the heart) is a curative. In case adverse gas ascends from the stomach caused by a grave deficiency, the above decoction is also applicable."

7 The incorrect application of a purgative will result in repeated diarrheas of undigested cereals several dozen times a day. Other possibilities are a gurgling sound in the abdomen, fullness and hardness at the esophagus. Nausea and restlessness are also observed. The reason for the just mentioned symptoms is a congealing of pathogenic heat, and is the adverse gas ascending from the stomach caused by a grave deficiency. *Gancao Xiexin Tang* (Decoction of Radix Glycyrrhizae for purging the heart) is a curative.

8 If a diaphoretic is used as treatment for the greater yin syndrome accompanied by diarrheas of undigested cereals, distension of the abdomen will certainly occur. In such a case, *Houpo Banxia Tang* (Decoction of Cortex Magnoliae Officinalis and Rhizoma Pinelliae) should be used.

9 After dispelling the syndrome of febrile disease caused by cold through perspiration, *Shengjiang Xiexin Tang* (Decoction of Rhizoma Zingiberis Recens for purging the heart) suits the following symptoms and signs: uneasiness of the stomach, fullness and hardness in the epigastrium, water stagnancy below the costal margin, and diarrhea with a gurgling sound in the abdomen.

10 After taking the purgative, the patient who had a febrile disease caused by cold had continuing diarrheas, fullness and hardness at the epigastrium. After the adoption of *Xiexin Tang* (Decoction for purging the heart) and other purgatives, continuing diarrheas occurred. *Lizhong Tang* was then given to stop the diarrheas, but the diarrheas became more serious. *Chishizhi Yuyuliang Tang* (Decoction of Halloysitum Rubrum and Limonitum) will be the curative.

11 I have said, "For the above-mentioned, the syndrome originating from yin, for which a purgative is given as a remedy, is the same disease which results from the stomach with a grave deficiency. *Huoxiang Zhengqi San* should be used rather than purgation with Radix et Rhizoma Rhei. Herba Ephedrae and Radix et Rhizoma Rhei are the drugs for a greater yin person, not the lesser yin person. Thus, it is impossible to adopt Herba Ephedrae and Radix et Rhizoma Rhei for a lesser yin person's disease, whether exterior or interior syndrome, to induce diaphoresis and purgative. A lesser yin person's disease with watery diarrheas and undigested food in the stool indicates that the congestion will be spontaneously cured. For watery diarrheas with undigested food in the stool of the greater yin disease, the following is recommended: *Gwakhyang Jeonggi San, Hyangsa Yangwi Tang* (Decoction for nourishing the stomach with Rhizoma Cyperi and Fructus Amomi) or *Gangchul Gwanjung Tang* (Decoction for relieving the middle with Rhizoma Zingiberis Recens and Rhizoma Atractylodis Macrocephalae) to warm the stomach and lower yin. For lesser yin disease, if watery diarrhea with undigested food in the stool appears, the following should be adopted: *Gwangye Buja Ijung Tang* (Decoction for regulating the middle with Cortex Cinnamomi and Radix Aconiti Lateralis Praeparata) to invigorate the Spleen and lower yin."

12 *Huoxiang Zhengqi San, Xiangsha Liujunzi Tang* (Decoction of six noble ingredients with Rhizoma Cyperi and Fructus Amomi), *Kuanzhong Tang* and *Suhe Yuan* are the variations of *Xiexin Tang* created by Zhang Zhongjing. It is comparable to that brilliant blue which comes from indigo blue. Ah! Although the blue is brilliant by itself, it would not be so were it not for the indigo blue. How can the blue be so blue?

13 Zhang Zhongjing said, "If a patient with *yindu* (yin type inflammatory swelling) of the febrile disease caused by cold had a bluish face and aching as if the patient were suffering a severe beating with sticks, within five days, the syndrome is curable. After seven days, it is difficult to cure."

14 Li Chan said, "When the disease of the three yin meridians becomes severe, it must change into yin type inflammatory swelling. The symptoms are coldness in the limbs, vomiting, diarrheas, no thirst, curling up while sleeping, and, in more serious cases, a sore throat, speaking incoherently in a state of unconsciousness, headaches, morbid perspiration on the head, intraocular pain, shying from light, a dark-green face, lips and nails, and severe ache of the body as if beaten by a club. This symptom includes a green, white or black face, coldness in the limbs, and somnolence."

15 I have said, "The above symptoms should be treated with *Renshen Guizhi Tang* or *Insam Buja Ijung Tang*."

16 Zhang Zhongjing said, "When a febrile disease caused by cold attacks straight into the yin meridian, in the beginning, there is no headache, no fever and no thirst, but there is intolerance to cold, curling up while sleeping, heaviness, a tendency to fall asleep, bluish lips, cold limbs, and either a feeble and expiring pulse or a hiding pulse. For the above condition, *Sini Tang* should be used. '*Sini*' means cold limbs."

17 Once I treated a lesser yin person with dry cholera, obstruction and rejection (dysuria and constipation with incessant vomiting) induced by cold attacking straight into the yin meridian. It was during the height of the hot summer weather. The lesser yin person's face color was sometimes green or white and also had four or five pellet-sized spots. His daily activities were almost as usual, but when he sat in the room, he leaned against the wall with general weakness and a tendency towards drowsiness. When he was asked of the cause, he said that he had had watery diarrhea one or two times several days before, after experiencing constipation for two days. Besides that, there were no other problems. Being asked of his diet, he said he had been eating barley meal. When he was treated with

Badou Ruyi Dan (Pills for alleviation with Semen Crotonis), sweat originating from the Renzhong point immediately covered his face, and he had loose stools one or two times after an hour and a half. I found that his green watery diarrhea was accompanied with some dregs when I saw his diarrhea at sunset. He had diarrheas ten or several more times at night. The next day, from early morning to nightfall, he had diarrheas ten or more times containing grains of barley like swollen yellow beans. Since his disease was induced by indigestion, I did not allow him to eat the following three days, except for one or two bowls of water boiled with burned rice everyday. On the early morning of the third day, his face looked somewhat bright, and his body showed general coldness. While sitting, his head and neck fell two to three inches from the ground, and he could not lift his head. His condition worsened. Examining the patient in detail, I found that his limbs, bladder, flank, abdomen were all cold as ice. The entire lower abdomen was hard as stone; however, the heat from his chest and abdomen upward to the Zhongwan region felt as if it could cauterize hands. His condition was a sight! On the early morning of the fifth day, there was an outbreak of vomiting of clear froth containing a bud of rice, after which the disease subsided considerably. He began to eat several bowls of thin rice gruel and took rice gruel in the next day. Since the patient was living in a poor mountain village, it was difficult for him to take the drugs that would warm the stomach and regulation. There was another lesser yin person who had diarrheas several times a day, and his diarrhea was like still clear water. He also had whole abdominal edema. At the beginning, he was treated with *Gyebugwakjin Ijung Tang* (Decoction of regulating the middle with Cortex Cinnamomi, Radix Aconiti Lateralis Praeparata, Herba Agastachis and Pericarpium Citri Reticulatae), in addition to 7.5g of Radix Ginseng and Cortex Cinnamomi each, and 3.75g to 7.5g of Radix Aconiti Lateralis Praeparata four times a day. A few days later, it was taken three times a day for ten or more days. There was watery diarrhea with undigested food in the stool. He had bowel movements 30 to 40 times continuously over a three day period, and the edema markedly decreased. There was another lesser yin child who had green watery diarrheas with a dark-green face and exhaustion to the point of near-sleep. He was treated with *Doksam Tang* (Decoction with a heavy dose of Radix Ginseng), in addition to 7.5g of Zingiberis Rhizoma Recens, 3.75g of Pericarpium Citri Reticulatae and 3.75g of Fructus Amomi. It was taken three or four times a day. After several days, he had diarrheas ten or more times, and was relieved by profuse sweating. It is considered that if the lesser yin person with dry cholera and obstruction and rejection had perspired at the Renzhong point, then he is on his way to being out of danger. When the patient with indigestion has massive diarrheas, he is further along in being saved from danger. When the patient vomits spontaneously, then he is saved from danger immediately. Not taking rice gruel or rice, but taking water boiled with burned rice or thin rice gruel is the best way of supporting healthy qi and inhibiting the pathogens. For the patient with indigestion to take warm water boiled with burned rice is good not only for digestion, but it can also be a substitute for regular foods. Though food is not ingested for two to four days, there is no need to worry.

18 Zhang Zhongjing said, "The symptoms and signs of the lesser yin disease are in general a feeble and weak pulse and a tendency for the patient to always fall asleep."

19 In case of the febrile disease caused by cold, if the patient cannot vomit and experiences fidgetiness, somnolence and diarrheas with thirst for five to six days, it will become the lesser yin disease. If the urine is clean, *Sini Tang* should be adopted.

20 In case of the lesser yin disease, *Fuzi Tang* (Decoction of Radix Aconiti Praeparata) is suitable for pain all over the body, cold limbs and arthralgia with a deep pulse.

21 In case of diarrhea, abdominal distension, and pain all over the body, we should warm the interior first and then treat the exterior. For warming the interior conditions, *Sini Tang* should be adopted. For treating the exterior conditions, *Guizhi Tang* should be adopted.

22 I have said, "The above symptoms should be treated with *Gwangye Buja Ijung Tang*."

23 Zhang Zhongjing said, "*Mahuang Fuzi Xixin Tang* (Decoction of Herba Ephedrae, Radix Aconiti Lateralis Praeparata and Herba Asari) act as curatives for a patient in the initial stages of the lesser yin disease with a fever and a deep pulse."

24 Lesser yin disease, the first or second day: When the patient has no abnormal sensation in the mouth and has chills over the back, *Fuzi Tang* should be adopted.

25 The reason why *Mahuang Fuzi Gancao Tang* (Decoction of Herba Ephedrae, Radix Aconiti Lateralis Praeparata and Radix Glycyrrhizae) was adopted to induce light perspiration on the second or third day in the lesser yin disease is that there were no symptoms or signs during this period. "No symptoms and signs" means an absence of vomiting, diarrhea and cold limbs.

26 If a patient has diarrhea with undigested cereals, a deep and slow pulse, a lightly flushed face and light perspiration, his illness will be gone following a period of vertigo and perspiration. The patient will then experience a light coldness in the limbs. This is caused by the deficiency of the lower portion, which can be seen from the symptom of *daiyang* (wearing yang) on the face.

27 The lesser yin disease with a slender, deep and speedy pulse would indicate that the disease is at the interior. Diaphoresis is prohibited for a patient having lesser yin disease that has coldness in the limbs, but without perspiration. If a diaphoretic is adopted for such a case, there will be bleeding, possibly from the mouth, nose, or eyes. It is termed "Lower coldness with upper exhaustion" and is a difficult case to treat.

28 I have said, "The greater yin disease and lesser yin disease which Zhang Zhongjing described are the same as the diarrhea of the lesser yin person with stomach qi asthenia. Greater yin disease with diarrhea is the usual symptom in serious cases, while lesser yin disease with diarrhea is dangerous for a patient in critical condition. If a doctor considers the two diarrheas as one and he is not seriously concerned with the lesser yin dis-

ease's diarrhea, then the patient cannot avoid death. The diarrhea in the greater yin disease is the diarrhea in the large intestine, and the diarrhea in the lesser yin disease is the diarrhea in the stomach. The diarrhea in the greater yin disease occurs when warm qi is dispelling cold qi, while the diarrhea in the lesser yin disease occurs when cold qi is suppressing warm qi."

29 In order for the lesser yin disease to disappear naturally, there must be a lightly flushed face and light perspiration. Following a period of vertigo and perspiration, there is relief. The ancients had seen this condition, so a patient having the lesser yin disease with only cold limbs, but without perspiration, was forced to sweat by Herba Ephedrae. The purpose was to help the patient to spontaneous recovery. However, unexpectedly, the drug moved his blood to come out of his mouth and nose. Thus, doctors became cautious and worried. We should not make light of the use of Herba Ephedrae for the lesser yin disease. Yet for the initial one or two days, or for the initial two or three days, a patient with lesser yin disease was given *Mahuang Fuzi Gancao Tang* to render light perspiration. But Herba Ephedrae is a harmful drug for the lesser yin disease. So although there are the initial symptoms for two to three days, Herba Ephedrae cannot be adopted to render perspiration. For this case, *Gwangye Buja Ijung Tang* should be used and Ramulus Cinnamomi can be substituted for Cortex Cinnamomi.

30 Since the initial symptom of the lesser yin disease can develop into a dangerous condition, we should make an early diagnosis and treatment at the initial stage of this disease to prevent the condition from worsening. Abdominal pain, spontaneous diarrhea without thirst and normal sensation in the mouth are the symptoms of the greater yin disease, while abdominal pain, spontaneous diarrhea with a feeling of thirst and with abnormal sensation in the mouth are the symptoms of the lesser yin disease. The lesser yin disease produces an aching of the body and arthralgia, which are symptomatic of the exterior syndrome. Though both the exterior and interior syndromes appear, the cold qi in the large intestine certainly surpasses the stomach warm qi and ascends. The greater yin disease has no aching of the body or arthralgia, which are symptomatic of

the exterior syndrome. This is the case in which the interior syndrome appears, but the exterior syndrome does not. The stomach warm qi surpasses the cold qi in the large intestine and descends.

31 Zhang Zhongjing said, "For the lesser yin disease with watery stools, pain in the epigastric region and a parched mouth, *Da Chengqi Tang* can be adopted."

32 Zhu Gong said, "Immediate purgation is recommended for the lesser yin disease with a dry mouth and throat, and thirst. Although it does not belong to the yang brightness disease, this disease should be purged, and the slow-acting laxative also can be adopted."

33 In the 『*Dongyuanshu*[1)]』 ("Book of Dongyuan"), Li Gao said, "The lesser yin disease should be diagnosed through the conditions of the mouth. The patient who has a normal sensation in the mouth should use warming drugs, and the patient who has a dry mouth should use purgatives. The lesser yin disease should be diagnosed by the colors of the diarrheas. The patient who has diarrhea without a greenish color should use warming drugs, and the one who has greenish diarrhea should use purgatives."

34 Li Chan said, "For dryness of the tongue and mouth or watery stool, and delirium followed by sudden difficulty in defecation, *Xiao Chengqi Tang* should be adopted. For cyanoses of the lips, cold limbs and dark-bluish nails, *Jiangfu Tang* (Decoction of Rhizoma Zingiberis Recens and Radix Aconiti Lateralis Praeparata) is suitable."

35 I have said, "For watery diarrhea, Semen Crotonis should be adopted as a purgative, and *Gwangye Buja Ijung Tang* as a warming drug. If there is watery stool accompanied with sudden difficulty in defecation, Semen Crotonis should be adopted first, and then *Gangchul Gwanjung Tang*."

36 There once was a ten year old lesser yin boy who was always too pensive and anxious. Therefore, he experienced abdominal pain and diarrhea every one or two days. He was treated with two to four packs of *Baikhao Ijung Tang* (Decoction for regulating the middle with Radix Aconiti Lateralis Praeparata), and when his condition worsened, one to two packs

of *Buja Ijung Tang* was administered. The diarrhea was subsequently always relieved. Another time, the boy was depressed for several days. Two packs of *Baikhao Ijung Tang* were taken as preventive treatment, but diarrhea with watery stool persisted. He continued to take six packs of *Baikhao Ijung Tang* a day, but in vain. He was immediately given six packs of *Buja Ijung Tang*. The clear, watery stool having changed to a dark color, he took two more packs, after which the dark watery stool ceased. Afterwards, he continued to take two to three packs for recuperation. Analyzing the above case, the initial diarrhea with clear watery stool was accompanied with cholera and obstruction and rejection. In this case, there was no doubt that treatment required eliminating the obstinate cold syndrome and indigestion with Semen Crotonis. The boy got diarrhea with clear watery stool in December, in his tenth year, and on February of the next year, he got the yang collapse disease again.

37 Zhu Gong said, "Ceaseless restlessness and coldness in the limbs is called *zangjue* (visceral shock)."

38 Li Chan said, "In case of visceral shock, the patient has unceasing restlessness, and seven to eight days after the onset of fever, he has a weak pulse, cold skin with restlessness and occasional vomiting and diarrhea with restlessness. This is induced by the shortage of the genuine visceral qi of the reverting yin. It was named visceral shock. Zhongjing was at a loss for a suitable treatment, and simply adopted cool *Sini Tang*. In case of the lesser yin disease, symptoms such as coldness in the limbs, vomiting, diarrhea and restlessness are difficult to cure. *Sanwei Shenyu Tang* is suitable."

39 I have said, "Lesser yin persons are at times unstably delighted, but as a result of a lack of ideas and power, they become annoyed and impatient. In the case of the febrile disease caused by cold in lesser yin disease, is the disease not due to a lack of ideas and powers, which results in symptoms such as nausea without vomiting, restlessness and tendency to fall asleep? Generally, unstable delight comes from avarice. How does a man contract the lesser yin disease from a lack of ideas and power? Why does he not have a generous mind? However, during the initial stage of febrile

disease caused by cold, if a patient manifesting symptoms of nausea without vomiting, restlessness in the mind and a tendency to fall asleep is treated early, he can be saved. If the patient displays symptoms such as unceasing restlessness and cold limbs, he is in a dangerous stage. What a pity for him! For these symptoms, he should take *Shenyu Tang* (Decoction of Radix Ginseng and Fructus Evodiae), *Sini Tang, Gwangye Buja Ijung Tang* and *Osuyu Buja Ijung Tang* (Decoction for regulating the middle with Fructus Evodiae and Radix Aconiti Lateralis Praeparata)."

40 Zhu Gong said, "Coldness on the body, a deep, slender and rapid pulse, restlessness, and an inability to drink water are the manifestations of yang being kept in the exterior by excessive yin in the interior. If the patient can drink water, he does not have this disease. In reverting yin disease, if the patient wants to drink water, he will recover after frequent drinking of small amounts of water."

41 Cheng Wuji[2)] said, "*Fan* (irritability) means that the patient feels restlessness in the chest, and *zao* (restlessness) means that the qi radiates from the heat outward. If there is irritability without restlessness, or irritability first and restlessness next, the patient will be curable. If there is restlessness without irritability, or restlessness first and irritability next, the patient will be incurable. Restlessness first and irritability next is similar to the feeling of restlessness and annoyance one has after getting angry; in this case, the yang is being kept in the exterior by excessive yin in the interior. Although the patient is thirsty enough to immerse himself in muddy water, he cannot drink any water at all. This action is a last-ditch attempt by the patient to replenish his qi, and can be characterized as a lamp being lit for the last time before going out."

42 Li Chan said, "If yang is kept in the exterior by excessive yin in the interior in a febrile disease caused by cold, the patient will experience coldness all over his body; but because of restlessness, he will want to jump into a well. He will have bluish lips and a dark face, thirst, as well as regurgitate water and pass diarrhea with black fluid. A deep, slender, and fast or impalpable pulse is a serious asthenic sign of yang being kept in the exte-

rior by excessive yin in the interior. *Pili San* (Powder of thunderbolt) is suitable, but if the patient experiences cold limbs, irritability and restlessness, he will not be cured."

43 I have said, "For the above symptoms, *Gwangye Buja Ijung Tang* and *Osuyu Buja Ijung Tang* should be adopted; *Pili San* is also suitable."

44 The conditions of visceral shock and yang being kept in the exterior by excessive yin in the interior are almost the same, and both are very critical. Once facing this crisis, it is very difficult to handle it. The only way to survive this illness is to adopt *Gwangye Buja Ijung Tang* and *Osuyu Buja Ijung Tang* before these symptoms manifest themselves.

45 Generally, we have to check whether the patient has *xinfan* (fidgetiness) or not at the onset of diarrhea in a lesser yin person's disease. In case the patient has fidgetiness, he should have thirst with an abnormal sensation in the mouth. In case he has no fidgetiness, he should have no thirst with a normal sensation in the mouth. When we observe the critical conditions in a lesser yin person's disease, we have to check whether restlessness is stabilized or not. When we check whether restlessness is stable or not, we should understand the state of the patient's mind so as to see if it is stable or not. A collected mind shows that restlessness is stabilized. A restless mind shows that restlessness is unstabilized. However, in the midst of an anxious state, if the patient feels temporary comfort, the illness can be cured. For the curable patient, the administration of Rhizoma Zingiberis and Radix Aconiti Lateralis Praeparata will prove effective.

46 Generally, if a lesser yin person has diarrhea three times a day, it will be more serious than having it once or twice a day. Four to five times are certainly more serious than two to three times, and four times a day is a sign of grave illness. One day's diarrhea is milder than two day's, and two day's diarrhea is milder than three to four day's. Frequent diarrhea that persists for more than three days is frequently very serious. If an ordinary lesser yin person has diarrhea two or three times a month, he is not in a mild stage. If he has dry stool three or four times a day, he is not in a mild stage. Even though the patient has diarrhea of fluid stools containing

undigested food several dozen times a day, his mouth will not be dry and his cool qi will be expelled from the exterior. If a patient has diarrhea with watery stool, he will certainly have blue water in the abdomen. If the patient has diarrhea with yellow water, it certainly will not be clear and certainly shows some dregs.

47 Zhang Zhongjing said, "On the seventh or eighth day of the febrile disease caused by cold, symptoms such as orange-yellowish skin, dysuria and slight abdominal distension belong to greater yin disease. *Yinchenhao Tang* (Decoction of Herba Artemisiae Scopariae) is suitable. In case of febrile disease caused by cold, if there is perspiration only over the head and neck and dysuria, the skin will turn yellowish."

48 Li Chan said, "Infectious epidemic diseases which cause jaundice are called epidemic jaundice. This is very fatal and urgent, and *Zhangdan Wan* (Pills for pestilential jaundice) is suitable."

49 I have said, "For treating the disease above, *Yinchen Jupi Tang* (Decoction of Herba Artemisiae Scopariae and Pericarpium Citri Reticulatae), *Yinchen Fuzi Tang* (Decoction of Herba Artemisiae Scopariae and Radix Aconiti Lateralis Praeparata), *Yinchen Sini Tang* (Decoction for warming cold limbs with Herba Artemisiae Scopariae), *Zhangdan Wan* or *Badou Wan* should be adopted."

50 In the 『*Yixue Gangmu*』, we read, "*Jiexiong* (accumulation of pathogen in the chest) without high fever is caused by *shuijie* (accumulation of fluid). If there is sweating on the head only, that is *shuijiexiong* (accumulation of fluid in the chest). *Xiao Banxia Tang* is suitable."

51 Gong Xin said, "For accumulation of pathogen in the chest due to excessive cold without fever, one should adopt *Sanwu Bai San* (Powder of three white drugs)."

52 I have said, "To treat the above symptoms, *Gyeji Banha Sainggang Tang* (Decoction of Ramulus Cinnamomi, Rhizoma Pinelliae and Rhizoma Zingiberis Recens), *Jeokbaikhao Gwanjung Tang* (Decoction for relieving middle with Radix Polygoni Multiflori rubra et alba), *Sanwu Bai San* or the *Padu Dan* should be adopted."

53 In a lesser yang person's disease, hardness in the epigastrium is named the accumulation of pathogen in the chest, which is treatable. In a lesser yin person's disease, hardness in the epigastrium is named *zangjie* (accumulation of yin cold in the viscera), which is untreatable. The drugs for accumulation of fluid in the chest and *hanshijiexiong* (locked chest due to excessive cold) mentioned in the 『*Yixue Gangmu*』 and 『*Yijian*』 are almost the same as that for a lesser yin person with the greater yin disease. Those are similar to Zhang Zhongjing's *Yinchenhao Tang*. They do not have actual masses, but experience a sensation of fullness in the epigastrium. The symptoms of Zhang Zhongjing's *Xiexin Tang* are a sensation of fullness and hardness in the epigastrium due to purgation of the febrile disease caused by cold. However, a sensation of fullness and hardness in the epigastrium after the diaphoretic treatment are simply sensations in the epigastrium or above the umbilicus area; there is not an actual solid mass in the epigastrium. If a lesser yin person has a hard mass on the right side of the epigastrium, he is untreatable.

54 Zhang Zhongjing asked himself, "Where there are accumulation of pathogen in the chest and accumulation of yin cold in the viscera, what are the differences and respective symptoms and signs?" He replied, "Tenderness (at the lower part of the chest and epigastrium), a pulse floating under the forefinger and deep under the middle finger are the symptoms and signs of accumulation of pathogen in the chest." And "What about accumulation of yin cold in the viscera?" he asked again. The reply was, "The symptoms and signs are similar to those of accumulation of pathogen in the chest, but with a normal intake of food and frequent loose bowels." A pulse floating under the forefinger and a feeble, deep and tense pulse under the middle finger are the symptoms and signs of accumulation of yin cold in the viscera. If the tongue's coating is white, moist and glossy, then it is considered to be a serious case. The patient used to have vital qi stagnancy in the chest. If it extends to the part near the navel and stretches to the lower abdomen and the genitals, the syndrome is termed accumulation of yin cold in the viscera and may result in death.

55 Zhu Gong said, "The symptoms and signs of accumulation of yin cold in

viscera are similar to those of accumulation of pathogen in the chest. Drinking and eating are as usual, there are occasional diarrhea, and a white coating on the tongue." There is a phrase for this, "Drinking and eating as usual, occasional diarrhea and white coating on the tongue. Since the pain of the abdomen and penis adjoins, he is going to die."

56 I have said, "There was a lesser yin person who had a solid and hard mass in the right side of the epigastrium, and most of the drugs given were useless. After the administration of *Badou Ruyi Dan*, the condition worsened and was accompanied by a shaking of the head and tremors that occurred for a short time, followed by death several months later. Another lesser yin person exhibiting the same symptoms and signs used *Badou Dan*. He perspired all over the body except for both sides of the Renzhong point and also died one year later. After this, I observed four or five people with solid and hard mass on the epigastrium. They died within six months or a year, even though they had been treated with drugs, or received acupuncture and moxibustion. It is the accumulation of yin cold in the viscera disease and lesser yin person's disease."

57 Zhang Zhongjing said, "The period of jaundice is 18 days. After ten days, recovery should begin; but if it becomes severe, it is difficult to manage. If it is generated from the yin area, the patient should vomit. If it generates from the yang area, the patient should shiver and get feverish."

58 Every jaundice with yellow-red colored urine is induced by dampness-heat, so one must adopt the treatment against dampness-heat. Clean urine that cannot come from fever means no fever. If there are the symptoms and signs of *xuhan* (deficiency-cold type), it should be treated as *xulao* (consumption).

59 The patient becomes unable to sleep when accompanied by abdominal distension, a pale and yellowish face, and restlessness.

60 Patients with jaundice used to get fever at sunset, but have chills, which are caused by overindulgence. The urgencies in the bladder, lower abdominal distension, yellowish discoloration of the whole body, black color on the forehead, and heat sensation under the feet are the symptoms

of black jaundice. The abdominal distension seems to contain fluid. There is tarry and occasionally loose stool that is caused by overindulgence. Abdominal distension is not a fluid disease; if the patient has abdominal distension, he cannot be easily cured.

61 Zhu Gong said, "Yin jaundice manifests itself as restlessness, impatience, shortness of breath, nausea, and no thirst. *Yinchen Jupi Tang* is available. For one who has jaundice of the febrile disease caused by cold accompanied by a weak pulse and cold body, *Yinchen Sini Tang* showed dramatic effects. For one who has jaundice of the febrile disease caused by cold accompanied by a deep, slender, slow and weak pulse, *Yinchen Fuzi Tang* showed a dramatic effect."

62 In the 『*Yixue Gangmu*』, we read, "A jaundice originating from dampness is accompanied by a dark yellowish discoloration, without pain on the body. A jaundice originating from heat, has a bright yellowish discoloration like orange and there is pain over the whole body."

63 Wang Haogu said, "If one fails to adopt a diaphoretic or a diuretic, he will get jaundice."

64 Zhu Zhenheng said, "If jaundice results from food accumulation, the accumulated food should be removed by purgative. For other cases, the diuretic method should be used. Once the urine is clean, the jaundice will spontaneously disappear."

65 Li Chan said, "A patient will die if jaundice persists more than ten days and is accompanied by abdominal distension, shortness of breath, severe thirst and a dark face."

66 In the 『*Maijing*[3)]』 ("Classic of Pulse"), Wang Shuhe[4)] said, "If one cannot detect a pulse near the wrist of a jaundice patient, who also has black, cold skin over the nose and mouth area, he is untreatable."

67 I have said, "Yin jaundice is a lesser yin person's disease and should be treated with Zhu's *Yinchen Jupi Tang* and *Yinchen Sini Tang*." However, I am not sure if jaundice from overindulgence, jaundice from heat, and

jaundice treated with a diuretic are a lesser yin person's disease. Since I have no experience in treating jaundice, it is impossible to say in detail. Feeling of fullness, jaundice and edema have the same origin, and they only have different degrees of severity. If it is necessary to induce urination, Rhizoma Zingiberis, Rhizoma Alpiniae Officinarum, Pericarpium Citri Reticulatae, Pericarpium Citri Reticulatae Viride, Rhizoma Cyperi, Semen Alpiniae Oxyphyllae, etc. can promote fluent urination in a lesser yin person. Herba Schizonepetae, Radix Saposhnikoviae, Rhizoma seu Radix Notopterygii, Radix Angelicae Pubescentis, Poria, Rhizoma Alismatis etc. can promote fluent urination in a lesser yang person.

3

General Remarks on the Lesser Yin Person*

1 I have said, "Fever and chills are symptomatic of the greater yang disease, while fever with no chills is symptomatic of the yang brightness disease. Although both diseases have the same symptom of fever, there are big differences in chills and the status and strength of the yang qi, which can be likened to the differences between high mountains and hills. Diarrhea with no thirst is a symptom of the greater yin disease. Diarrhea with thirst is a symptom of the lesser yin disease. Although both diseases share the symptom of diarrhea, there are big differences in thirst and the conditions of cold qi, which can be likened to the clouds in the sky and the puddles. So the symptoms of *Gwakhyang Jeonggi San* and *Hyangsa Yangwi Tang* can be thought of running horses on the plain. However, the symptoms for *Doksam Palmul Tang* and *Gyebu Ijung Tang* (Decoction for regulating middle with Ramulus Cinnamomi and Radix Aconiti Lateralis Praeparata) can be thought of climbing a high mountain with a short walking stick. In case of a lesser yin person, one must distinguish whether he has yang brightness or lesser yin disease. Such diseases are very serious, like the treacherous byways of a high mountain. The patient must attempt good cultivation and take care, as though he were walking on a wide road and leaving behind a world of illusions."

---

* 少陰人泛論

2 The perspiration of the greater yang disease is a sign that heat qi pushing out the cold qi. The perspiration of the yang brightness disease is a sign that cold qi is attacking heat qi. The diarrhea of the greater yin disease is a sign that warm qi is kicking out cool qi. The diarrhea of the lesser yin disease is a sign of cool qi pushing out warm qi.

3 There are two auspicious symptoms in a lesser yin person's disease. They are perspiration from the Renzhong point and the ability to drink water.

4 There are two critical symptoms in a lesser yin person's disease. They are fever with profuse sweating and watery diarrhea.

5 There are six major symptoms in a lesser yin person's disease. The first one is the lesser yin disease; the second is the yang brightness disease; the third is yin type inflammatory swelling syndrome of the greater yin disease; the fourth is the reverting yin syndrome of the greater yang disease; the fifth is jaundice of the greater yin disease; and the last is the excess of the stomach and intestines of the greater yang disease.

6 Following fever with sweating, a patient's condition should improve. If it worsens, it must be the yang brightness disease. After relaxing the bowels with diarrhea, the disease should be relieved. If it gets worse after relaxing the bowels with diarrhea, it must be the lesser yin disease. Since the yang brightness and the lesser yin disease are induced by the situations in which the pathogen attacks healthy qi, we should treat the situation immediately. After chills and sweating, the illness will leave; but if the illness seems half cured, it could develop into reverting yin syndrome. After abdominal pain and diarrhea, the disease will leave; but if the illness seems half cured, it could develop into the yin type inflammatory swelling disease. Since both are diseases in which healthy qi and the pathogen confront each other, we should adopt the medicine quickly. If a disease is relieved after just one bout of perspiration when the patient has fever, it is a mild condition of the greater yang disease. If indigestion is relieved after just one bout of purgation, it is a mild condition of the greater yin disease. It is not necessary to take medicine for a mild condition of the greater yang and greater yin diseases, as they become relieved

naturally. However, if fever lasts for three days, even though diaphoresis is used, it could be a serious condition of the greater yang disease; and if indigestion lasts for three days, even though purgative methods are used, it could be a serious condition of the greater yin disease. Although the serious conditions of greater yang and greater yin diseases cannot be judged as mild cases, if the patients take two to three packs of suitable medicine, they can be relieved spontaneously. If fever lasts for six days even though a diaphoresis is used, and indigestion lasts for six days even though a purgative is used, the patient's condition belongs to the excess of the stomach and intestines and the jaundice of the greater yang and the greater yin disease. Since the excess of the stomach and intestines and the jaundice of the greater yang and the greater yin disease are induced by the blocking and congestion of healthy qi and the pathogen, the patient should take a massive dosage of medicine.

7 A case of either the greater yang or greater yin disease lasting for six or seven days can develop into a dangerous or serious condition, and certainly can become a critical condition within 10 days. The yang brightness and lesser yin diseases start as serious conditions and become critical in two to three days. Therefore, one should be careful from the onset of the yang brightness and lesser yin diseases. In the case of the greater yang and greater yin diseases, the patient should be observed for approximately four to five days.

8 Since the developments of the greater yang and greater yin diseases are moderate and last long, there are many complications. Since the developments of yang brightness and lesser yin diseases are urgent and do not last long, there are few complications. Therefore, it is necessary to use drugs between the first and second days of the yang brightness and lesser yin diseases. It is also necessary to use drugs between the fourth and fifth days of the greater yang and greater yin diseases. Since the reverting yin of greater yang and yin type inflammatory swelling of greater yin disease can develop into the critical stage within six to seven days, one should be more careful.

9 For the dangerous conditions of yang brightness disease and greater yang disease, *Doksam Palmul Tang* and *Bojung Ikgi Tang* are appropriate. If the patient does not take them three or four times a day or for a few days continuously, he will not be cured. For the dangerous conditions of lesser yin disease and greater yin disease, *Doksam Buja Ijung Tang* and *Gyebugwakjin Ijung Tang* (Decoction for regulating the middle with Ramulus Cinnamomi, Radix Aconiti Lateralis Praeparata, Herba Agastachis and Pericarpium Citri Reticulatae) are suitable. If he does not take them three or four times a day or for a few days continuously, he will not be cured. When the patient's condition is dangerous, he has to take the drugs four times a day. When the patient's condition is half-well, he has to take the drugs three times a day. When the patient's condition sees no change, he has to take the drugs twice a day. When a patient's condition improves slightly, he has to take the drugs three times over two days, or once one day and twice the other day. When a patient's condition gets much better, he has to take the drugs once a day. The medicine should also be taken once for two to five days. When one falls ill, one should take the medicine. If nothing is wrong, one should not take the medicine. One should take heavy medication when one has a serious problem, and mild medication for mild problems. However, if one likes to take heavy medication for mild problems and takes the drugs when nothing is wrong, his visceral qi will be weakened, and his sickness will worsen.

10 Though rich foods can stimulate our appetites, if we indulge in them every day, they will prove harmful to our eating habits. Though sheepskin can protect against coldness, if we wear it every day, it will become cold. If rich foods and sheepskin can lose their effectiveness, what of medicine? The hazards of taking medicine everyday are one hundred times more harmful than no administration. Generally, if one gets sick and one's symptoms are identified, one should take the medicine. If one has no problem, though the symptoms have been identified, one should refrain from taking medicine. We can guess that taking tobacco made of opium, mercury, wild Radix Ginseng and Cornu Cervi Pantotrichum repeatedly will shorten lives.

11 For the hematemesis of a lesser yin person, *Doksam Palmul Tang* should be taken. For nasopharyngeal pains, *Doksam Gwangye Ijung Tang* (Decoction for regulating the middle with Radix Ginseng and Cortex Cinnamomi) should be taken.

12 I once treated a lesser yin person who had become an overeater. He began consuming twice the amount he had been eating, until one month later, his belly swelled up and he died. A lesser yin person's diabetes belongs to swelling, and is a dangerous condition. He should be treated immediately with *Gunggwichongso Ijung Tang* (Decoction for regulating the middle with Rhizoma Chuanxiong, Radix Angelicae Sinensis, Bulbus Allii Fistulosi and Folium Perillae).

13 I once treated a lesser yin person with edema. After he had taken sliced roe liver five times, his edema was relieved. Another lesser yin person also took roe liver, and saw his vision improve and energy level increase. However, a lesser yang person with asthenia took a slice of roe liver and vomited blood until he died.

14 I once met a lesser yin person with general edema who had been advised by a doctor to take half a spoonful of natural salt water every day. In four or five days, his edema was greatly relieved; and one month later, the illness was cured.

15 Once, there was a lesser yin person who had been suffering from nasopharyngeal pain for several years. A doctor advised him to take gold snake liquor, and after drinking it, he was cured. The ingredient of the liquor is a gold-colored serpent.

16 Once, there was a lesser yin patient with dysentery. He was told to take redneck snake soup, and after eating it, he was cured. One should take the head and tail off from the redneck snake, and put it into a double silk pocket and hang it on the wooden bars of a jar. Cook the snake with five bowls of water into one bowl of soup. To prevent poisoning from direct contact with the snake's bone, it is better to put the snake into a pocket. Snake bones are toxic.

17 I witnessed that a lesser yin person with dysentery who had been cured by taking three big garlic cloves and half a spoonful of honey boiled together for three days.

18 Once, there was a lesser yin person with a mammary abscess of open sores and pus for seven to eight months. A doctor advised her to use a patch of wild Radix Ginseng and Fel Ursi, 0.375g each. The patient was immediately relieved. Using a patch of Radix Ginseng powder also cured another lesser yin person with whole-body swelling.

19 I once saw a lesser yin person with *neiyong* (internal carbuncle) near the breast. A doctor taught her to take out pus with a heated needle. He said, "An internal carbuncle manifests itself through fever with chills, like a febrile disease caused by cold, and severe pain in the settled portion. If we identify the existence of pus through the observation of the region, we should use a heated needle."

20 I once saw a lesser yin person with *beiyong* (back carbuncle). He was told by a doctor to be operated upon with a heated knife. The doctor said, "It is good to get rid of a carbuncle with a heated knife as soon as possible. If we hesitate, then the whole back will be hardened. It is of no use to regret about it then."

21 I witnessed a lesser yin person with hemiplegia. He was taught to take iron-enriched water and he was cured.

22 Once I saw a lesser yin child with *funue* (chronic malaria with splenomegaly). A doctor advised him to take toasted 0.225g of finely powdered Arsenicum with the decoction of Radix Glycyrrhizae in the morning when it occurred, and he was cured. The doctor said, "Yellow-din must be used and it must be toasted. The weight cannot be less or more than 0.225g. If more than 0.225g, there will be side effects. If less, it is useless. This drug was tested and used many times. If the malaria recurs after relief from this drug, we cannot use it again. If we use it again, the disease will worsen, so we may only use the drug once." According to the doctor, children who recover after one treatment and no recurrence are lesser yin children. If not, they

are not lesser yin children. This medicine is only to be adopted for a lesser yin child with chronic malaria with splenomegaly, and not for ordinary malaria. When he has chills, two to three packs of *Cheongung Gyeji Tang* (Decoction of Rhizoma Chuanxiong and Ramulus Cinnamomi) should be adopted for a lesser yin person with ordinary malaria over a two-day period; he will certainly be cured. If a patient has fullness in the abdomen and constipation, though he has malaria, he may also be given Semen Crotonis.

23 We cannot say that every drug is bad, but Arsenicum Trioxidum for lesser yin person and Pedicellus Melo for greater yin person are the worst drugs. It is very dangerous to adopt Arsenicum Trioxidum for every disease in the lesser yin person; it must only be used to cure malaria in the lesser yin person. However, this is a cure in name only: the medicine is actually useless, and doctors should beware. It is better to take Ramulus Cinnamomi, Radix Ginseng and Radix Paeoniae Alba three or four times to treat malaria. Arsenicum Trioxidum is not only useless, but hazardous as well, is it not? Pedicellus Melo is dangerous for every disease of the greater yin person, except in curing phlegm. It is thus useless, and doctors should beware. It is better to take Radix Platycodi, Radix Ophiopogonis and Fructus Schizandrae for three or four times for removing the phlegm. Pedicellus Melo is not only useless, but hazardous as well, is it not? Those two drugs can be used externally, but not orally.

24 There was once a lesser yin person who had had a stroke, curled tongue and aphagia. A doctor inserted a needle into the Hegu (LI 4) point, and the patient was cured as if by miracle. We can see that acupuncture can also get wonderful results when a drug has no immediate effects. It is of the opinion that there are certain points along the four constitutions that have wondrous effects upon the qi's up-down and slow-fast flow. As physicians, we must take this into account, and I wait and hope to see future doctors who have faithful hospitality and are pleased to save their patients.

3-1

Twenty Three Prescriptions for the Lesser Yin Person's Disease from Zhang Zhongjing's 『*Shanghanlun*』

1 Decoction of Ramulus Cinnamomi (*Guizhi Tang* 桂枝湯)

· Ramulus Cinnamomi 11.25 g
· Radix Paeoniae Alba 7.5 g
· Radix Glycyrrhizae 3.75 g
· Fructus Jujubae 2 pcs.
· Rhizoma Zingiberis Recens 3 slices

2 Decoction for regulating the middle (*Lizhong Tang* 理中湯)

· Radix Ginseng 7.5 g
· Rhizoma Zingiberis 7.5 g
· Rhizoma Atractylodis Macrocephalae 7.5 g
· Radix Glycyrrhizae (stir-baked with adjuvant) 3.75 g

3 Decoction of Rhizoma Zingiberis and Radix Aconiti Lateralis Praeparata (*Jiangfu Tang* 薑附湯)

· Rhizoma Zingiberis (stir-baked at high temperature) 37.5 g
· Radix Aconiti Lateralis Praeparata (stir-baked at high temperature) 18.75g

Stew and take the decoction. When 18.75g of Radix Aconiti Lateralis Praeparata is used in its raw form, it is called *Baitong Tang* (白通湯).

4 **Decoction of four drugs for favorable condition and regulating the middle** (*Sishun Lizhong Tang* 四順理中湯)

- Radix Ginseng 7.5 g · Rhizoma Zingiberis 7.5 g
- Rhizoma Atractylodis Macrocephalae 7.5 g
- Radix Glycyrrhizae (stir-baked with adjuvant) 7.5 g

5 **Decoction of Ramulus Cinnamomi and Radix Ginseng** (*Guizhi Renshen Tang* 桂枝人蔘湯)

- Radix Glycyrrhizae (stir-baked with adjuvant) 6.75 g
- Rhizoma Atractylodis Macrocephalae 5.625 g
- Ramulus Cinnamomi 6.75 g · Radix Ginseng 5.625 g
- Rhizoma Zingiberis 5.625 g

6 **Decoction for warming cold limbs** (*Sini Tang* 四逆湯)

- Radix Glycyrrhizae (stir-baked with adjuvant) 22.5 g
- Rhizoma Zingiberis Recens (stir-baked at high temperature) 18.75 g
- Radix Aconiti Lateralis Praeparata (crude) 1 pc.

Chop up the above ingredients and make two packs. Stew and take the decoction.

7 **Decoction of Rhizoma Pinelliae and Cortex Magnoliae Officinalis** (*Houpo Banxia Tang* 厚朴半夏湯)

- Cortex Magnoliae Officinalis 11.25 g
- Rhizoma Pinelliae 5.625 g · Radix Ginseng 5.625 g
- Radix Glycyrrhizae 2.625 g

8 **Powder of Rhizoma Pinelliae** (*Banxia San* 半夏散)

- Rhizoma Pinelliae (detoxicated with ginger decoction) 7.5 g
- Radix Glycyrrhizae (stir-baked) 7.5 g
- Ramulus Cinnamomi 7.5 g

9 **Decoction of Halloysitum Rubrum and Limonitum Cum Terra** (*Chishizhi Yuyuliang Tang* 赤石脂禹餘粮湯)

- Halloysitum Rubrum 9.375 g · Limonitum Cum Terra 9.375 g
- Halloysitum Rubrum 9.375 g · Limonitum Cum Terra 9.375 g

10 Decoction of Radix Aconiti Lateralis Praeparata (*Fuzi Tang* 附子湯)

- Rhizoma Atractylodis Macrocephalae 15 g
- Radix Paeoniae Alba 11.25 g · Poria (white) 11.25 g
- Radix Aconiti Lateralis Praeparata (stir-baked at high temperature) 7.5 g
- Radix Ginseng 1 pc.

11 Decoction of Herba Ephedrae, Radix Aconiti Lateralis Praeparata and Herba Asari (*Mahuang Fuzi Xixin Tang* 麻黃附子細辛湯)

- Herba Ephedrae 7.5 g · Herba Asari 7.5 g
- Radix Aconiti Lateralis Praeparata (stir-baked at high temperature) 3.75 g

12 Decoction of Herba Ephedrae, Radix Aconiti Lateralis Praeparata and Radix Glycyrrhizae (*Mahuang Fuzi Gancao Tang* 麻黃附子甘草湯)

- Herba Ephedrae 11.25 g · Radix Glycyrrhizae 11.25 g
- Radix Aconiti Lateralis Praeparata (stir-baked at high temperature) 3.75 g

13 Decoction for warming cold limbs with Radix Angelicae Sinensis (*Danggui Sini Tang* 當歸四逆湯)

- Radix Paeoniae Alba 7.5 g · Radix Angelicae Sinensis 7.5 g
- Ramulus Cinnamomi 5.625 g · Herba Asari 3.75 g
- Medulla Tetrapanacis 3.75 g · Radix Glycyrrhizae 3.75 g

14 Decoction of Rhizoma Pinelliae for purging the heart (*Banxia Xiexin Tang* 半夏瀉心湯)

- Rhizoma Pinelliae (detoxicated with ginger decoction) 7.5 g
- Radix Ginseng 5.625 g · Radix Glycyrrhizae 5.625 g
- Radix Scutellariae 5.625 g · Rhizoma Zingiberis 3.75 g
- Rhizoma Coptidis 1.875 g · Fructus Jujubae 2 pcs
- Rhizoma Zingiberis Recens 3 slices

15 Decoction of Rhizoma Zingiberis Recens for purging the heart (*Shengjiang Xiexin Tang* 生薑瀉心湯)

· Rhizoma Zingiberis Recens	7.5 g	· Rhizoma Pinelliae	7.5 g
· Radix Ginseng	5.625 g	· Rhizoma Zingiberis	5.625 g
· Rhizoma Coptidis	3.75 g	· Radix Glycyrrhizae	3.75 g
· Radix Scutellariae	1.875 g	· Fructus Jujubae	3 pcs

16 Decoction of Radix Glycyrrhizae for purging the heart (*Gancao Xiexin Tang* 甘草瀉心湯)

· Radix Glycyrrhizae	7.5 g	· Rhizoma Zingiberis	5.625 g
· Radix Scutellariae	5.625 g	· Radix Ginseng	3.75 g
· Fructus Jujubae	3 pcs.		
· Rhizoma Pinelliae (detoxicated with ginger decoction)			3.75 g

17 Decoction of Herba Artemisiae Scopariae (*Yinchenhao Tang* 茵蔯蒿湯)

· Herba Artemisiae Scopariae	37.5 g	· Rhizoma et Radix Rhei	18.75 g
· Fructus Gardeniae	7.5 g		

Stew Herba Artemisiae Scopariae in water until half of the water remains. Add the remaining two drugs and stew until the water decreases again by half. Take the decoction for two days. This is only for the patient who has difficult in urination and whose urine is bloody. Abdominal distension will be reduced, and jaundice will disappear with urination.

18 Decoction of Didang (*Didang Tang* 抵當湯)

· Hirudo (stir-baked)	10 pcs.
· Tabanus (stir-baked, remove the legs and wings)	10 pcs.
· Rhizoma et Radix Rhei (steamed)	11.25 g
· Semen Persicae (with the tip)	10 pcs.

19 Decoction for purgation with Semen Persicae (*Taoren Chengqi Tang* 桃仁承氣湯)

· Radix et Rhizoma Rhei	11.25 g	· Ramulus Cinnamomi	7.5 g
· Natrii Sulfas	7.5 g	· Radix Glycyrrhizae	3.75 g

· Semen Persicae (with the tip) 10 pcs.

20 Bolus of Fructus Cannabis (*Maren Wan* 麻仁丸)

· Radix et Rhizoma Rhei (steamed) 150 g
· Fructus Aurantii Immaturus 7.5 g
· Cortex Magnoliae Officinalis 75 g
· Semen Armeniacae Amarum 46.875 g
· Radix Paeoniae Rubra 75 g · Fructus Cannabis 56.25 g

Make the bolus with honey, as big as the seed of an empress tree. Take 50 boli on an empty stomach with warm water.

21 Purgative method with honey (蜜導法)

This is used for the weak and elderly who cannot take drugs. Pour the powdered Fructus Gleditsiae into boiling honey, and from the mixture make suppositories. Insert the suppository into the anus in order to loosen the stool.

22 Decoction for potent purgation (*Da Chengqi Tang* 大承氣湯)

· Radix et Rhizoma Rhei 15 g · Natrii Sulfas 7.5 g
· Cortex Magnoliae Officinalis 7.5 g
· Fructus Aurantii Immaturus 7.5 g

First stew Cortex Magnoliae Officinalis and Fructus Aurantii Immaturus with two large glasses of water, and then stew until one glass of water remains. Remove the dregs and add Rhizoma et Radix Rhei. Stew the remaining amount and remove the dregs. Add Natrii Sulfas and boil it again. Take it while it is warm.

23 Decoction for mild purgation (*Xiao Chengqi Tang* 小承氣湯)

· Radix et Rhizoma Rhei 15 g
· Cortex Magnoliae Officinalis 5.625 g
· Fructus Aurantii Immaturus 5.625 g

Chop up the three drugs and make a pack. Stew it and take the decoction.

3-2

Thirteen Prescriptions and Six Other Prescriptions Containing Semen Crotonis for the Lesser Yin Person's Disease Mentioned in the Writings of Famous Doctors in the Song, Yuan and Ming Dynasties

1 Decoction of ten powerful tonics (*Shiquan Dabu Tang* 十全大補湯)

· Radix Ginseng	3.75 g	· Radix Paeoniae Alba	3.75 g
· Radix Astragali	3.75 g	· Cortex Cinnamomi	3.75 g
· Poria (white)	3.75 g	· Rhizoma Chuanxiong	3.75 g
· Radix Angelicae Sinensis	3.75 g	· Fructus Jujubae	2 pcs.
· Rhizoma Atractylodis Macrocephalae	3.75 g		
· Radix Glycyrrhizae (stir-baked with adjuvant)	3.75 g		
· Radix Rehmanniae Praeparata	3.75 g		
· Rhizoma Zingiberis Recens	3 slices		

This prescription from Wang Haogu's 『*Haizangshu*』 is for consumptive patients.

In accordance with results from recent studies, Poria (white), Radix Rehmanniae Praeparata Should be excluded from this prescription, and Fructus Amomi and Pericarpium Citri Reticulatae should be added.

2 Decoction for tonifying the middle and replenishing qi (*Buzhong Yiqi Tang* 補中益氣湯)

· Radix Astragali	5.625 g	· Radix Ginseng	3.75 g
· Radix Bupleuri	1.125 g	· Rhizoma Cimicifugae	1.125 g

· Fructus Jujubae	2 pcs.
· Radix Angelicae Sinensis	2.625 g
· Pericarpium Citri Reticulatae	2.625 g
· Radix Glycyrrhizae (stir-baked with adjuvant)	3.75 g
· Rhizoma Atractylodis Macrocephalae	3.75 g
· Rhizoma Zingiberis Recens	3 slices

This prescription from Li Gao's 『*Dongyuanshu*』 is for patients suffering from exhaustion, asthenia, fever, irritability, spontaneous perspiration and weariness.

In accordance with results from recent studies, the dosage of Radix Astragali should be increased to 11.25g, Rhizoma Cimicifugae and Radix Bupleuri should be excluded, and Herba Agastachis and Folium Perillae must be added.

3 Decoction of Rhizoma Cyperi and Fructus Amomi Rotundus with six noble ingredients (*Xiangsha Liujunzi Tang* 香砂六君子湯)

· Rhizoma Cyperi	3.75 g	· Poria (white)	3.75 g
· Radix Glycyrrhizae	1.875 g	· Radix Aucklandiae	1.875 g
· Rhizoma Pinelliae	3.75 g	· Radix Ginseng	1.875 g
· Fructus Amomi	1.875 g	· Fructus Jujubae	2 pcs.

· Rhizoma Atractylodis Macrocephalae	3.75 g
· Pericarpium Citri Reticulatae	3.75 g
· Fructus Amomi Rotundus	3.75 g
· Semen Alpiniae Oxyphyllae	3.75 g
· Cortex Magnoliae Officinalis	3.75 g
· Rhizoma Zingiberis Recens	3 slices

This prescription, from Gong Xin's 『*Yijian*』 ("Mirror of Medicine") is for patients with loss of appetite, slowness of digestion and fullness of stomach after meal.

In accordance with results from recent studies, Poria (white) should be excluded from this prescription, and Radix Polygoni Multiflori (white) must be added.

4 Powder of smoothing the flow of qi with Radix Amomi Aucklandiae (*Muxiang Shunqi San* 木香順氣散)

· Radix Linderae	3.75 g	· Rhizoma Cyperi	3.75 g
· Fructus Aurantii	3.75 g	· Rhizoma Pinelliae	3.75 g
· Fructus Amomi	1.875 g	· Cortex Cinnamomi	1.125 g
· Rhizoma Zingiberis	1.125 g	· Fructus Jujubae	2 pcs.
· Pericarpium Citri Reticulatae Viride			3.75 g
· Pericarpium Citri Reticulatae			3.75 g
· Cortex Magnoliae Officinalis			3.75 g
· Radix Amomi Aucklandiae			1.875 g
· Radix Glycyrrhizae (stir-baked with adjuvant)			1.125 g
· Rhizoma Zingiberis Recens			3 slices

These prescriptions, from Gong Xin's 『*Wanbing Huichun*』[1] ("Recovery from All Ailments") is for patients who have been attacked by qi. This disease occurs when a person is fighting and is so overwhelmed by anger that he loses consciousness. The above drug should be taken, after Rhizoma Zingiberis Recens decoction is administered and the patient regains consciousness.

5 Storax pill (*Suhexiang Yuan* 蘇合香元)

· Radix Aucklandiae	75 g	· Moschus	75 g
· Flos Caryophylli	75 g	· Benzoinum	75 g
· Lignum Santali Albi	75 g	· Fructus Chebulae	75 g
· Rhizoma Cyperi	75 g	· Fructus Piperis Longi	75 g
· Cornu Rhinoceri	75 g	· Olibanum	37.5 g
· Borneolum	37.5 g		
· Rhizoma Atractylodis Macrocephalae			75 g
· Lignum Aquilariae Resinatum			75 g
· Cinnabaris			75 g

(Use half of the Cinnabaris for coating the boli. Mix Storax oil with Benzoinum paste)

Make the above drugs into powder and mix them with the Benzoinum paste and honey. Pound 1000 times in a mortar. Make 40 boli from 37.5g of the resulting mixture. Two or three boli should be taken with spring water or warm water.

This prescription from the 『*Jufang*』[2] ("Formularies of the Bureau of People's Welfare Pharmacies") is for patients suffering from all manner of qi-related diseases: qi attack, reversed flow of qi, stagnation of qi, pain due to qi disorders.

In the 『*Benshifang*』 ("Effective Prescriptions") by Xu Shuwei said, "This prescription should be used for the cases, where excessive joy impairs yang, sudden anger impairs yin, and melancholy results from stuffiness, which, if serious, reverses the flow of qi. If used for apoplexy, many patients will die."

In the 『*Dexiaofang*』, Wei Yilin said, "The patient who is affected by wind has a floating pulse, fever and abundant expectoration in the mouth. The patient who is attacked by qi has a deep and sinking pulse, cold body, and dry mouth."

In accordance with results from recent studies, Moschus, Cornu Rhinoceri, Cinnabaris, Borneolum and Olibanum should be excluded from this prescription, and Herba Agastachis, Fructus Foeniculi, Cortex Cinnamomi, Faeces Trogopterorum and Rhizoma Corydalidis must be added.

6 Powder of Herba Agastachis for restoring qi (*Huoxiang Zhengqi San* 藿香正氣散)

· Herba Agastachis	5.625 g	· Folium Perillae	3.75 g
· Pericarpium Arecae	1.875 g	· Rhizoma Pinelliae	1.875 g
· Radix Glycyrrhizae	1.875 g	· Radix Platycodi	1.875 g
· Poria (white)	1.875 g	· Fructus Jujubae	2 pcs.
· Cortex Magnoliae Officinalis			1.875 g
· Rhizoma Atractylodis Macrocephalae			1.875 g
· Pericarpium Citri Reticulatae			1.875 g
· Radix Angelicae Dahuricae			1.875 g
· Rhizoma Zingiberis Recens			3 slices

This prescription, from Gong Xin's 『*Yijian*』 is for patients affected by Cold.

In accordance with results from recent studies, Radix Platycodi, Radix Angelicae Dahuricae and Poria (white) should be excluded from this prescription, while Cortex Cinnamomi, Rhizoma Zingiberis and Fructus Alpiniae Oxyphyllae must be added.

7 Powder of Rhizoma Cyperi and Folium Perillae (*Xiangsu San* 香蘇散)

· Rhizoma Cyperi	5.625 g	· Folium Perillae	3.75 g
· Rhizoma Atractylodis	1.875 g	· Rhizoma Pinelliae	1.875 g
· Radix Glycyrrhizae	1.875 g	· Radix Platycodi	1.875 g
· Poria (white)	1.875 g	· Fructus Jujubae	2 pcs.
· Cortex Magnoliae Officinalis			1.875 g
· Rhizoma Atractylodis Macrocephalae			1.875 g
· Pericarpium Citri Reticulatae			1.875 g
· Radix Angelicae Dahuricae			1.875 g
· Rhizoma Zingiberis Recens			3 slices

This prescription, from Wei Yilin's 『*Dexiaofang*』 is for patients suffering from four seasons' epidemic febrile diseases.

In the 『*Jufang*』, we read, "Once upon a time, there was an old man. He gave this prescription to a man. There were many patients who suffered from epidemic febrile disease in that city. Everyone who took that medicine recovered."

8 Decoction of Ramulus Cinnamomi and Radix Aconiti Lateralis Praeparata (*Guizhi Fuzi Tang* 桂枝附子湯)

· Ramulus Cinnamomi	11.25 g	· Radix Paeoniae Alba	7.5 g
· Fructus Jujubae	2 pcs.		1.875 g
· Radix Aconiti Lateralis Praeparata (stir-baked at high temperature)			11.25 g
· Radix Glycyrrhizae (stir-baked with adjuvant)			3.75 g
· Rhizoma Zingiberis Recens			3 slices

This prescription from Li Chan's 『*Yixue Rumen*』 is for patients with continuous sweating and stiffness of the limbs.

9 Decoction for warming cold limbs with Herba Artemisiae Scopariae (*Yinchen Sini Tang* 茵蔯四逆湯)

· Herba Artemisiae Scopariae	37.5 g
· Radix Aconiti Lateralis Praeparata (dehydrated)	3.75 g
· Rhizoma Zingiberis Recens (stir-baked at high temperature)	3.75 g
· Radix Glycyrrhizae (stir-baked with adjuvant)	3.75 g

This prescription cures yin type jaundice with incessant cold sweating.

10 Decoction of Herba Artemisiae Scopariae and Radix Aconiti Lateralis Praeparata (*Yinchen Fuzi Tang* 茵蔯附子湯)

· Herba Artemisiae Scopariae	37.5 g
· Radix Aconiti Lateralis Praeparata (dehydrated)	3.75 g
· Radix Glycyrrhizae (stir-baked with adjuvant)	3.75 g

This prescription cures yin type jaundice with cold body.

11 Decoction of Herba Artemisiae Scopariae and Pericarpium Citri Reticulatae (*Yinchen Jupi Tang* 茵蔯橘皮湯)

· Herba Artemisiae Scopariae	37.5 g		
· Pericarpium Citri Reticulatae	3.75 g		
· Rhizoma Atractylodis Macrocephalae	3.75 g		
· Rhizoma Pinelliae	3.75 g	· Rhizoma Zingiberis Recens	3.75 g

This prescription cures the yin type jaundice with asthma, vomiting and no thirst.

The above three prescriptions originate from Zhu Gong's『*Huorenshu*』(“Book for Saving Life”).

12 Decoction of three drugs including Radix Ginseng and Fructus Evodiae (*Sanwei Shenyu Tang* 三味蔘萸湯)

· Fructus Evodiae	11.25 g	· Radix Ginseng	7.5 g
· Rhizoma Zingiberis Recens	4 slices	· Fructus Jujubae	2 pcs.

This prescription cures reverting yin syndrome with vomiting of frothy sputum, lesser yin syndrome with cold limbs, irritability and restlessness, and yang brightness syndrome with a tendency to vomit after eating.

13 Powder of thunderbolt (*Pili San* 霹靂散)

· Radix Aconiti Lateralis Praeparata	1 pcs.

Bake it well at high temperature and bury it in cold ashes for 30 minutes. Take out from the ashes and cut it into many pieces. Stew them with 3.75g of old tea leaves in one glass of water until six-tenths of the liquid remains.

Remove the dregs, add half a spoonful of honey and take it when it cools down. After a short time, the patient's irritability will cease, and he will fall asleep and perspire. Recovery follows.

This prescription is for patients whose yang is being kept in the exterior by excessive yin in the interior. The above two prescriptions originate from Li Chan's 『*Yixue Rumen*』.

14 Warm and white pills (*Wenbai Yuan* 溫白元)

· Fructus Evodiae	18.75 g	· Radix Platycodi	18.75 g
· Radix Bupleuri	18.75 g	· Radix Asteris	18.75 g
· Rhizoma Coptidis	18.75 g	· Cortex Cinnamomi	18.75 g
· Poria (red)	18.75 g	· Radix Ginseng	18.75 g

- · Radix Aconiti (stir-baked at high temperature) 93.75 g
- · Rhizoma Apori Graminei 18.75 g
- · Rhizoma Zingiberis (stir-baked at high temperature) 18.75 g
- · Radix Rubiae (stir-baked) 18.75 g
- · Spina Gleditsiae (stir-baked with adjuvant) 18.75 g
- · Cortex Magnoliae Officinalis 18.75 g
- · Semen Crotonis Pulveratum 18.75 g

Pound the above drugs and make pills with honey as big as the seed of an empress tree. Take three to seven pills with the decoction of Rhizoma Zingiberis Recens.

This prescription from the 『*Jufang*』 is for patients with abdominal mass, hypochondriac lump, jaundice, distension of the abdomen, ten types of disease due to water retention, nine types of heart-related pain, eight types of disease due to hypochondriac obstruction, five types of gonorrhea and chronic malaria.

In the 『*Yijian*』, Gong Xin says, "This medicine is for patients who have an abdominal mass as though pregnant, weight loss, fatigue, and sometimes extreme mood swings as if insane. This drug will bring spontaneous relief. When used for chronic diseases, it will cause the patient to discharge stool containing worm-, snake- or pus-like elements."

15 Pills for pestilential jaundice (*Zhangdan Wan* 瘴疸丸)

- Herba Artemisiae Scopariae 37.5 g
- Fructus Gardeniae 37.5 g
- Radix et Rhizoma Rhei 37.5 g
- Natrii Sulfas 37.5 g
- Radix Dichroae 15 g
- Carapax Trionycis 15 g
- Semen Armeniacae Amarum 22.5 g
- Fructus Crotonis Pulveratum 15 g
- Semen Sojae Praeparatum 7.5 g

Pound the drugs into a powder and make the pills with rice cake as big as the seed of empress tree. Three to five pills are to be taken with warm water.

This prescription from Wei Yilin's 『*Dexiaofang*』 is also called *Yinchen Wan*. It cures epidemic febrile diseases, endemic malaria, jaundice and dampness-heat disease.

16 Pills for removing stagnancy of indigested food with Rhizoma Sparganii (*Sanling Xiaoji Wan* 三棱消積丸)

- Rhizoma Sparganii 26.25 g
- Rhizoma Zedoariae 26.25 g
- Fructus Foeniculi 18.75 g
- Massa Medicata Fermentata 26.25 g
- Semen Crotonis (with skin, stir-baked with rice and then remove the rice) 18.75 g
- Pericarpium Citri Reticulatae Viride 18.75 g
- Pericarpium Citri Reticulatae 18.75 g
- Flos Caryophylli (skin) 11.25 g
- Fructus Alpiniae Oxyphyllae 11.25 g

Pound the drugs into a powder and make the pasted pills with vinegar as big as the seed of an empress tree. 30~40 pills are taken with the decoction of Rhizoma Zingiberis Recens.

This prescription from 『*Dongyuanshu*』 written by Li Gao, treats the patient who suffers from indigestion induced by raw and cold food, with a stuffness-fullness sensation.

17 Secretly prescribed pills for removing stagnancy (*Mifang Huazhi Wan* 秘方化滞丸)

· Rhizoma Sparganii 18 g · Radix Aucklandiae 9.375 g
· Flos Caryophylli 9.375 g · Rhizoma Coptidis 9.375 g
· Rhizoma Edoariae (roasted in hot ashes with Rhizoma Sparganii) 18 g
· Rhizoma Pinelliae (fermented) 9.375 g
· Pericarpium Citri Reticulatae Viride 9.375 g
· Pericarpium Citri Reticulatae (only pink portion) 9.375 g
· Semen Crotonis 22.5 g
(preserve in vinegar for one night and stew until dried)

Pound the drugs into a powder with Fructus Mume and some wheat flour and make pasted pills as big as an oat. Take five to ten pills. In order to facilitate bowel movement, take with hot water. To eliminate abdominal mass, taken with the decoction of Cortex Fraxini. To bine the bowels, take with cold water.

This prescription originated from『*Danxi Xinfa*』written by Zhu Zhen-heng. It regulates the flow of all kinds of qi, removes all kinds of abdominal mass and makes the obstinate chronic abdominal mass spontaneously. It quickly removes the mass whether the mass appeared suddenly or a short time ago. It has the function of clearing blockage by using natural laws and has the wonder of reinforcing and reducing by regulating yin and yang.

18 Powder of three white drugs (*Sanwu Bai San* 三物白散)

· Radix Platycodi 11.25 g
· Fritillariae Cirrhosae Hulbus 11.25 g
· Semen Crotonis 3.75 g
(remove husk, stew the seeds and mash to form a greasy pulp)

Pound the drugs into a powder, mix 2g of the drugs with hot water and have the patient take it. If the patient is weak, the dosage should be reduced by half. In case the patient vomits or loose stool is desired, give a cup of hot rice gruel. In case of ceaseless diarrhea, a cup of cold rice gruel should be given.

19 Pills for alleviation (*Ruyi Dan* 如意丹)

· Semen Arecae	18.75 g	· Radix Ginseng	18.75 g
· Radix Bupleuri	18.75 g	· Fructus Evodiae	18.75 g
· Radix Rubiae	18.75 g	· Poria (white)	18.75 g
· Rhizoma Coptidis	18.75 g	· Radix Asteris	18.75 g
· Cortex Cinnamomi	18.75 g	· Radix Platycodi	18.75 g
· Spina Gleditsiae			18.75 g
· Radix Aconiti (stir-baked at high temperature)			30 g
· Rhizoma Zingiberis Recens			18.75 g
· Cortex Magnoliae Officinalis			18.75 g
· Radix Angelicae Sinensis			18.75 g
· Rhizoma Acori Graminei			18.75 g
· Semen Crotonis Pulveratum			9.375 g

Pound the drugs into powder and make pills with honey as big as the seed of empress tree and coat with Cinnabaris. Take five to seven pills with warm water.

It can cure all kinds of epidemic febrile diseases and possessedness. The above two prescriptions originated from Li Chan's 『*Yixue Rumen*』.

I have said that the above six prescriptions originated from the experiments of ancient doctors, and all of them use the effectiveness of Semen Crotonis. The purposes of its use are not different from one another. Generally, in a lesser yin person's disease, it must be used. Do not use the drug in an imprudent manner, nor be afraid of using it. I have set down my experiences with these six prescriptions. Someone who knows the principles well will obtain good results, but it is not to be used in an imprudent manner.

3-3

Twenty Four Newly Created Prescriptions for the Lesser Yin Person's Disease

1 Decoction of Radix Astragali, Ramulus Cinnamomi and Radix Aconiti Lateralis Praeparata

(*Hwanggi Gyeji Buja Tang*: *Huangqi Guizhi Fuzi Tang* 黃芪桂枝附子湯)

· Ramulus Cinnamomi	11.25 g	· Radix Astragali	11.25 g
· Radix Paeoniae Alba	7.5 g	· Fructus Jujubae	2 pcs.
· Radix Angelicae Sinensis	3.75 g		

· Radix Glycyrrhizae (stir-baked with adjuvant) 3.75 g
· Radix Aconiti Lateralis Praeparata (stir-baked at high temperature) 3.75~7.5 g
· Rhizoma Zingiberis Recens 3 slices

2 Decoction of Radix Ginseng, Ramulus Cinnamomi and Radix Aconiti Lateralis Praeparata

(*Insam Gyeji Buja Tang*: *Renshen Guizhi Fuzi Tang* 人蔘桂枝附子湯)

· Radix Ginseng	15 g	· Ramulus Cinnamomi	11.25 g
· Radix Paeoniae Alba	7.5 g	· Radix Astragali	7.5 g
· Radix Angelicae Sinensis	3.75 g	· Fructus Jujubae	2 pcs.

· Radix Glycyrrhizae (stir-baked with adjuvant) 3.75 g
· Radix Aconiti Lateralis Praeparata (stir-baked at high temperature) 3.75~7.5 g
· Rhizoma Zingiberis Recens 3 slices

3 Decoction for ascending yang and replenishing qi with Radix Aconiti Lateralis Praeparata

(*Seungyang Ikgi Buja Tang*: *Shengyang Yiqi Fuzi Tang* 升陽益氣附子湯)

- Radix Ginseng 7.5 g
- Radix Paeoniae Alba 7.5 g
- Ramulus Cinnamomi 7.5 g
- Radix Polygoni Multiflori 3.75 g
- Ramulus Cinnamomi 3.75 g
- Radix Astragali 7.5 g
- Fructus Jujubae 2 pcs.
- Radix Angelicae Sinensis 3.75 g
- Radix Glycyrrhizae (stir-baked with adjuvant) 3.75 g
- Radix Aconiti Lateralis Praeparata (stir-baked at high temperature) 3.75~7.5 g
- Rhizoma Zingiberis Recens 3 slices

4 Decoction of Radix Ginseng, Cortex Cinnamomi and Radix Aconiti Lateralis Praeparata

(*Insam Gwangye Buja Tang*: *Renshen Guangui Fuzi Tang* 人蔘官桂附子湯)

- Radix Ginseng 18.75~37.5 g
- Radix Astragali 11.25 g
- Radix Angelicae Sinensis 3.75 g
- Cortex Cinnamomi 11.25 g
- Radix Paeoniae Alba 7.5 g
- Fructus Jujubae 2 pcs.
- Radix Glycyrrhizae (stir-baked with adjuvant) 3.75 g
- Radix Aconiti Lateralis Praeparata (stir-baked at high temperature) 7.5~9.375 g
- Rhizoma Zingiberis Recens 3 slices

The above four prescriptions are used for yang collpase, which is a critical disease. If the yang collapse patient's urine is clean and fluent, there is a possibility of recovery. The patient should take 3.75g of Radix Aconiti Lateralis Praeparata twice a day. If he is in critical condition, with reddish and difficult urination, then there is little chance for recovery. The patient should take 7.5g of Radix Aconiti Lateralis Praeparata two or three times a day. However, in general, before facing the critical condition, 3.75g of Radix Aconiti Lateralis Praeparata should be taken. The same amount is also used when the patient is no longer in critical condition. If the patient is nursing himself, 3.75g of Radix Aconiti Lateralis Praeparata should be taken twice a day.

5 Decoction for ascending yang and replenishing qi

(*Seungyang Ikgi Tang*: *Shengyang Yiqi Tang* 升陽益氣湯)

· Radix Ginseng	7.5 g	· Ramulus Cinnamomi	7.5 g
· Radix Paeoniae Alba	7.5 g	· Radix Astragali	7.5 g
· Radix Polygoni Multiflori	3.75 g	· Cortex Cinnamomi	3.75 g
· Radix Angelicae Sinensis	3.75 g	· Fructus Jujubae	2 pcs.
· Radix Glycyrrhizae (stir-baked with adjuvant)			3.75 g
· Rhizoma Zingiberis Recens			3 slices

6 Decoction for tonifying the middle and replenishing qi

(*Bojung Ikgi Tang*: *Buzhong Yiqi Tang* 補中益氣湯)

· Radix Ginseng	11.25 g	· Radix Astragali	11.25 g
· Radix Angelicae Sinensis	3.75 g	· Herba Pogostemonis	1.125 g
· Folium Perillae	1.125 g	· Fructus Jujubae:	2 pcs.
· Radix Glycyrrhizae (stir-baked with adjuvant)			3.75 g
· Rhizoma Atractylodis Macrocephalae			3.75 g
· Pericarpium Citri Reticulatae			3.75 g
· Rhizoma Zingiberis Recens			3 slices

7 Decoction of Radix Astragali and Ramulus Cinnamomii

(*Hwanggi Gyeji Tang*: *Huangqi Guizhi Tang* 黃芪桂枝湯)

· Ramulus Cinnamomi	11.25 g	· Radix Paeoniae Alba	7.5 g
· Radix Astragali	7.5 g	· Fructus Aurantii	3.75 g
· Radix Polygoni Multiflori	3.75 g		
· Radix Angelicae Sinensis	3.75 g		
· Radix Glycyrrhizae (stir-baked with adjuvant)			3.75 g
· Rhizoma Zingiberis Recens			3 slices
· Fructus Jujubae			2 pcs.

8 Decoction of Rhizoma Chuanxiong and Ramulus Cinnamomi

(*Cheongung Gyeji Tang*: *Chuanxiong Guizhi Tang* 川芎桂枝湯)

· Ramulus Cinnamomi 11.25 g
· Radix Paeoniae Alba 7.5 g
· Rhizoma Chuanxiong 3.75 g
· Rhizoma Atractylodis 3.75 g
· Pericarpium Citri Reticulatae 3.75 g
· Radix Glycyrrhizae (stir-baked with adjuvant) 3.75 g
· Rhizoma Zingiberis Recens 3 slices
· Fructus Jujubae 2 pcs.

9 Powder of Rhizoma Chuanxiong, Radix Angelicae Sinensis, Rhizoma Cyperi and Folium Perillae

(*Gunggwi Hyangso San*: *Xionggui Xiangsu San* 芎歸香蘇散)

· Rhizoma Cyperi 7.5 g
· Folium Perillae 3.75 g
· Rhizoma Chuanxiong 3.75 g
· Radix Angelicae Sinensis 3.75 g
· Rhizoma Atractylodis 3.75 g
· Radix Allii: 5 stems
· Pericarpium Citri Reticulatae 3.75 g
· Radix Glycyrrhizae (stir-baked with adjuvant) 3.75 g
· Rhizoma Zingiberis Recens 3 slices
· Fructus Jujubae 2 pcs.

10 Powder of Herba Agastachis for restoring qi

(*Gwakhyang Jeonggi San*: *Huoxiang Zhengqi San* 藿香正氣散)

· Herba Agastachis 5.625 g
· Folium Perillae 3.75 g
· Rhizoma Atractylodis 1.875 g
· Rhizoma Pinelliae 1.875 g
· Pericarpium Arecae 1.875 g
· Ramulus Cinnamomi 1.875 g
· Rhizoma Zingiberis 1.875 g
· Radix Glycyrrhizae 1.875 g
· Rhizoma Atractylodis Macrocephalae 1.875 g
· Pericarpium Citri Reticulatae 1.875 g
· Pericarpium Citri Reticulatae Viride 1.875 g
· Fructus Alpiniae Oxyphyllae (stir-baked with adjuvant) 1.875 g
· Rhizoma Zingiberis Recens 3 slices
· Fructus Jujubae 2 pcs.

11 Decoction of eight noble ingredients

(*Palmul Gunja Tang*: *Bawu Junzi Tang* 八物君子湯)

· Radix Ginseng	7.5 g	· Radix Astragali	3.75 g
· Radix Paeoniae Alba	3.75 g	· Rhizoma Chuanxiong	3.75 g
· Radix Angelicae Sinensis	3.75 g	· Fructus Jujubae	2 pcs.
· Rhizoma Atractylodis Macrocephalae			3.75 g
· Pericarpium Citri Reticulatae			3.75 g
· Radix Glycyrrhizae (stir-baked with adjuvant)			3.75 g
· Rhizoma Zingiberis Recens			3 slices

If Radix Polygoni Multiflori is substituted for Radix Ginseng in this prescription, it is named *Baikhao Gunja Tang* (白何烏君子湯).

If one uses 3.75g of both Radix Ginseng and Radix Astragali, and adds 3.75g each of Radix Polygoni Multiflori and Ramulus Cinnamomi to the remaining drugs, it is named *Sibjeon Daibo Tang*.

If one uses 3.75g each of Radix Ginseng and Radix Astragali, it is named *Doksam Palmul Tang* (獨蔘八物湯).

12 Decoction of eight noble ingredients with Rhizoma Cyperi

(*Hyangbuja Palmul Tang*: *Xiangfuzi Bawu Tang* 香附子八物湯)

· Rhizoma Cyperi	7.5 g	· Radix Angelicae Sinensis	7.5 g
· Radix Paeoniae Alba	7.5 g	· Radix Polygoni Multiflori	3.75 g
· Rhizoma Chuanxiong	3.75 g	· Fructus Jujubae	2 pcs.
· Rhizoma Atractylodis Macrocephalae			3.75 g
· Pericarpium Citri Reticulatae			3.75 g
· Radix Glycyrrhizae (stir-baked with adjuvant)			3.75 g
· Rhizoma Zingiberis Recens			3 slices

I once obtained good results in treating a woman who had a dry throat and parched tongue with a mild headache as a consequence of her anxiety impairing her spleen.

13 Decoction of Ramulus Cinnamomi, Rhizoma Pinelliae and Rhizoma Zingiberis Recens

(*Gyeji Banha Sainggang Tang*: *Guizhi Banxia Shengjiang Tang* 桂枝半夏生薑湯)

- Rhizoma Zingiberis Recens 11.25 g · Ramulus Cinnamomi 7.5 g
- Rhizoma Pinelliae 7.5 g · Radix Paeoniae Alba 3.75 g
- Rhizoma Atractylodis Macrocephalae 3.75 g
- Pericarpium Citri Reticulatae 3.75 g
- Radix Glycyrrhizae (stir-baked with adjuvant) 3.75 g

This prescription cures vomiting brought on by deficiency-cold and accumulation of water in the chest.

14 Decoction of Rhizoma Cyperi and Fructus Amomi Rotundus for nourishing the stomach

(*Hyangsa Yangwi Tang*: *Xiangsha Yangwei Tang* 香砂養胃湯)

- Radix Ginseng 3.75 g · Radix Paeoniae Alba 3.75 g
- Rhizoma Pinelliae 3.75 g · Rhizoma Cyperi 3.75 g
- Rhizoma Zingiberis 3.75 g · Fructus Crataegi 3.75 g
- Fructus Amomi 3.75 g · Fructus Amomi Rotundus 3.75 g
- Rhizoma Zingiberis Recens 3 slices · Fructus Jujubae 2 pcs.
- Rhizoma Atractylodis Macrocephalae 3.75 g
- Radix Glycyrrhizae (stir-baked with adjuvant) 3.75 g
- Pericarpium Citri Reticulatae 3.75 g

15 Decoction for relieving the middle with Radix Polygoni Multiflori Rubra et Alba

(*Jeokbaikhao Gwanjung Tang*: *Chibaihewu Kuanzhong Tang* 赤白何烏寬中湯)

- Rhizoma Zingiberis 3.75 g · Rhizoma Cyperi 3.75 g
- Fructus Alpiniae Oxyphyllae 3.75 g · Fructus Jujubae 2 pcs.
- Radix Polygoni Multiflori (white) 3.75 g
- Radix Polygoni Multiflori (red) 3.75 g
- Rhizoma Alpiniae Officinarum 3.75 g
- Pericarpium Citri Reticulatae Viride 3.75 g
- Pericarpium Citri Reticulatae 3.75 g

This prescription is for patients experiencing exhaustion in all four limbs, difficult urination, impotency and the strong possibility of edema. If Cortex Magnoliae Officinalis, Fructus Aurantii Immaturus, Radix Aucklandiae and Pericarpium Arecae, 1.875g each, are added, it will promote the normal flow of qi in the meridian. After the appearance of an edema, one should calm the patient for 100 days and give him two packs of this prescription every day; the edema will disappear. If Radix Ginseng is substituted for Radix Polygoni Multiflori Rubra in this prescription, it is named *Insam Baikhao Gwanjung Tang* (人蔘白何烏寬中湯). If Radix Angelicae Sinensis is substituted for Radix Polygoni Multiflori Rubra in this prescription, it is named *Danggwi Baikhao Gwanjung Tang* (當歸白何烏寬中湯).

There is an old prescription that consists of Rhizoma Zingiberis, Rhizoma Alpiniae Officinarum, Pericarpium Citri Reticulatae Viride and Pericarpium Citri Reticulatae in equal dosage. When it is made into pills or a decoction, it is named *Kuanzhong Tang*. I have treated lesser yin person experiencing discomfort in urinating, impotency, general exhaustion and weakness with the above, and obtained good results in all cases. In the case where 3.75g each of Faeces Trogopterorum and Fructus Alpiniae Oxyphyllae are added to the *Kuanzhong Wan*, it will relieve the abdominal pain miraculously.

16 Decoction with garlic and honey (*Sanmil Tang*: *Suanmi Tang* 蒜蜜湯)

- · Radix Paeoniae Alba 3.75 g
- · Ramulus Cinnamomi 3.75 g
- · Fructus Papaveris 3.75 g
- · Garlic 5 roots
- · Honey: half of a spoon
- · Fructus Jujubae 2 pcs.
- · Radix Polygoni Multiflori (white) 3.75 g
- · Rhizoma Atractylodis Macrocephalae 3.75 g
- · Herba Artemisiae Scopariae 3.75 g
- · Fructus Alpiniae Oxyphyllae 3.75 g
- · Limonitum Cum Terra 3.75 g
- · Rhizoma Zingiberis Recens 3 slices

This prescription treats dysentery.

17 Paste of chicken and Radix Ginseng (*Gyesam Go*: *Jishen Gao* 鷄蔘膏)

- · Radix Ginseng 3.75 g
- · Cortex Cinnamomi 3.75 g
- · Chicken 1

Stew and take the decoction. It may be flavored with black pepper and honey. This prescription has a long tradition of treating malaria and dysentery miraculously. I once cured a case of chronic malaria, first using Semen Crotonis as a purgative drug, and then *Gyesam Go* for several days. It also cured chronic malaria. Often, a cinnamon core is substituted for Cortex Cinnamomi.

18 Pellet of Semen Crotonis (*Padu Dan*: *Badou Dan* 巴豆丹)

· Semen Crotonis 1 grain (remove husk)

Take a half-grain or whole grain of Semen Crotonis with warm water. While the other drugs are being stewed, Semen Crotonis can directly affect the stomach and intestine. After the effect of Semen Crotonis has almost cleared, the decoction is taken and it will go together with Semen Crotonis. This will clear the contents in the stomach and intestines and raise the normal qi. After defecation, take Semen Crotonis continuously.

A whole grain can induce diarrhea, while a half-grain can eliminate retained stool.

19 Decoction of Radix Ginseng and Pericarpium Citri Reticulatae (*Insam Jinpi Tang*: *Renshen Chenpi Tang* 人蔘陳皮湯)

· Radix Ginseng 37.5 g · Fructus Amomi 3.75 g
· Rhizoma Zingiberis Recens 3.75 g · Fructus Jujubae 2 pcs.
· Pericarpium Citri Reticulatae 3.75 g

If Rhizoma Zingiberis (stir-baked at high temperature) is substituted for Rhizoma Zingiberis Recens and 3.75g of Cortex Cinnamomi is added in this prescription, it will warm the stomach and expel the cold more efficiently. I once treated a baby, only several months old, who had chronic infantile convulsions due to yin type inflammatory swelling. I administered the drug for several days, and the infant recovered. However, I did not subsequently have the baby take the medicine continuously, and he suffered a relapse from which he never recovered.

20 Decoction of Radix Ginseng and Fructus Evodiae

(*Insam Osuyu Tang*: *Renshen Wuzhuyu Tang* 人蔘吳茱萸湯)

· Radix Ginseng	37.5 g	· Fructus Evodiae	11.25 g
· Rhizoma Zingiberis Recens	11 g	· Radix Paeoniae Alba	3.75 g
· Radix Angelicae Sinensis	3.75 g	· Ramulus Cinnamomi	3.75 g

21 Decoction for regulating the middle with Cortex Cinnamomi and Radix Aconiti Lateralis Praeparata

(*Gwangye Buja Ijung Tang*: *Guangui Fuzi Lizhong Tang* 官桂附子理中湯)

· Radix Ginseng	11.25 g	· Cortex Cinnamomi	7.5 g
· Radix Paeoniae Alba	3.75 g		

- · Rhizoma Atractylodis Macrocephalae 7.5 g
- · Rhizoma Zingiberis (stir-baked at high temperature) 7.5 g
- · Pericarpium Citri Reticulatae 3.75 g
- · Radix Glycyrrhizae (stir-baked with adjuvant) 3.75 g
- · Radix Aconiti Lateralis Praeparata (stir-baked at high temperature) 3.75~7.5 g

22 Decoction for regulating the middle with Fructus Evodiae and Radix Aconiti Lateralis Praeparata

(*Osuyu Buja Ijung Tang*: *Wuzhuyu Fuzi Lizhong Tang* 吳茱萸附子理中湯)

· Radix Ginseng	7.5 g	· Cortex Cinnamomi	7.5 g
· Radix Paeoniae Alba	3.75 g	· Fructus Evodiae	3.75 g
· Fructus Foeniculi	3.75 g	· Fructus Psoraleae	3.75 g

- · Rhizoma Atractylodis Macrocephalae 7.5 g
- · Rhizoma Zingiberis (stir-baked at high temperature) 7.5 g
- · Pericarpium Citri Reticulatae 3.75 g
- · Radix Glycyrrhizae (stir-baked with adjuvant) 3.75 g
- · Radix Aconiti Lateralis Praeparata (stir-baked at high temperature) 3.75~7.5 g

23 Decoction for regulating the middle with Radix Polygoni Multiflori Alba and Radix Aconiti Lateralis Praeparata

(*Baikhao Buja Ijung Tang*: *Baihewu Fuzi Lizhong Tang* 白何烏附子理中湯)

· Radix Polygoni Multiflori Alba	7.5 g
· Rhizoma Atractylodis Macrocephalae (stir-baked)	7.5 g
· Radix Paeoniae Alba (stir-baked to just dry)	7.5 g
· Ramulus Cinnamomi	7.5 g
· Rhizoma Zingiberis (stir-baked at high temperature)	7.5 g
· Pericarpium Citri Reticulatae	3.75 g
· Radix Glycyrrhizae (stir-baked with adjuvant)	3.75 g
· Radix Aconiti Lateralis Praeparata (stir-baked at high temperature)	3.75 g

24 Decoction for regulating the middle with Radix Polygoni Multiflori Alba

(*Baikhao Ijung Tang*: *Baihewu Lizhong Tang* 白何烏理中湯)

· Radix Paeoniae Alba	7.5 g
· Ramulus Cinnamomi	7.5 g
· Radix Polygoni Multiflori Alba	7.5 g
· Rhizoma Atractylodis Macrocephalae	7.5 g
· Rhizoma Zingiberis (stir-baked at high temperature)	7.5 g
· Pericarpium Citri Reticulatae	3.75 g
· Radix Glycyrrhizae (stir-baked with adjuvant)	3.75 g

If you have Radix Ginseng, use it; if none is available, use Radix Polygoni Multiflori Alba instead.

The properties and flavor of Radix Polygoni Multiflori Alba and Radix Ginseng are similar, but compared to Radix Polygoni Multiflori Alba, Radix Ginseng is lacking in cooling and dispersing properties. Its warming and tonifying properties, however, are superior, so there are differences between the two. In case of a critical syndrome or a dangerous disease, if it is not possible to use more than 7.5g of Radix Ginseng, then Radix Polygoni Multiflori Alba should be used instead. Since there have been few cases of the use of Radix Polygoni Multiflori Alba in prescriptions of the past, and also because the medicine remains so unfamiliar, Radix Polygoni Multiflori Alba is rarely used. This medicine, however, should not be ignored as a tonifying drug. An old prescription, *Heren Yin*, is used with 18.75g of Radix Polygoni Multiflori Alba to treat malaria. The drugs below for a lesser yin person should be prepared as follows. Radix Aconiti Lateralis Praeparata should be stir-baked at high temperature; Radix Glycyrrhizae should be stir-baked with adjuvant; Rhizoma Zingiberis should be stir-baked at high temperature or used raw; Radix Astragali should be stir-baked with adjuvant or used raw.

If a person falls ill in a remote or secluded place, it is better to use a simple recipe than to leave him untreated. For yang brightness disease, though it is a simple recipe, we can use Radix Astragali, Ramulus Cinnamomi, Radix Ginseng and Radix Paeoniae. For lesser yin disease, though it is a simple recipe, we can use Radix Aconiti Lateralis Praeparata, Radix Paeoniae, Radix Ginseng and Radix Glycyrrhizae. For greater yang disease, though it is a simple recipe, we can use Folium Perillae, Radix Allii, Radix Astragali and Ramulus Cinnamomi. For greater yin disease, though it is a simple recipe, we can use Rhizoma Atractylodis Macrocephalae, Rhizoma Zingiberis, Pericarpium Citri Reticulatae and Herba Pogostemonis. If the complete prescription is not available, use a simple recipe first. If the complete prescription is available, one should not hesitate to treat the patient. We must only use the drugs appropriate to that prescription; to use inappropriate drugs is unacceptable.

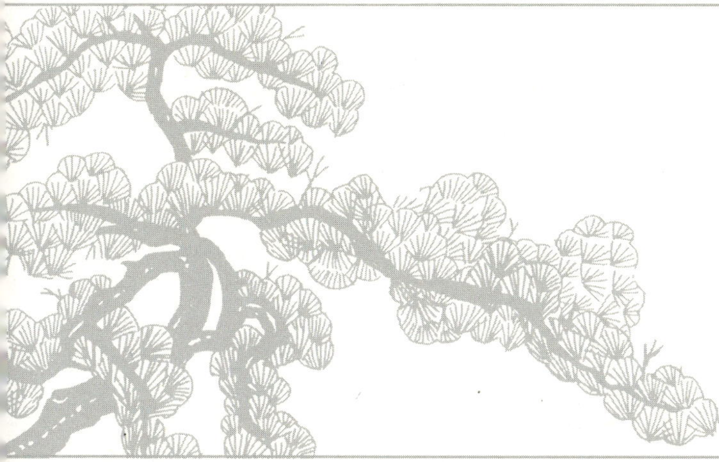

PART / III

1

Discourse on the Soyang (Lesser Yang) Person's Exterior Cold Disease Induced from the Spleen Affected by Cold*

1 Zhang Zhongjing said, "For the symptoms and signs of the greater yang disease such as a floating and tense pulse, fever, chills, aching of the body and restlessness without sweating, *Da Qinglong Tang* (Big blue dragon decoction) is suitable."

2 I have said, "Symptoms and signs such as fever, chills, aching of the body, a floating and tense pulse, and irritability and restlessness without sweating are related to the lesser yang person's exterior cold disease induced from the Spleen affected by cold. For this disease, *Da Qinglong Tang* should not be adopted, but rather *Hyeongbang Paidok San* (Antiphlogistic powder of Herba Schizonepetae and Radix Saposhnikoviae) should be used."

3 Zhang Zhongjing said, "The symptoms and signs of the lesser yang disease are bitterness in the mouth, a parched throat and vertigo."

4 Vertigo and bitterness in the mouth with a parched tongue belong to the lesser yang disease.

5 Bitterness in the mouth, deafness and fullness in the chest are the symptoms and signs of the febrile disease caused by wind of the lesser yang disease.

---

* 少陽人脾受寒表寒病論

6 Bitterness in the mouth, a parched throat, vertigo, deafness and fullness in the chest and costal region, or alternate attacks of chills and fever and nausea are the symptoms of the lesser yang disease. Avoid using an emetic or purgative; rather, regulate with *Xiao Chaihu Tang* (Minor Bupleurum Decoction).

7 I have said, "*Xiao Chaihu Tang* should not be used; instead, we ought to use *Hyeongbang Paidok San, Hyeongbang Dojeok San* (Powder for treating dark urine with Herba Schizonepetae and Radix Saposhnikoviae) and *Hyeongbang Sabaik San* (Powder for expelling Lung-heat with *Herba* Schizonepetae and Radix Saposhnikoviae)."

8 The lesser yang disease mentioned by Zhang Zhongjing with the symptoms of bitterness in the mouth, a parched throat, fullness of the chest and the costal region or alternate attacks of chills and fever is the disease in which the lesser yang person's Kidney yin qi is besieged by the evil heat, and the Spleen yin qi is blocked by the evil heat. As a result, the Spleen yin qi cannot descend to connect with the Kidney yin, and congeals in the vertebra to become an obstinate disease.Vomiting is due to the ascending of the exogenous evil cold surrounding the internal heat, and the alternate attacks of chills and fever are due to the Spleen yin qi going down occasionally, even though on the whole, the Spleen yin qi can not go down when it tries. Bitterness in the mouth, a parched throat, vertigo and deafness are due to the yin qi's descent being blocked in the vertebra. This induces chills without fever and deafness. Bitterness in the mouth, a parched throat and vertigo are ordinary symptoms; however, deafness indicates a serious condition. The agitation in the chest and the costal region develops into an accumulation of pathogen in the chest. Fullness of the costal region is not a serious condition, however, fullness in the chest is a serious symptom. The ancients treated this kind of disease with diaphoretics, emetics and purgatives. These types of treatments caused deteriorated cases such as delirium, and are dangerous. Therefore, Zhang Zhongjing designed *Xiao Chaihu Tang* to clear away phlegm and to eliminate sputum, and tried to regulate it evenly by mixing up warm and cold drugs together in order to prevent aggravating the disease and achieve spontaneous relief. Speaking from the perspective of the diaphoretic,

emetic and purgative methodology, this decoction must be valued as an excellent drug. *Xiao Chaihu Tang*, however, is not a prescription that can regulate the functional relations of the internal organs and prevent the illness from getting worse. This illness is as tragic today as it was in the past. How can *Xiao Chaihu Tang* be applied to deafness, sensation of fullness in the chest and the symptoms induced by the evil wind? Is Gong Xin's *Jingfang Baidu San* not the most suitable prescription for a lesser yang person's exterior cold disease? To treat the above symptoms, if the interior heat is cleared out and the exterior yin is lowered, the phlegm and fluid that has been retained will be dispersed spontaneously and an accumulation of pathogen in the chest will not form. Clearing away phlegm and eliminating sputum are not helpful in lowering yin and dispersing phlegm; it might even cause an accumulation of pathogen in the chest to mutate into another disease.

9 Zhu Gong said, "If a patient perspires in droplets above the waist, and perspires but a little from the waist down, he will not recover."

10 I have said, "In the lesser yang person's disease, whether exterior or interior disease, the patient can be relieved after there is perspiration on the palms of the hands and the soles of the feet. If there is no sweating on the palms and the soles, he will not recover, even though he might be sweating all over his body."

11 In the lesser yang person's exogenous febrile disease caused by cold, some patients get well after repeated pain with sweating. This disease is not a case of repeated pain with sweating induced by repeated invasion of wind and cold. Originally, the disease is the same as the disease of a lesser yang person with symptoms of headache, stiff neck, alternate attacks of chills and fever, deafness, and a sensation of fullness in the chest. If the exogenous pathogen is deeply congealed, the disease will be relieved after three bouts of pain. Whether sweating for the first, second or third time, we have to apply two packs of *Hyeongbang Paidok San* or *Hyeongbang Dojeok San* or *Hyeongbang Sabaik San* a day until the symptoms disappear. Afterwards, we must apply ten or more packs to prevent a relapse.

12 Zhang Zhongjing said, "A lesser yang disease with the following symptoms, such as a clammy body with perspiration, hardness and fullness at the epigastrium, a referred pain below the costal margin, nausea with shortness of breath, and no chills may indicate that the interior syndrome is still dominating, even after the exterior syndrome is gone. *Shizao Tang* (Decoction of ten Fructus Jujubae) can be taken. If the decoction's purgative action is in vain, the patient will experience abdominal distension and general edema of the whole body."

13 When a purgative is given to the patient whose exterior syndrome caused by cold has not been cleared away, he will feel pain in a part of the diaphragm because of compression, and fullness and hardness in the chest. This indicates that an accumulation of pathogen in the chest is taking shape. *Da Xianxiong Tang* (Decoction for severe phlegm-heat pattern in the chest) will be the curative.

14 Though the patient is thirsty for water, he will still regurgitate any ingested water; this is called *shuini* (water regurgitation). *Wuling San* (Powder of five drugs with Poria) will be the curative.

15 Du Ren[1)] said, "The domination of the interior syndrome manifests itself in the phlegm and the pathogenic dryness congealing in the middle-*jiao*. Its symptoms include headaches, retching and sweating. These are due to the phlegm in the diaphragm. Without *Shizao Tang*, one can not heal this illness."

16 Gong Xin said, "Hardness and pain in the epigastrium (which one cannot even touch), thirst, delirium, constipation, and a deep and forceful pulse are due to the major accumulation of phlegm-heat in the chest. *Da Xianxiong Tang* as a purgative should be adopted. If the patient becomes more irritated after taking the drug, he will die. The minor accumulation of phlegm-heat in the chest manifests itself only in the epigastrium. *Xiao Xianxiong Tang* (Decoction for mild phlegm-heat pattern in the chest) should be used."

17 I have said, "The above three syndromes that Zhang Zhongjing mentioned

are all accumulations of pathogen in the chest. The tenderness in the chest, thirst and delirium are the most serious symptoms along with an accumulation of pathogen in the chest. Regurgitating any ingested water, feeling of fullness in the epigastrium, retching and shortness of breath are secondary ones. Generally, an accumulation of pathogen in the chest induces vomiting just after drinking medicine or water. Only the powder of Radix Euphorbiae Kansui taken with saliva, and drinking some warm water to rinse the mouth will not cause the patient to vomit. I had an experience curing an accumulation of pathogen in the chest. The patient took the powder of Radix Euphorbiae Kansui with warm water. The patient vomited until the sixth time and his bowels relaxed. On the second day, he vomited water again, so he took Radix Euphorbiae Kansui and was cured after one bout of diarrhea. Since an accumulation of pathogen in the chest is generally a serious disease, we should use Radix Euphorbiae Kansui and *Hyeongbang Dojeok San* to stop it. When there are only symptoms of retching and shortness of breath, but no vomiting of drugs, we do not have to use Radix Euphorbiae Kansui. If we use *Hyeongbang Dojeok San* with Poria and Rhizoma Alismatis, 3.75g each, two or three packs a day, then the patient will be cured. Thirst and delirium are signs of the most dangerous conditions. Immediately apply Radix Euphorbiae Kansui and take three or four packs of *Jihwang Baikho Tang* (White tiger decoction with Radix Rehmanniae) to stop it. The patient must then take *Jihwang Baikho Tang* everyday. Zhang Zhongjing said, 'When a purgative is to be given to a patient whose exterior syndrome caused by cold has not been cleared away,' the necessary purgative is *Da Chengqi Tang*, not *Xianxiong Tang* or *Shizao Tang*. Using Radix Euphorbiae Kansui is better than using either *Shizao Tang* or *Xianxiong Tang*. For an accumulation of pathogen in the chest, we generally use 1.125g of Radix Euphorbiae Kansui, and for the major accumulation of pathogen in the chest, we use 1.875g of Radix Euphorbiae Kansui. *Gamsu Cheonil Dan* (Tianyi pills with Radix Euphorbiae Kansui) also can be adopted. For curing a patient with symptoms of thirst, delirium and irritability with restlessness to death mentioned by Gong Xin, the delirium will disappear through purgation with *Shizao Tang*; *Baihu Tang* will cure irritability with restlessness.

18 Radix Euphorbiae Kansui is a drug for removing the accumulation of fluid in the chest in the exterior cold disease. Gypsum Fibrosum is a drug for relaxing the bowels in the interior heat disease. For the exterior disease, Radix Euphorbiae Kansui can be used, but not Gypsum Fibrosum. For the interior disease, Gypsum Fibrosum can be used, but not Radix Euphorbiae Kansui. For symptoms such as waving of hands and feet, thirst and diarrhea, Gypsum Fibrosum should be used. For symptoms such as arthralgia with numbness, cold knees and constipation, Radix Euphorbiae Kansui should be used.

19 There are symptoms, such as hardness and fullness in the lower abdomen in the exogenous febrile disease, caused by cold in the lesser yin person, and the accumulation of pathogens in the epigastrium in the exogenous febrile disease caused by cold in the lesser yang person. These two symptoms are both due to the struggle, lasting for several days, between the healthy qi and the pathogen induced by the deficiency of the exterior qi of both yin and yang, and the unevenness of the interior qi.

20 In his 『*Shanghan Shiquanlun*』[2] ("Ten Pieces of Advice on Exogenous Febrile Disease"), Li Zijian[3] said, "When there is abdominal pain in the exogenous febrile disease caused by cold which belongs to the heat syndrome, be careful in giving drugs of a warm nature." He said, "We should differentiate the yin and yang syndromes when the patient shows symptoms of spontaneous diarrhea in the exogenous febrile disease caused by cold. Do not make thoughtless prescriptions for taking drugs of warm nature or anti-diarrheal drugs."

21 Zhu Zhenheng said, "For the yang syndrome of the exogenous febrile disease caused by cold with symptoms and signs such as fever, fast pulse, restlessness with thirst and spontaneous diarrhea, *Chailing Tang* (Decoction of Radix Bupleuri and Poria) should be adopted."

22 The Banryongsan elder said, "A lesser yang person with symptoms of fever, headache and diarrhea should be treated with *Jeoryeong Chajeonja Tang* (Decoction of Polyporus and Semen Plantaginis) and *Hyeongbang*

Sabaik San. The symptoms of chills, abdominal pain and diarrhea should be treated by *Hwalseok Gosam Tang* (Decoction of Talcum and Radix Sophorae Flavescentis) and *Hyeongbang Jihwang Tang* (Decoction of Radix Rehmanniae Praeparata with Herba Schizonepetae and Radix Saposhnikoviae). These diseases are called *mangyin* (yin collapse) disease."

23 If a lesser yang person has a fever, headache and diarrhea, his diarrhea may stop for no reason one to four days later. However, if his fever and headache are not relieved, and he becomes constipated, then his condition is dangerous, and he will become delirious.

24 If a patient barely has a bowel movement in the twenty four hours following diarrhea or has of a small amount of loose bowels three to five times in one day. And he still has the symptoms of fever and headache, this indicates constipation. If these symptoms occur before delirium, delirium will occur a few days later. If these symptoms occur after delirium, endogenous Wind stirring will occur.

25 If a lesser yang person vomits suddenly, there will be some strange symptoms. We should apply *Hyeongbang Paidok San* immediately. If the patient has a fever, a headache and diarrhea, Gypsum Fibrosum will be suitable for these symptoms. If the patient displays symptoms of chills, headache and diarrhea, Rhizoma Coptidis and Radix Sophorae Flavescentis will be suitable.

26 I once treated a lesser yang baby under a year of age. He vomited suddenly, and then had diarrhea, fever, headache, waving of his hands and feet, rolling his body. He also experienced thirst and diarrhea several times. After taking six packs of *Hyeongbang Sabaik San* for two days, the diarrhea stopped, and the fever and headache were gone, too. He took six more packs and fully recovered.

27 A lesser yang person displaying symptoms of fever, headache, waving of hands and feet and thirst are in a serious danger. Though he has diarrhea, we must use Gypsum Fibrosum. Whether he has diarrhea or not, we must

use *Hyeongbang Sabaik San* with Rhizoma Coptidis and Fructus Trichosanthis, 3.75g each, or use *Jihwang Baikho Tang*.

28 If a lesser yang person has symptoms of fever and headache, his condition is no more than a mild one; but if he also has diarrhea, he is in danger. We must use *Hyeongbang Sabaik San* two or three times per a day. Once the symptoms such as fever and headache are cleared away, then he can be saved.

29 If a lesser yang person has symptoms of chills, abdominal pains and diarrhea three to five times a day, he should take *Hwalseok Gosam Tang*. If he displays symptoms of chills and abdominal pains without diarrhea for two or three days, or has one bout of diarrhea, he should take *Hwalseok Gosam Tang* or *Sukjihwang Gosam Tang* (Decoction of Radix Rehmanniae Praeparata and Radix Sophorae Flavescentis).

30 I have seen a lesser yang person who had been suffering from continuous abdominal pain, and he was cured after taking sixty packs of *Liuwei Dihuang Tang* (Decoction of six drugs with Radix Rehmanniae Praeparata). I also have seen a lesser yang person who had had abdominal pain for more than ten years. Each time, it had lasted five to six, three to four, or one or two months; and each time it occurred, he took ten or more packs of *Hwalseok Gosam Tang* to stop the pain. During those periods where he experienced no pain, the patient tried to calm himself down and avoid sorrow and anger. He subsequently recovered within a year. I also have seen a lesser yang boy who always had indigestion and a feeling of hardness and fullness in the abdomen. He sometimes had abdominal pain and lumbago, and, later, facial hemiparalysis occurred. From the start, he took two hundred packs of *Dokhwal Jihwang Tang* (Decoction of Radix Rehmanniae Praeparata with Radix Angelicae Pubescentis) and tried to ease his mind by avoiding sorrow and anger. He subsequently recovered his health within one hundred days.

31 An ancient doctor said, "There is no headache that is due to cold, and there is no abdominal pain that is due to heat." However, this is not true. Why? Since the lesser yin person originally has excessive cold inside, his headache also cannot be induced by heat, but by cold. Since the lesser

yang person originally has excessive heat inside, his abdominal pain also cannot be induced by cold, but by heat. Another ancient doctor also said, "Too much perspiration causes yang collapse, and too much purgation causes yin collapse." That is true. Why? Although the lesser yin's nature is cold, because his yang is defeated and expelled by the yin excess, the defeated yang outwardly induces fever and profuse sweating. This is called the yang collapse disease. Conversely, although the lesser yang's nature is heat, because his yin is defeated and forced inwardly by the yang excess, the defeated yin inwardly induces an aversion to cold and diarrhea. This is called the yin collapse disease. If there is no drug administration, or no emergency management, the patient will die.

32 The yang collapse implies that the yang descends instead of ascends. The yin collapse implies that the yin ascends instead of descends. Due to the excessive yin expelling yang out of the upper part of the body, the yang is inhibited by yin and cannot ascend to the diaphragm and descend to the large intestine and circulate outside the bladder. As a result, fever with restlessness over the back and sweating occurs. The fever and sweating are not induced by an overabundance of yang. This is the so-called state of ice within and charcoal outside, and is the sign of dying yang. Due to excessive yang expelling yin out of the lower part of the body, yin is obstructed by yang and cannot descend to the bladder and ascend to the paravertebral musculature of the back and circulate inside the diaphragm. As a result, the stomach and intestine become averse to cold, and diarrhea occurs. The aversion to cold and diarrhea are not induced by an overabundance of yin. This is the so-called state of charcoal within and ice outside, and is the sign of dying yin.

33 A lesser yin patient will definitely be cured if his yang qi ascends and induces perspiration on the Renzhong point on the first day. If his perspiration does not cease on the second or third day and he is not cured, there is no doubt that the yang cannot ascend and is exhausted. A lesser yang patient will definitely be cured if his yin qi descends and induces diarrhea, with sweat on the palms and soles on the first day. If there is continuous diarrhea in the second or third day and no sign of recovery,

there is no doubt that the yin cannot descend and is exhausted. Generally, a doctor who understands the medical theories can predict the symptoms of yang collapse and yin collapse before they occur. Those diseases are easy to perceive on the first and second day, and on the third day it is as clear as daylight, so that even those less knowledgeable can discern the symptoms. On the fourth day, it is somewhat late; and on the fifth day, the patient will be in the dangerous state. Therefore, the drugs must be taken before the second or third day.

34 If a lesser yin person who is usually restless with profuse perspiration falls ill, he will certainly get yang collapse. A lesser yang person who usually has a cold body with frequent diarrhea falls ill, he will certainly get yin collapse. It is advisable for those who are susceptible to yang collapse or yin collapse to take the preventive drugs reinforcing yin or yang. It is very difficult to save a patient who contracts yang collapse or yin collapse and whose condition has become dangerous.

35 For a lesser yin person, the recovery from the disease shows itself through sweating on the Renzhong point first. Then with one bout of sweating, the patient feels his chest refreshed and becomes active. However, in yang collapse, sweating occurs on and off on the Renzhong point, and after several bouts of sweating, the patient feels restlessness in the chest and the qi becomes depressed. For a lesser yang person, the recovery from the disease shows itself through sweating on the palms and soles first. With one round of diarrhea, the exterior qi becomes clear and refreshes the mind. In yin collapse, there is no sweating on the palms and soles, and after several rounds of diarrhea, the exterior qi becomes cold and dizziness occurs.

36 Both an excess of the stomach and intestine of the lesser yin person and an accumulation of pathogen in the chest of the lesser yang person are produced by the conflicts between healthy qi and the pathogen, and those of yin and yang as well. They become dangerous as time passes. The yang collapse in the lesser yin person and the yin collapse in the lesser yang person are produced by the conflicts between healthy qi and the pathogen, and the conflicts between yin and yang which are unable to

match each other. They are already serious at the onset and become dangerous later. We can liken these cases to war. During the first day's battle, the enemy defeats our army and we lose a number of troops. During the second and third day's battle, our army is again defeated, with yet more losses. If we analyzed those three day's battles, we would surmise that a fourth and fifth day's battle would lead to the loss of all remaining troops. In the same way, we must not tarry in administering the medication after the illness's third day.

37 I call myself the Banryongsan elder because of my residence near this hill. Thus, the phrases "I have said" in this book are uttered by the Banryongsan elder. When writing about yin collapse and yang collapse, I cite myself as the Banryongsan elder to emphasize that yang collapse and yin collapse are most dangerous diseases whose study is worthwhile.

38 There was not much experience or medications for the yin collapse disease previously, although Li Zijian and Zhu Danxi[4)]'s books mention it a little; however, neither physician's experiences are clear or conclusive. It may be that death came so quickly that it was difficult to obtain knowledge and experience.

39 Zhang Zhongjing said, "Before the greater yang disease evanesces, it changes into the lesser yang disease. Then the following symptoms and signs such as hardness and fullness below the costal region, retching, anorexia, and alternate attacks of chills and fever appear. If the pulse is deep and tense before an emetic or purgative is adopted, *Xiao Chaihu Tang* will be the curative. When delirium appears after the adoption of an emetic, purgative, or diaphoretic, it means that the *Xiao Chaihu Tang* syndromes disappear and are followed by something worse. Therapy should be done according to the relevant diagnosis."

40 The exogenous febrile disease caused by cold with a tight and slender pulse, headache and fever would indicate that the syndrome is in the lesser yang disease. Diaphoresis is prohibited, as its adoption will cause delirium.

41 I once treated a lesser yang person suffering from the exterior febrile dis-

ease caused by cold and who exhibited symptoms of mania and delirium. It was the Qingming (Pure Brightness: fifth solar term) season in 1875. He got the febrile disease caused by cold and had more chills than fever. Four to five days later, dyspnea and shortness of breath were noted in the afternoon. At that time, I lacked experience. I only knew that the lesser yang person should be treated with *Liuwei Dihuang Tang* (Decoction of six drugs containing Radix Rehmanniae Praeparata), so I dared not use any other drugs. After taking a pack of *Liuwei Dihuang Tang*, his shortness of breath was cured, but several days later, the symptoms such as mania, delirium and shortness of breath recurred. He took a pack of *Liuwei Dihuang Tang* again, and there was a slight improvement for the shortness of breath. He then experienced continuous mania for three days and shortness of breath again in the afternoon, so he was given *Liuwei Dihuang Tang*. There was no relief for his shortness of breath, however, and shortly after the endogenous Wind stirring; the patient developed a curled tongue, a closed mouth, and difficulty in speech. I thereupon found out that *Liuwei Dihuang Tang* was ineffective and gave him a pack of *Baihu Tang* immediately. I fed the patient through the nose to the throat using a bamboo tube. The curled tongue and closed mouth persisted, but he gave off mild bowel sounds. After taking three packs of the drugs continuously, he gave loud bowel sounds like breaking wind. Three men helped him to take the drugs, and even they could not handle the patient due to his strength. Like this, he continued taking 300g of Gypsum Fibrosum from noon till midnight. Later, the patient's abdomen got fuller, and opisthotonos developed. After the opisthotonos, the patient sweated and slept. At dawn the next day, the patient took a pack of *Baihu Tang*. After sunrise, he passed loose stool and recovered. Later, he contracted an eye disease, and it, too, was cured after the application of Gypsum Fibrosum and Cortex Phellodendri 3.75g each twice a day, for seven or eight days. At the time, I had yet to understand the importance of examining stool and did not consider the duration of constipation. After reflecting on the case, I concluded that the constipation from the exterior cold disease had resulted in this disease.

42 Later, a lesser yang person who had the febrile disease caused by cold with more fever than chills got *yangdu* (yang type inflammatory swelling) with eruptions due to his eating pheasant as suggested by others. I prescribed three packs of *Baihu Tang*, but the patient only took half a pack. Several days later, delirium occurred and turned very serious. When I was asked to see the patient again, I noticed that he was in a coma and showed signs of the endogenous Wind stirring. He also exhibited symptoms of deafness, delirium, and white coating on the tongue. Later, at my house, I found that there were only 600g of Gypsum Fibrosum and 37.5g of Talcum in the drug box, so I immediately decocted 37.5g of Gypsum Fibrosum and 3.75g of Talcum and gave it to him. I did the same the following day. He had no bowel movement for but a day, and on the third day, I decided to refrain from giving him Gypsum Fibrosum–his family was worried about the side effects of the heavy doses. On the fourth day, his family hurriedly asked me to see the patient again. I found that the patient had had no bowel movement for two nights and one day, and he was speaking incoherently and could not drink water due to trismus. I decocted 75g of Gypsum Fibrosum and forced him to take it. Half of the decoction was regurgitated, and after a while, he could move his jaw; his speech, however, was still unclear. I continued to give him 37.5g of Gypsum Fibrosum. Since I was worried that he might have an endogenous Wind stirring which would make him unable to swallow in the afternoon, and in order to prevent that situation, I gave the medicine to him in the morning. He afterwards continued to take the medicine for five to six days, and the total amount of Gypsum Fibrosum that he had taken was 530g. For the last several days, he had mania and his speech became loud, and his illness was relieved. Several months later, the patient was able to walk in the house garden.

43 Later, another lesser yang person who first suffered from headache, fever and exterior cold disease for eight or nine days came to my house. After he had taken Rhizoma Coptidis, Fructus Trichosanthis, Rhizoma seu Radix Notopterygii and Radix Saposhnikoviae etc., there had been a little improvement, but his later mania persisted for three days. His family

regarded it as a common disease and did not pay much attention to it; they only used Rhizoma Coptidis and Fructus Trichosanthis. After the delirium continued for several days, the patient began to take one pack of *Jiwhang Baikho Tang*. The next afternoon, the endogenous Wind stirred, and I immediately decocted three packs of *Dihuang Baihu Tang* to prevent serious endogenous Wind stirring, but they were difficult to swallow. The day after, he took *Baihu Tang* with 37.5g of Gypsum Fibrosum before noon to prevent endogenous Wind stirring. After continuing treatment for three days more, the patient could stand and sit, urinate and defecate by himself; his health was much improved. Unfortunately, his illness worsened due to incomplete treatments, and in the end, he could not be saved. It is regrettable that this patient took two packs of *Baihu Tang* only in the morning to prevent from the endogenous Wind stirring, but did not continue to take medications in the afternoon, too. According to the above three patients' cases, for mania and delirium, *Baihu Tang* should be given not only once before noon to prevent endogenous Wind stirring, but five to ten additional doses per day. It would be better not to wait for the delirium to occur, but to administer when the mania shows itself. It is better to observe and detect the signs of oncoming mania rather than wait for mania to occur.

44 Later, there was a seventeen year old lesser yang girl who had previously suffered from a lack of vital energy and abdominal pain due to indigestion. One day, she suddenly had a headache, chills with fever and indigestion. A doctor prescribed her three *Suhe Wan* and ordered her to take them with a ginger decoction. She then had diarrhea over ten times a day for more than ten days. The patient felt seriously thirsty, and had insomnia and occasional delirium. It was November 23, 1875. I prescribed Radix Rehmanniae and Gypsum Fibrosum, 225g each, and 113g of Rhizoma Anemarrhenae for that night. The diarrhea decreased by half in frequency. The next day, I prescribed two packs of *Hyeongbang Jihwang Tang* and added 15g of Gypsum Fibrosum to be taken orally. She then slept soundly and had smooth urination that day. It is clear that the pharmaceutical power of this decoction is ten times more effective than *Zhimu Baihu Tang*

(White tiger decoction with Rhizoma Anemarrhenae), so I proceeded to use it for several days, twice in the day and twice at night. The diarrhea ceased completely, but she was sweating over the preauricular region. Suddenly, the delirium turned into mania. Her family stopped her treatment for two days out of fear, and she lapsed into a dangerous state. She had no perspiration over the head, but had dysuria, oliguria, coldness of the mouth and lips, and was unconscious. These symptoms were sinister signs. I was forced to use *Hyeongbang Jihwang Tang* and added 37.5g of Gypsum Fibrosum, ten packs a night, to be taken orally. The patient urinated three bowls at night. Mania persisted, but she regained consciousness. The next day, she took six packs, and four to six packs continuously for the next five days. The mania disappeared, and the patient fell asleep easily, if somewhat fitfully. After taking three to four packs a day for five days continuously, she had sweat in the preauricular region and fell asleep within half an hour, and was able to take rice gruel. Afterwards, I added 3.75g of Gypsum Fibrosum to the decoction, for two packs a day. When she had no bowel movement, I added 15g of Gypsum Fibrosum. By the 23rd of December, her critical condition had stabilized, and she was able to stand up in the room. She had taken a total of 1687.5g of Gypsum Fibrosum for a month. Later, she walked for a mile to see me on the fifteenth of next January. She continued to take *Hyeongbang Jihwang Tang* with 3.75g of Gypsum Fibrosum added until March.

45 I have said, "The lesser yang person's diseases are mainly due to the fire-heat; thus, it progresses rapidly. The initial symptoms must not be taken lightly. Generally, if a lesser yang person has a headache from the exterior disease, and constipation from the interior disease, he is already in a serious condition. Only one to three packs of inappropriate medications for a serious disease can kill the patient; and if one to three packs, normally suitable medication for a critical condition, are not used, the patient can not be saved, either."

2

Discourse on the Lesser Yang Person's Interior Febrile Disease Induced from the Stomach Affected by Heat*

1 Zhang Zhongjing said, "In the greater yang disease, after eight to nine days, the patient has fever and chills with malaria, but more fever than chills. If there is a feeble pulse and chills, they are the symptom of a deficiency both in the yin and the yang. For such a case, neither a diaphoretic, nor a purgative, nor an emetic should be used. A flushed face, which indicates the color of heat, and an itchy skin caused by a lack of light perspiration, signifies that the syndrome is not gone. *Guima Geban Tang* (Combination of half *Guizhi Tang* and half *Mahuang Tang*) will disperse the remaining syndrome."

2 In the greater yang disease, when the patient has fever and chills with malaria, but more fever than chills, with a feeble pulse, it is a disease of yang collapse. A diaphoretic should not be adopted if there is no itching. *Guipi Geban Tang* (Combination of half *Guizhi Tang* and half *Yuepi Tang*) can be adopted.

3 I have said, "In this syndrome, if stool is passed within twenty four hours, *Hyeongbang Sabaik San* should be used. If not, *Jihwang Baikho Tang* should be used."

---

* 少陽人胃受熱裏熱病論

4 Zhang Zhongjing said, "For the yang brightness syndrome, *Zhuling Tang* (Decoction of Polyporus) is suitable when there is dysuria and a floating pulse with thirst."

5 A combination of the three yang diseases displays symptoms such as headaches, a dirty face, delirium and incontinence. It manifests itself through fever both in the interior and the exterior. When there is spontaneous perspiration, restlessness with thirst, abdominal pain and a heavy feeling in movement, *Baihu Tang* can be adopted.

6 I have said, "The yang brightness syndrome is the only apparent fever with no chills. A combination of the three yang diseases means that the greater yang, lesser yang and yang brightness diseases are simultaneously complicated. For this case, we should use *Zhuling Tang* and *Baihu Tang*. The ancient prescription of *Zhuling Tang* is no better than the recent practice of prescribing *Jeoryeong Chajeonja Tang*. Similarily, the ancients' *Baihu Tang* is no better than the new prescription of *Jihwang Baikho Tang*. If the yang brightness disease has symptoms such as dysuria and constipation, it is suitable to use *Jihwang Baikho Tang*."

7 Zhu Gong said, "Yang syncope is the disease which shows fever and headache, and looks like yang syndrome externally in the initial stage, with syncope not appearing until the fourth or fifth day. Syncope is suddenly accompanied with fever within half a day. There never is syncope until the heat qi is localized deeply. It is a serious fever if the fever suddenly occurs when syncope is mild. The pulse can only be detected when pressed deeply, and the pulse is slippery. This means that there is a fever inside which may lead to symptoms, including drinking large amounts of water, waving of hands and feet, restlessness with insomnia, constipation, reddish urine and coma. *Baihu Tang* should be used."

8 I have said, "For the interior febrile disease of a lesser yang person, *Jihwang Baikho Tang* would be the best drug. Before adopting this decoction, we must monitor a patient's bowel movements. If he has not passed anything for one day, we may use it; if he has not passed anything for two days, we must use it. Generally, if a lesser yang person cannot pass stool

for one day, his stomach-heat has been already congealed. If there was no bowel movement for two days in the lesser yang person, he has a serious fever. If there is no bowel movement within three days and nights, his condition is dangerous. It is reasonable to adopt the drug when the patient has had no bowel movement for over a day or two. One should not, however, allow this constipation to last a third day and night; and if there is delirium and constipation, do not let the symptoms persist for more than one day and night."

9 If the stomach of a lesser yang person receives the heat, his feces will be dry. If his Spleen receives the cold, diarrhea will be induced. If there is yin collapse with diarrhea for two to three days and constipation for one day and night, the clean yin will be exhausted, and the patient's condition will be in danger. If there is the stomach-heat syndrome with constipation for three days and nights and perspiration, the clean yang will be exhausted, and the patient's condition will be in danger.

10 If a lesser yang person with constipation takes three to four packs of *Baihu Tang*, he will recover, though he will not have had any bowel movement that day. If he takes two to three packs continuously the next day, he will certainly have a bowel movement.

11 When attempting to identify a lesser yang person disease, whether it is the exterior or interior syndrome, and whether aggravated or relieved, it is important that one examines the stool. If the feces are dry at first and loose later, and there is no difficulty in bowel movement, the lesser yang person is in good health. If his bowel movements cease after passing a large amount of loose stool, once or twice, his illness will be relieved. Ordinarily, smooth stool, once or twice, indicates that the patient's condition has not changed. No bowel movement for more than one day and night, or small amount of loose stools three to five times for one day and night indicates that his stool will be constipated. This stool indicates a bad prognosis, which we must prevent.

12 At the onset of the lower abdomen cold syndrome of a lesser yin person's

interior cold disease, symptoms such as borborygmus and diarrhea are easily detected, and a treatment should be adopted as early as possible. At the onset of the chest-phrenic fever syndrome of a lesser yang person's interior febrile disease, symptoms such as restlessness in the chest cannot be easily detected, and a treatment is usually adopted at a later stage. If a lesser yang person had marked restlessness in the chest that can be easily identified, it is very difficult to treat, because such a symptom indicates that his condition is already serious. Generally, for the exterior disease of the lesser yang person, we can easily understand that headache is one of the initial symptoms. If there are other symptoms, such as thirst and reddish urine, we must be cautious; and if there are other symptoms, such as diarrhea and waving of hands and feet, we must practice prudence here, as well. As for the interior disease of the lesser yang person, it is clear that no bowel movement for more than one day and night belongs to the initial symptom of the interior disease. If a patient has had no bowel movement for more than three days and nights, he is in danger. A patient, who suffers from diseases such as back carbuncle, brain carbuncle, swelling of the lips, diphtheria and laryngopharyngeal disease, is already in danger from onset. The macule due to yang type inflammatory swelling, multiple erysipelas and jaundice also indicates a dangerous condition from onset. The illnesses of the face, eyes, mouth, nose and teeth are serious when they occur. Generally, *Hyeongbang Paidok San* should be used for headache induced by the exterior disease, and *Baikho Tang* should be used for the interior disease of a lesser yang person who has had no bowel movement for more than one day and night.

13 Wang Haogu said, "There are three types of thirst disease whose names are *xiaoke* (polydipsia), *xiaozhong* (polyphagia) and *xiaoshen* (polyuria). Restlessness in the chest and reddish tongue and lips are caused by the ascending heat qi. This thirst, called polydipsia, is characterized by an imbibing of a large amount of fluids and frequent urination in small quantities, and belongs to the upper-*jiao*. Hyperphagia, over-appetite and emaciation are caused by the accumulation of heat in the middle-*jiao*. This results in a thirst in which the restlessness in the chest is mild, urination is frequent, and the urine tastes sweet; it belongs to the middle-*jiao*.

This thirst is called polyphagia, and is characterized by emaciation of the thigh and knee joint, soreness and pain in the joints, drinking small amounts of water, and a large quantity of turbid urine. These are all caused by the latency of the heat in the lower-*jiao*. This disease is called polyuria, and one symptom is a leakage of sperm without sexual intercourse induced by the over-consumption of five mineral stones that causes the exhaustion of the essential qi and the remainder of mineral heat. This thirst is called *qiangzhong* (persistent erection). Polydipsia is mild, polyphagia is serious, and polyuria even more so. The persistent erection is a fatal disease where death is welcome relief."

14 Zhu Zhenheng said, "*Baihu Tang* should be adopted for diabetes involving the upper-*jiao*, which manifests itself as a red and fissured tongue, and polyposia with severe thirst. *Huanglian Zhudu Wan* (Pills of Rhizoma Coptidis and pig stomach) should be adopted for diabetes involving the middle-*jiao*, whose symptoms include polyposia with emaciation, spontaneous sweating, constipation and frequent urination. *Liuwei Dihuang Tang* should be adopted for diabetes stemming from the lower-*jiao*, whose symptoms are restlessness with much drinking of water, oily urine, and dry and thin legs."

15 In the『*Yixue Gangmu*』, we read, "Polyposia with thirst is diabetes involving the upper-*jiao*. Polyposia with polyphasia is diabetes involving the middle-*jiao*; and thirst with frequent and oily urination is diabetes involving the lower-*jiao*."

16 Wei Yilin said, "If a person overindulgent in sensual pleasures takes a mineral stone while his essential qi is already exhausted and only the evil heat remains, he will display symptoms of polyphagia, emaciation, oily urine and persistent erection with spontaneous ejaculation. This is the most serious type among the three diabetic diseases."

17 I have said, "Diabetes is induced by a person's own mean and narrow mind. A hard, hasty, shallow and unoriginal mind makes it difficult for the large intestine qi to ascend. Hence, gradually, the qi is exhausted, and the disease is formed. If the clean yang in the stomach ascends and cannot

nourish the head, face and four limbs, diabetes involving the upper-*jiao* will be formed. If the clean yang in the large intestine ascends and cannot nourish the stomach, diabetes involving the middle-*jiao* will be formed. Originally, diabetes involving the upper-*jiao* was serious, but diabetes involving the middle-*jiao* is twice as serious as diabetes involving the upper-*jiao*. Diabetes involving the middle-*jiao* is a dangerous disease, but diabetes involving the lower-*jiao* is twice as dangerous as diabetes involving the middle-*jiao*. *Yanggyeok Sanhwa Tang* (Decoction for cooling diaphragm and dispersing fire) should be used for diabetes involving the upper-*jiao*, *Indongdeung Jigolpi Tang* (Decoction of Caulis Lonicerae and Cortex Lycii) should be used for diabetes involving the middle-*jiao*, and *Sukjihwang Gosam Tang* (Decoction of Radix Rehmanniae Praeparata and Radix Sophorae Flavescentis) should be used for diabetes involving the lower-*jiao*. Sufferers should be generous and broad-minded. To be generous means to be slow-paced, and as a result, a person's clean yang will ascend and flow. To be narrow-minded means to be in a hurry; his clean yang will be exhausted in the lower part."

18 Stable emotion with a peaceful mind will raise the yang qi and spread this qi to the face, head and limbs. This qi is called primordial qi and clean yang. The exertion of the mind will lower and concentrate the yang qi. This will lead to the stagnated heat on the face, head, and limbs. This qi is called the fire qi and the consuming yang.

19 Wei Yilin said, "Since diabetes must try to prevent the formation of carbuncles, it is advisable to take the root, stem, flower or leaf of the Caulis Lonicerae without consideration of amounts."

20 Li Gao said, "If a diabetic patient is able to eat food, he will get a carbuncle on the nape and back in the late stages; and if a patient can not eat food, he will have abdominal distension or tympanites."

21 In the 『*Dongui Uibang Yuchui*』[1)] ("Classified Collection of Eastern Medical Prescriptions"), we read, "Diabetes can lead to carbuncles, fluid imbalance or total blindness."

22 I have said, "Carbuncles and optic diseases are developed from diabetes involving the middle-*jiao*. Since diabetes involving the middle-*jiao* is already dangerous, we should treat it when it is still involving the upper-*jiao*. In the case of diabetes involving the middle-*jiao*, we should treat it immediately. Diabetes involving the lower-*jiao* may be regarded as virtually fatal."

23 Wang Haogu said, "One child sweated at night for seven years. He took many drugs, but did not experience any improvement. He took *Liangge San* (Powder for cooling diaphragm) for three days, and then he recovered from his illness."

24 I have said, "If the lesser yang person's large intestine clean yang flows up to the stomach and nourishes the head, face and limbs, there will be no sweating. The sweating of the lesser yang person is induced by the weakness of yang. Here, recovery by *Liangge San* means that the disease is diabetes involving the upper-*jiao*, and is but a mild case."

25 In the 『*Dongui Uibang Yuchui*』, we read, "Generally, the diabetic patient drinks water frequently, and certainly has symptoms such as dizziness and cold back with vomiting. These symptoms are caused by his asthenia."

26 Gong Xin said, "Generally, yin deficiency syndrome shows chills and fever every day in the afternoon, which is relieved after slight sweating. If we treat it as malaria, it can not be cured."

27 Sun Simiao[2)], in his 『*Qianjinfang*』[3)] ("Essential Prescriptions Worth a Thousand Gold Pieces") said, "There are three things which diabeties should avoid: drinking, overindulging in sensual pieasures and eating salty food and noodles. If he avoids them, he may recover from his illness without taking drugs."

28 I have said, "Even though the ascending qi of the interior yang is exhausted in diabetes involving the upper-*jiao* and diabetes involving the middle-*jiao*, their descending qi of the exterior yin is still strong; so though the diseases are dangerous, the patient can manage for a long time. Afternoon fever and insatiable thirst show yin deficiency, and the two

with a cold back and vomiting indicates that their yin and yang of both the exterior and interior are totally exhausted. Their condition is in as much danger as though they were suffering diabetes involving the lower-*jiao*. However, if they can maintain good psychosomatic cultivation and proper administration of drugs, six to seven out of ten will stay alive. If, however, they neglect psychosomatic cultivation and simply rely upon the drugs, they will be unable to cure the patient. *Dokhwal Jihwang Tang* (Decoction of Radix Rehmanniae Preparata with Radix Angelicae Pubescentis) and *Sibimi Jihwang Tang* (Decoction of twelve drugs containing Radix Rehmanniae Preparata) should be adopted."

29 In the undivided third line of the Xu in the 『*Ijing*』[4] ("Classic of Changes"), we read, "The third line of the Xu, undivided, shows its subject in the mud (close by the stream). He thereby invites the approach of the enemy. "It says in the Great Symbolism",'He is waiting in the mud'. This tells us that calamity is close at hand in the outer trigram.'He himself invites the approach of the enemy" tell us that if he be reverent and careful, he will not be bested." If we say, quoting the meaning above, "Though a patient has afternoon fever caused by yin deficiency, cold back and vomiting, which is dangerous, his death will depend upon other factors. If he cleans and purifies his mind, respects his body and takes the proper medicine, he will recover."

3

General Remarks on the Lesser Yang Person*

1 For the lesser yang person's disease, there are five major symptoms: stroke, hematemesis, vomiting, abdominal pain, and indigestion with feeling of fullness. All of these five symptoms have the same cause, and there are different degrees of each symptom. Another group of five symptoms is edema, dyspnea, accumulation of pathogen in the chest, dysentery and alternate attacks of chills and fever with fullness in the chest and costal region. These all have the same cause, but different intensities in expression.

2 There is no way to cure the hemiplegia or monoplegia of the upper limbs induced by stroke in a lesser yang person. If the stroke is severe, the patient will die, and if it is mild, he can survive. Since there is no guarantee the patient will recover, he should take drugs from time to time and hope for the best.

3 If a lesser yang person has hematemesis, he must control his hard and irritable temper; not fight with others; eat a simple diet; take the proper drug, and cultivate himself like a Buddhist. After 100 days, his illness will somewhat improve; after 200 days, it will be much improved; one year

---

* 少陽人泛論

later, he will have all but recovered; and three years later, he will have fully recovered. If he does not follow this direction, the illness will recur. If this happens, all prior efforts will have been in vain, and the patient must begin anew. If he follows the directions for ten or twenty years, he will have a long life.

4 Generally, a lesser yang person will sometimes experience slight bleeding in the nasal cavity or in the sputum. Even though it is slight, it is still hematemesis. If there is bleeding in the mouth and cold phlegm, though there be no vomiting, it still belongs to vomiting. A young man contracting this illness will die shortly. This is caused by negligence. These two symptoms are very serious and dangerous, so the patient must take medicine. After ridding the patient of the root of his illness, his life can be saved.

5 A stroke is so serious in nature that we cannot expect to cure it; hematemesis, however, is milder, and the patient's chances of recovery are high. These two diseases can be cured first, by taking care of oneself, and second, by taking medicine. However, for symptoms such as vomiting, abdominal pain and indigestion with a feeling of fullness, a patient must take medicine as well as care of himself, if he expects to recover.

6 For stroke and vomiting, *Dokhwal Jihwang Tang* should be adopted; and for hematemesis, *Sibimi Jihwang Tang*.

7 Edema is a disease that has to be treated quickly. If not, the patient will be in danger. The more quickly he takes medicine, the more easily he will recover; if not, he will die. From outward appearances, this disease seems to progress slowly and not pose much of a threat to a person's health, but it is not so. It must be treated within four or five days, and must not last more than ten days. In the beginning, the patient of edema takes *Moktong Daian Tang* (Decoction for greatly stabilizing with Caulis Akebiae) or *Hyeongbang Jihwang Tang* added Caulis Akebiae, then once more afterwards. In six or seven days, the edema will be cured. Following recovery, he must take one or two packs of the above decoction (*Hyeongbang Jihwang Tang* added Caulis Akebiae) everyday for 100 days, to clean the

urine and to prevent the disease from recurring. If it recurs, recovery will prove difficult. After the relief from edema, the patient should not take much food. If he takes too much, the disease will recur. In cases of edema, reddish urine is a sign of malignancy. If the urine is clean, the edema will be successfully treated, but if it is red, edema will occur.

8 If a lesser yang person who has diabetes involving the middle-*jiao* has abdominal distension, he will definitely develop tympanites, which is incurable. A lesser yang person with tympanites, just as a lesser yin person with *zangjie* (accumulation of yin cold in the viscera), dies within five months to a year. In a lesser yin person with accumulation of yin cold in the viscera, though his exterior yang warm qi is almost exhausted, his interior yin warm qi stands out strongly. In a lesser yang person with tympanites, though his interior yang cool qi is almost exhausted, his exterior yin cool qi stands out strongly. Both may live with their respective disease for quite a long time before dying.

9 For shortness of breath due to a febrile disease caused by cold in a lesser yang person, first, 0.375g of Cinnabaris should be used with warm water, and just after decocted Herba Schizonepetae, Radix Saposhnikoviae, Fructus Trichosanthis, etc. should be taken. There is no time to wait for the decoction.

10 Since the effect of Cinnabaris is very strong, it must not be used many times. The medicine is good for emergencies only. It must be boiled into soup. After the stomach and intestine are filled with it, it can tonify and invigorate yin and yang.

11 When compared to accumulation of pathogen in the chest, dysentery is regarded as a mild disease. However, when dysentery is close in seriousness to edema, it is regarded as a serious disease. When compared to abdominal pain, vomiting is a deteriorated case. However, when vomiting is close in seriousness to stroke, it is regarded as a malignant disease.

12 For dysentery in a lesser yang person, *Hwanglyeon Cheongjang Tang* (Decoction for clearing the intestines with Rhizoma Coptidis) should be adopted.

13 There is a type of malaria which has a three-day cycle of one day on and two days off in a lesser yang person: it is malaria with general debility. It must be treated slowly, not hastily. When the malaria is off, the patient should take two packs of *Dokhwal Jihwang Tang* during the morning and the evening. When it starts again, he should take two packs of *Hyeongbang Paidok San* continuously when he feels chilly. If the patient accepts the standard of taking 40 packs of *Dokhwal Jihwang Tang* and 20 packs of *Hyeongbang Paidok San* within a month, the disease will be cured.

14 For the lesser yang person, the swelling inside the throat and outside the neck and cheeks is called diphtheria. In two or three days, it will kill the patient. Swelling in the raphe of the upper lip is called swollen lips. Swelling that looks like hulled millet around both sides of the raphe is also dangerous. When the above two diseases are still mild in the initial stage, the patient should take *Yanggyeok Sanhwa Tang* and *Yangdok Baikho Tang* (White tiger decoction for yang type inflammatory swelling). If serious, nasal fumigation with mercury should be adopted. If there is perspiration over the neck and cheeks after fumigation into the nose, the patient will be cured. If there is no fumigant, he should take a pill mixed with 0.5625g of Calomelas, Olibanum, Myrrha, Radix Euphorbiae Kansui, 1.875g each, with starch at once.

15 If a lesser yang child eats much, but remains thin, he should take *Luhui Feier Wan* (Children's weight-gaining pills with Aloe) or *Indongdeung Jigolpi Tang*.

16 I once observed a lesser yang person with *duzhong* (poisonous swelling) on his shoulder. He had no sensation of heat when boiled sesame oil was poured on the swelling and the skin and flesh was burnt. A doctor taught him to place a piece of bull's horn on the coal and let the smoke into the swelling. The poisonous pus was flushed and the swelling cured.

17 I once observed a seventy year old lesser yang person who had a carbuncle on the nape of his neck. A doctor had told him to patch it with a powdered swellfish's egg, and he recovered immediately. Since swellfish's

eggs are very poisonous, pigs or dogs die immediately when they eat them. When they are hung in a tree, birds do not dare eat them.

18 I once treated a lesser yang person with a carbuncle resembling a serpent's head. A swellfish's egg was made into powder; a small amount was placed on the adhesive plaster, and the dressing was changed daily. After five or six days, we could see the effects: new flesh had grown quickly, but there was too much of it. I covered all the new flesh with whetstone powder, the excess flesh disappeared, and the patient recovered. I have also used this drug for several days to treat scrofula resembling a lotus seed pot. It is also good for burns and dog or insect bites.

19 I once treated a sixty year old lesser yang person with monoplegia of the upper limb due to a stroke. I told him to take 0.1875g of Calomelas, but his condition worsened. I prescribed *Gyeongbun Gamsu Yongho Dan* (Dragon-tiger pills with Calomelas and Radix Euphorbiae Kansui) for a twenty year old lesser yang person who had a slight monoplegia of the lower limb with numbness. After two or three administrations, he recovered.

20 I once treated a lesser yang person with a throat problem. He could not drink at all and had no bowel movement for three days. All signs pointed to a serious problem, so I prescribed *Gamsu Cheonil Hwan* (Tianyi pills with Radix Euphorbiae Kansui). He recovered immediately.

21 I once treated a seventy year old lesser yang person who had had no bowel movement for four to seven days and coldness, but no strength in his feet, although he could eat as usual. I prescribed *Gyeongbun Gamsu Yongho Dan*, and he immediately had a bowel movement. Several days later, however, the constipation recurred, and I told him to take this prescription several times more. Later, he was able to have normal bowel movements every day, and his disease was cured. He lived to the age of eighty.

22 I once observed a lesser yang person with heavy bleeding in his central incisors ridge, and immediately recognized his condition as dangerous. A doctor taught him how to apply new cotton soaked in boiled sesame oil to his ridge, and the bleeding stopped.

23 I once observed a lesser yang person who experienced facial nerve paralysis after combing his hair every day for several months. There were three more lesser yang persons suffering from the same illness, so I concluded that it is not good for a lesser yang person to comb his hair every day. I once knew an eighty year old greater yin person who combed his hair every day, who affirmed that combing was a pleasant activity in which he had been indulging for forty years.

3-1

Ten Prescriptions for the Lesser Yang Person's Disease from Zhang Zhongjing's『*Shanghanlun*』

1 White tiger decoction (*Baihu Tang* 白虎湯)

· Gypsum Fibrosum 18.75 g
· Radix Glycyrrhizae 2.625 g
· Rhizoma Anemarrhenae 7.5 g
· Semen Oryzae Sativae 9.375 g

2 Decoction of Polyporus (*Zhuling Tang* 猪苓湯)

· Polyporus 3.75 g
· Rhizoma Alismatis 3.75 g
· Colla Corii Asini 3.75 g
· Poria (red) 3.75 g
· Talcum 3.75 g

3 Powder of five drugs containing Poria (*Wuling San* 五苓散)

· Rhizoma Alismatis 9.375 g
· Polyporus 5.625 g
· Poria (red) 5.625 g
· Cortex Cinnamomi 1.875 g
· Rhizoma Atractylodis Macrocephalae 5.625 g

4 Minor decoction of Radix Bupleuri (*Xiao Chaihu Tang* 小柴胡湯)

· Radix Bupleuri 11.25 g
· Radix Ginseng 5.625 g
· Radix Glycyrrhizae 1.875 g
· Radix Scutellariae 7.5 g
· Rhizoma Pinelliae 5.625 g

5 Big blue dragon decoction (*Da Qinglong Tang* 大青龍湯)

· Gypsum Fibrosum	15 g	· Herba Ephedrae	11.25 g
· Ramulus Cinnamomi	7.5 g	· Radix Glycyrrhizae	3.75 g
· Semen Armeniacae Amarum	3.75 g	· Fructus Jujubae	2 pcs.
· Rhizoma Zingiberis Recens	3 slices		

6 Combination of half *Guizhi Tang* and half *Yuepi Tang* (*Guipi Geban Tang* 桂婢各半湯)

· Gypsum Fibrosum	7.5 g	· Herba Ephedrae	3.75 g
· Ramulus Cinnamomi	3.75 g	· Radix Paeoniae Alba	3.75 g
· Radix Glycyrrhizae	1.125 g	· Fructus Jujubae	2 pcs.
· Rhizoma Zingiberis Recens			3 slices

7 Decoction for mild phlegm-heat pattern in the chest (*Xiao Xianxiong Tang* 小陷胸湯)

· Rhizoma Pinelliae (detoxicated with ginger decoction)	18.75 g
· Rhizoma Coptidis	9.375 g
· Fructus Trichosanthis	(1/4 of large one)

8 Decoction for severe phlegm-heat pattern in the chest (*Da Xianxiong Tang* 大陷胸湯)

· Radix et Rhizoma Rhei	11.25 g	· Natrii Sulfas	7.5 g
· Radix Euphorbiae Kansui	1.875 g		

9 Decoction of ten Fructus Jujubae (*Shizao Tang* 十棗湯)

· Flos Genkwa (stir-baked to just dry)
· Radix Euphorbiae Kansui
· Radix Euphorbiae Pekinensis (stir-baked)

Pound equal amounts of the drugs into a powder. Stew ten dates (Fructus Jujubae) in one glass of water until half a glass remains. Remove the dregs and add 3.75g of the above powder for a strong patient and 1.875g for a weak patient. If loose stool is observed, serve the patient rice gruel for tonifying.

10 Pill for invigorating Kidney qi (*Shenqi Wan* 腎氣丸)

This prescription consists of *Liuwei Dihuang Tang* and Fructus Schizandrae.

3-2

Nine Prescriptions for the Lesser Yang Person's Disease Mentioned in the Writings of Famous Doctors in the Yuan and Ming Dynasties

1 Powder for removing heat from the diaphragm (*Liangge San* 凉膈散)

Drug	Dose	Drug	Dose
· Fructus Forsythiae	7.5 g	· Radix et Rhizoma Rhei	3.75 g
· Natrii Sulfas	3.75 g	· Radix Glycyrrhizae	3.75 g
· Herba Menthae	1.875 g	· Radix Scutellariae	1.875 g
· Fructus Gardeniae	1.875 g		

The original source of this prescription is the『*Jufang*』. It cures irritability, oral sores, conjunctival congestion and dizziness due to congestion of heat in the chest.

In accordance with recent studies, Radix et Rhizoma Rhei, Radix Glycyrrhizae and Radix Scutellariae must be excluded from this prescription.

2 Pills of Rhizoma Coptidis and pig stomach (*Huanglian Zhudu Wan* 黃連猪肚丸)

Drug	Dose	Drug	Dose
· Male pig stomach	1 pc.	· Rhizoma Coptidis	187.5 g
· Flour (stir-baked)	87.5 g	· Radix Trichosanthis	150 g
· Poria	150 g	· Radix Ophiopogonis	75 g

Pound the above drugs into a powder. Put the powder into a male pig stomach and stitch it up. Stew and pulverize, then make the pills as big as the seed of an empress tree.

The original source of this prescription is the『Dexiaofang』, compiled by Wei Yilin. This cures a prolonged erection of the penis with involuntary emission.

In accordance with the results of recent studies, Radix Ophiopogonis is the medicinal ingredient for the Lung in this prescription. Normally, the Lung raises the vital energy, while the Kidney lowers it, though both organs are separate. With five medicinal ingredients aimed at the Kidney, it would seem that Radix Ophiopogonis is unnecessary for the Lung, but that is not so. On the contrary, one should appreciate its properties.

3 Decoction of six drugs containing Radix Rehmanniae Praeparata

(*Liuwei Dihuang Tang* 六味地黃湯)

· Rhizoma Dioscoreae	7.5 g	· Fructus Corni	3.75 g
· Rhizoma Alismatis	5.625 g	· Cortex Moutan	5.625 g
· Radix Rehmanniae Praeparata	15 g	· Poria (white)	5.625 g

The original source of this prescription is the『Yixue Zhengzhuan』("Orthodox Medical Record")[1] compiled by Yu Tuan[2]. It cures consumption.

In accordance with the results of recent studies, Rhizoma Dioscoreae in this prescription is the medicinal ingredient for the Lung.

4 Pills of Radix Rehmanniae and Radix Rehmanniae Praeparata

(*Shengshou Dihuang Wan* 生熟地黃丸)

· Radix Rehmanniae	37.5 g	· Radix Scrophulariae	37.5 g
· Gypsum Fibrosum	37.5 g		
· Radix Rehmanniae Praeparata			37.5 g

Make the pasted pills as big as the seed of an empress tree. Take 50~70 pills on an empty stomach with tea.

The original source of this prescription is the『Yixue Rumen』, compiled by Li Chan. It cures weak eyesight.

5 Powder for promoting diuresis (*Daochi San* 導赤散)

· Caulis Akebiae	3.75 g	· Talcum	3.75 g
· Cortex Phellodendri	3.75 g	· Poria (red)	3.75 g
· Radix Rehmanniae	3.75 g	· Fructus Gardeniae	3.75 g
· Radix Glycyrrhizae	3.75 g	· Fructus Aurantii	1.875 g
· Rhizoma Atractylodis Macrocephalae			1.875 g

The original source of this prescription is the 『*Jufang*』. It cures irritability, oral sores, conjunctival congestion and dizziness due to congestion of heat in the chest.

In accordance with recent studies, Radix et Rhizoma Rhei, Radix Glycyrrhizae and Radix Scutellariae must be excluded from this prescription.

6 Antiphlogistic Powder of Herba Schizonepetae and Radix Saposhnikoviae (*Jingfang Baidu San* 荊防敗毒散)

· Radix Bupleuri	3.75 g	· Radix Peucedani	3.75 g
· Poria (red)	3.75 g	· Herba Schizonepetae	3.75 g
· Radix Saposhnikoviae	3.75 g	· Fructus Aurantii	3.75 g
· Radix Platycodi	3.75 g	· Rhizoma Chuanxiong	3.75 g
· Radix Ginseng	3.75 g	· Radix Glycyrrhizae	3.75 g
· Rhizoma seu Radix Notopterygii			3.75 g
· Radix Angelicae Pubescentis			3.75 g
· Herba Menthae			a small amount

This cures an exogenous febrile disease and all seasonal epidemic disease; a fever, a rigidity of the nape with a headache and arthrodynia of the limbs.

In accordance with the results of recent studies, Fructus Aurantii, Radix Platycodi, Rhizoma Chuanxiong, Radix Ginseng and Radix Glycyrrhizae have to be excluded from this prescription.

7 Children's weight-gaining pills (*Feier Wan* 肥兒丸)

- Rhizoma Picrorhizae 18.75 g
- Radix Ginseng 13.125 g
- Fructus Crataegi 13.125 g
- Aloe (calcined) 9.375 g
- Fructus Quisqualis 16.875 g
- Rhizoma Coptidis 13.125 g
- Poria (white) 11.25 g
- Massa Fermentata Medicinalis 13.125 g
- Fructus Hordei Germiniatus 13.125 g
- Rhizoma Atractylodis Macrocephalae 11.25 g
- Radix Glycyrrhizae (stir-baked with adjuvant) 11 g

Pound the above drugs into a powder and with glutinous millet paste and make the pills as big as mung beans. Take 20～30 pills with thin rice gruel.

This prescription is good for infantile malnutrition.

In accordance with the results of recent studies, Radix Ginseng, Rhizoma Atractylodis Macrocephalae, Fructus Crataegi and Radix Glycyrrhizae have to be excluded from this prescription. About Fructus Quisqualis, since we lack experience concerning this drug, we are not clear on the medicine's properties. Thus, Fructus Quisqualis should not be spoken of lightly.

8 Detoxicating decoction (*Xiaodu Yin* 消毒飲)

- Fructus Arctii 7.5 g
- Herba Schizonepetae 3.75 g
- Radix Glycyrrhizae (crude) 1.875 g
- Radix Saposhnikoviae 1.875 g

This cures pea-like skin sores which are not very pronounced and appear mainly and densely on the chest. Quickly give this decoction three or four times; some results are remarkable. The original source of the above three prescriptions is the『*Yijian*』, complied by Gong Xin.

In accordance with the results of recent studies, Radix Glycyrrhizae has to be excluded from this prescription.

9 Calomelas-fumigating method (*Shuiyin Xunbi Fang* 水銀熏鼻方)

- Graphite 3.75 g
- Cinnabaris 3.75 g
- Calomelas 3.75 g
- Olibanum 1.875 g

- Myrrha 1.875 g
- Sanguis Draconis 1.125 g
- Realgar 1.125 g
- Lignum Aquilariae Resinatum 1.125 g

Pound equal amounts of the drugs into a powder. Roll up into seven cigarette-like shapes. Make seven of them. Place lamp burning scented oil on the table. The patient should lie in his bed with his whole body under a coverlet with his legs stretched. The patient has to hold cold water in his mouth and change it frequently in order to prevent damage to his mouth. Fumigate three times the first day and once a day from then on.

The original source of this prescription is Zhu Zhenheng's 『*Danxi Xinfa*』. It is a miraculous cure against syphilitic skin lesions.

I have said that Calomelas has the effect of eliminating accumulated heat, refreshing the mind and vision, restraining the yang qi, and leading the yin qi back to the lower-*jiao*. This is the best among the drugs for a lesser yang person needing to restrain yin and reinforce yang. This method can be used only once as an emergency measure. It cannot be used continuously to reinforce yin. To use a metaphor, one must attack the first time where the enemy dwells with the power to root out a high mountain or the strength to carry a cauldron on one's shoulder. A second attack, however, in which the enemy has already been scattered, can lead to an attack on friendly forces. One must use this prescription for patients who have diphtheria.

A lesser yang person with monoplegia or hemiplegia of the lower limbs has to take 0.1875g or 0.375g of Calomelas powder for three days. Irrespective of the consequences, this cannot be used over three days in amounts exceeding 0.1875g or 0.375g a day. The patient must avoid cold air and take other precautions. The patient with monoplegia of the upper limbs, hemiplegia and facial palsy must not take this medicine; if he does, he will die.

An acute disease must be tackled immediately, but a chronic one need not be. Calomelas is so dangerous that we should not use it to cure a disease immediately. A chronic disease is only cured gradually; if it is cured quickly, the patient will most assuredly suffer a relapse from which recovery is difficult. There is the patient who has to take this medicine for three days and the patient who has to take it at one, two or three day intervals, for three cycles continuously.

I have treated lesser yang people who have had diseases of the throat, eyes and nose, and arthralgia of the lower limbs.

I gave them mercury for three or four days, either through fumigation or orally; all recovered. They were not allowed to expose themselves to cold air or chilly weather for at least one month afterwards, not even to wash their faces, change their clothes or comb their hair. Violating these prohibitions might have meant death. Remind the patient not to stay in a chilly room, or he will die. Nor let him stay in a warm room; if he cannot endure the fever with dysphoria, he might open the window, expose himself to cold air, and die.

I have witnessed a patient die in ten days after initial recovery because he had changed into new clothes; another died twenty days after initial recovery as a result of combing his hair. Another who had a disease of the throat died one night suddenly in a warm room because he had been exposed to the cold wind after fumigation of the nose two times on the first day and one time on the second. It is said that it is forbidden to give soybean sauce to a patient taking mercury, because soybean sauce made from fermented soybeans can neutralize the poison of the mercury. However, I believe it to be harmless, since the severe poison is easily neutralized.

3-3

Seventeen Newly Created Prescriptions for the Lesser Yang Person's Disease

1 Antiphlogistic powder of Herba Schizonepetae and Radix Saposhnikoviae

(*Hyeongbang Paidok San*: *Jingfang Baidu San* 荊防敗毒散)

· Radix Bupleuri	3.75 g	· Radix Peucedani	3.75 g
· Herba Schizonepetae	3.75 g	· Radix Saposhnikoviae	3.75 g
· Poria (red)	3.75 g	· Radix Rehmanniae	3.75 g
· Cortex Lycii	3.75 g	· Semen Plantaginis	3.75 g
· Rhizoma seu Radix Notopterygii			3.75 g
· Radix Angelicae Pubescentis			3.75 g

This prescription is for patients experiencing headaches and alternating attacks of chills and fever.

2 Powder for treating dark urine with Herba Schizonepetae and Radix Saposhnikoviae

(*Hyeongbang Dojeok San*: *Jingfang Daochi San* 荊防導赤散)

· Radix Rehmanniae	11.25 g	· Caulis Akebiae	7.5 g
· Radix Scrophulariae	5.625 g	· Fructus Trichosanthis	5.625 g
· Radix Peucedani	3.75 g	· Herba Schizonepetae	3.75 g
· Rhizoma seu Radix Notopterygii			3.75 g
· Radix Angelicae Pubescentis			3.75 g
· Radix Saposhnikoviae			3.75 g

This prescription is for patients experiencing headaches and fever with dysphoria in the chest.

3 Powder for expelling Lung-heat with Herba Schizonepetae and Radix Saposhnikoviae

(*Hyeongbang Sabaik San*: *Jingfang Xiebai San* 荊防瀉白散)

· Radix Rehmanniae	11.25 g	· Poria	7.5 g
· Rhizoma Alismatis	7.5 g	· Rhizoma Anemarrhenae	3.75 g
· Herba Schizonepetae	3.75 g	· Radix Saposhnikoviae	3.75 g
· Rhizoma seu Radix Notopterygii			3.75 g
· Radix Angelicae Pubescentis			3.75 g

This prescription is for patients experiencing headaches and irritation of the bladder.

4 Decoction of Polyporus and Semen Plantaginis

(*Jeoryeong Chajeonja Tang*: *Zhuling Cheqianzi Tang* 猪苓車前子湯)

· Rhizoma Alismatis	7.5 g	· Poria	7.5 g
· Polyporus	5.625 g	· Semen Plantaginis	5.625 g
· Rhizoma Anemarrhenae	3.75 g	· Gypsum Fibrosum	3.75 g
· Herba Schizonepetae	3.75 g	· Radix Saposhnikoviae	3.75 g
· Rhizoma seu Radix Notopterygii			3.75 g
· Radix Angelicae Pubescentis			3.75 g

This prescription is for patients experiencing headaches with abdominal pain and diarrhea.

5 Decoction of Talcum and Radix Sophorae

(*Hwalseok Gosam Tang*: *Huashi Kushen Tang* 滑石苦蔘湯)

· Rhizoma Alismatis	7.5 g	· Poria	7.5 g
· Talcum	7.5 g	· Radix Sophorae	7.5 g
· Rhizoma Coptidis	3.75 g	· Cortex Phellodendri	3.75 g
· Herba Schizonepetae	3.75 g	· Radix Saposhnikoviae	3.75 g
· Rhizoma seu Radix Notopterygii			3.75 g
· Radix Angelicae Pubescentis			3.75 g

This prescription is for patients experiencing abdominal pain without diarrhea.

6 Decoction of Radix Rehmanniae Praeparata with Radix Angelicae Pubescentis

(*Dokhwal Jihwang Tang*: *Duhuo Dihuang Tang* 獨活地黃湯)

· Fructus Corni 7.5 g
· Poria 5.625 g
· Rhizoma Alismatis 5.625 g
· Cortex Moutan 3.75 g
· Radix Rehmanniae Praeparata 15 g
· Radix Angelicae Pubescentis 3.75 g
· Radix Saposhnikoviae 3.75 g

This prescription is for patients experiencing indigestion and a feeling of fullness in the chest and upper abdomen.

7 Decoction of Radix Rehmanniae Praeparata with Herba Schizonepetae and Radix Saposhnikoviae

(*Hyeongbang Jihwang Tang*: *Jingfang Dihuang Tang* 荊防地黃湯)

· Fructus Corni 7.5 g
· Poria 7.5 g
· Rhizoma Alismatis 7.5 g
· Semen Plantaginis 3.75 g
· Herba Schizonepetae 3.75 g
· Radix Saposhnikoviae 3.75 g
· Radix Rehmanniae Praeparata 7.5 g
· Rhizoma seu Radix Notopterygii 3.75 g
· Radix Angelicae Pubescentis 3.75 g

For coughing, add Radix Peucedani. For blood problems, add Radix Scrophulariae and Cortex Moutan. For migraine, add Rhizoma Coptidis and Fructus Arctii. For indigestion and a feeling of fullness in the chest and abdomen, add Cortex Moutan. For internal fire, add Gypsum Fibrosum. For headaches, dysphoria with fever and blood problems, use Radix Rehmanniae instead of Radix Rehmanniae Praeparata, add Gypsum Fibrosum and remove Fructus Corni.

Herba Schizonepetae, Radix Saposhnikoviae, Rhizoma seu Radix Notopterygii and Angelicae Radix Pubescentis are all drugs tonifying and nourishing yin. Herba Schizonepetae and Radix Saposhnikoviae are very effective in clearing away heat from the chest and dispelling the wind. Rhizoma seu Radix Notopterygii and Radix Angelicae Pubescentis have the effect of greatly tonifying the genuine yin of the bladder.

Whether he suffers from a headache, abdominal pain, a feeling of fullness in the chest and upper abdomen, or diarrhea, it is my experience that a weak patient taking hundreds of packs of this medicine will recover; it is very effective medicine.

8 Decoction of twelve drugs containing Radix Rehmanniae Praeparata

(*Sibimi Jihwang Tang*: *Shierwei Dihuang Tang* 十二味地黃湯)

- Fructus Corni 7.5 g
- Rhizoma Alismatis 5.625 g
- Cortex Lycii 3.75 g
- Fructus Lycii 3.75 g
- Semen Plantaginis 3.75 g
- Radix Saposhnikoviae 3.75 g
- Poria (white) 5.625 g
- Cortex Moutan 3.75 g
- Radix Scrophulariae 3.75 g
- Fructus Rubi 7.5 g
- Herba Schizonepetae 3.75 g
- Radix Rehmanniae Praeparata 15 g

9 White tiger decoction with Radix Rehmanniae

(*Jihwang Baikho Tang*: *Dihuang Baihu Tang* 地黃白虎湯)

- Gypsum Fibrosum 18.75-37.5 g
- Rhizoma Anemarrhenae 7.5 g
- Radix Angelicae Pubescentis 3.75 g
- Radix Rehmanniae 15 g
- Radix Saposhnikoviae 3.75 g

10 White tiger decoction for yang type inflammatory swelling

(*Yangdok Baikho Tang*: *Yangdu Baihu Tang* 陽毒白虎湯)

- Gypsum Fibrosum 18.75-37.5 g
- Rhizoma Anemarrhenae 7.5 g
- Radix Saposhnikoviae 3.75 g
- Radix Rehmanniae 15 g
- Herba Schizonepetae 3.75 g
- Fructus Arctii 3.75 g

This prescription is for patients with macula caused by yang type inflammatory swelling and constipation.

11 Decoction for cooling the diaphragm and dispersing fire

(*Yanggyeok Sanhwa Tang*: *Liangge Sanhuo Tang* 凉膈散火湯)

- Radix Rehmanniae 7.5 g
- Fructus Forsythiae 7.5 g
- Herba Menthae 3.75 g
- Gypsum Fibrosum 3.75 g
- Herba Schizonepetae 3.75 g
- Caulis Lonicerae 7.5 g
- Fructus Gardeniae 3.75 g
- Rhizoma Anemarrhenae 3.75 g
- Radix Saposhnikoviae 3.75 g

This prescription is for patients suffering from diabetes involving the upper-*jiao*.

12 Decoction of Caulis Lonicerae and Cortex Lycii

(*Indongdeung Jigolpi Tang*: *Rendongteng Digupi Tang* 忍冬藤地骨皮湯)

- Caulis Lonicerae 15 g
- Cortex Lycii 7.5 g
- Cortex Phellodendri 3.75 g
- Radix Sophorae 3.75 g
- Rhizoma Anemarrhenae 3.75 g
- Fructus Lycii 3.75 g
- Herba Schizonepetae 3.75 g
- Flos Lonicerae 3.75 g
- Fructus Corni 7.5 g
- Rhizoma Coptidis 3.75 g
- Radix Scrophulariae 3.75 g
- Radix Rehmanniae 3.75 g
- Fructus Gardeniae 3.75 g
- Fructus Rubi 3.75 g
- Radix Saposhnikoviae 3.75 g

This prescription is for patients suffering from diabetes involving the middle-*jiao*.

13 Decoction of Radix Rehmanniae Praeparata and Radix Sophorae

(*Sukjihwang Gosam Tang*: *Shudihuang Kushen Tang* 熟地黃苦參湯)

- Fructus Corni 7.5 g
- Rhizoma Alismatis 5.625 g
- Cortex Phellodendri 3.75 g
- Poria (white) 7.5 g
- Rhizoma Anemarrhenae 3.75 g
- Radix Sophorae 3.75 g
- Radix Rehmanniae Praeparata 15 g

This prescription is for patients suffering from diabetes involving the lower-*jiao*.

14 Decoction for greatly stabilizing with Caulis Akebia

(*Moktong Daian Tang*: *Mutong Daan Tang* 木通大安湯)

· Caulis Akebiae	18.75 g	· Radix Rehmanniae	18.75 g
· Poria (red)	7.5 g	· Rhizoma Alismatis	3.75 g
· Semen Plantaginis	3.75 g	· Rhizoma Coptidis	3.75 g
· Radix Saposhnikoviae	3.75 g	· Herba Schizonepetae	3.75 g
· Rhizoma seu Radix Notopterygii			3.75 g

This prescription is for patients suffering from edema. Edema is hard to cure in a lesser yang person. From beginning to end of the treatment, a lesser yang person must take one hundred or more packs. Rhizoma Coptidis and Rhizoma Alismatis are expensive; the poor cannot afford them.

15 Decoction for clearing intestine with Rhizoma Coptidis

(*Hwanglyeon Cheongjang Tang*: *Huanglian Qingchang Tang* 黃連淸腸湯)

· Radix Rehmanniae	15 g	· Caulis Akebiae	7.5 g
· Poria	7.5 g	· Rhizoma Alismatis	7.5 g
· Polyporus	3.75 g	· Semen Plantaginis	3.75 g
· Rhizoma Coptidis	3.75 g	· Radix Saposhnikoviae	3.75 g
· Rhizoma seu Radix Notopterygii			3.75 g

This prescription is for patients suffering from dysentery. If gonorrhea is observed, exclude 7.5g of Caulis Akebiae and add 3.75g of Herba Schizonepetae.

16 Powder beneficial to vitality with Cinnabaris

(*Jusa Igwon San*: *Zhusha Yiyuan San* 朱砂益元散)

· Talcum	7.5 g	· Rhizoma Alismatis	3.75 g
· Radix Euphorbiae Kansui	1.875 g	· Cinnabaris	0.375 g

Pound the drugs into powder and let the patient take it with warm water or with water drawn from the well at daybreak. This can be used also to dispel summer-heat.

17 Tianyi pills with Radix Euphorbiae Kansui

(*Gamsu Cheonil Hwan*: *Gansui Tianyi Wan* 甘遂天一丸)

· Radix Euphorbiae Kansui 3.75 g · Calomelas 0.375 g

Make ten pills with a flour paste and coat them with *Cinnabaris*. If the pills are old and dried out, they will become hard and difficult to swallow. If this happens, wrap the pills in two or three layers of paper and pulverize them. Let the patient take them with water drawn from the well at daybreak. After three or four hours, if the patient does not have diarrhea, give two more pills. Diarrhea three to four times is desirable, but diarrhea five or six times is undesirable. To prevent the latter, prepare a thin gruel, and after two or three bouts of diarrhea, serve the gruel to the patient. If the preparation is not given, the patient will experience qi exhaustion and will not survive. In order to cure an accumulation of pathogen in the chest and immediate vomiting after drinking water, make ten pills from 3.75g of Radix Euphorbiae Kansui and 2.0g of Calomelas. It is called *Gyeongbun Gamsu Yongho Dan* (*Jingfen Gansui Longhu Dan*). Make ten pills from Calomelas and Radix Euphorbiae Kansui in equal amounts; this is called *Gyeongbun Gamsu Jawung Dan* (*Jingfen Gansui Cixiong Dan*). Make thirty pills from 3.75g of Calomelas, Olibanum, Myrrha and Radix Euphorbiae Kansui, 1.875g each; this is called *Yuhyang Molyak Gyeongbun Hwan (Ruxiang Moyao Jingfen Wan)*. Calomelas causes perspiration, and Radix Euphorbiae Kansui purges water. To obtain desirable results, use 0.375g of Calomelas–even 0.1875g is of use. Exactly 0.5625g of Radix Euphorbiae Kansui is efficient, but 0.2625g or 0.30g is not. Calomelas and Radix Euphorbiae Kansui are both drugs containing poison, so one should never use either in excess of 0.375g; the seriousness of the illness one is treating will determine exactly what amount is needed. If one wishes to dispel fire in the head, let Calomelas be the principle ingredient; for eliminating water in the chest, make Radix Euphorbiae Kansui the principle ingredient. The above drugs prescribed for the lesser yang person should not be stir-baked, stir-baked at high temperature, stir-baked with adjuvant, or roasted in hot ashes.

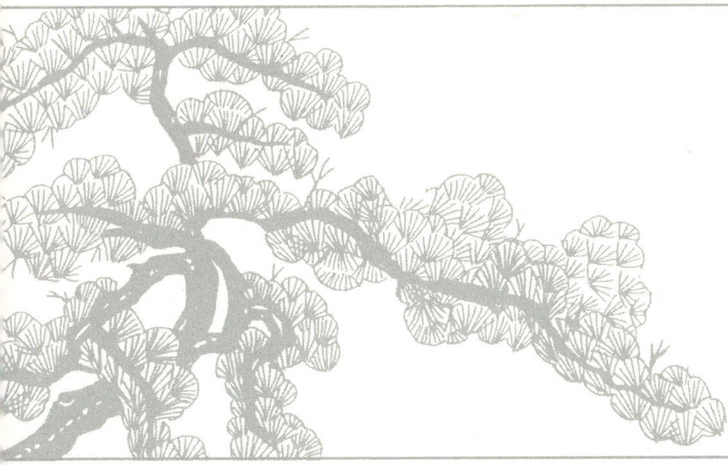

PART IV

1

Discourse on the Taieum (Greater Yin) Person's Exterior Cold Disease Induced from the Epigastrium Affected by Cold*

1 Zhang Zhongjing said, "*Mahuang Tang* (Decoction of Herba Ephedrae) suits a patient having the greater yang disease caused by cold with headache and fever, aching of the body and lumbago, arthralgia, chills, no perspiration, and cough."

This comment noted that the symptoms of febrile disease caused by cold, such as headaches and aches in the body, lower back and joints, were later called the greater yang disease caused by cold. These symptoms are all caused by bad circulation of the *ying* (nutrient) blood.

2 I have said, "The above disease is a mild case of the upper back exterior disease caused by cold in a greater yin person, and can be cured by *Mahuang Tang*. Among decoctions, Ramulus Cinnamomi and Radix Glycyrrhizae are not necessary; however, *Mahwang Balpyo Tang* (Decoction for diaphoresis with Herba Ephedrae) is suitable for this."

3 Zhang Zhongjing said, "As for the febrile disease caused by cold, on the fourth or fifth day: If *jue* (coldness) is observed, first there must have been a fever. Extreme coldness will lead to a high fever. When coldness is slight, the fever will also be slight. For the febrile disease caused by cold,

* 太陰人胃脘受寒表寒病論

coldness lasts for four days, followed by fever for three days. After that, coldness again prevails for five days. More chills than fever would indicate an aggravation of the syndrome. For the febrile disease caused by cold, coldness lasts for three days after the prevalence of a four day fever. The symptom of more fever than chills foretells recovery."

4 I have said, "The above mentioned coldness means the sensation of chills without fever, but it does not mean cold limbs. Fever after coldness for four to five days indicates a severe condition in the greater yin person's exterior syndrome caused by cold. In this syndrome, he has fever and sweating which starts from the hairline to the forehead. The fever recurs, and there is sweat on the eyebrows after several days. The fever recurs once again, and there is sweat on the cheeks for the next several days. The fever recurs once more, and there is sweat on the lips and jaw for the next several days, before another recurrence of fever, where there is sweat on the chest for several more days. As mentioned above, to the eyebrows there are several bouts of sweating on the forehead, to the cheeks there are several bouts of sweating on the eyebrows, to the lip and jaw there are several bouts of sweating on the cheeks, and directly to the chest just after one bout of sweating on the lips and jaw. This disease, which takes about twenty days of six or seven repeated sensations of coldness and then is relieved, is called long-term infectious disease. Generally, the greater yin person's disease, in which sweating begins on the forehead and eyebrows, and is not relieved until after several bouts of sweating, is a long-term infectious disease."

5 The greater yin person who has coldness for six or seven days without fever and perspiration will die. If he has coldness for two or three days with fever and perspiration, the illness will be a mild case. However, if he had coldness for four or five days with fever and little perspiration on his forehead, the illness is called the long-term infectious disease and is a serious case. This disease is caused by the exertion of the mind, which induces the Stomach duct to become asthenic, and the exterior of body cannot resist the cold and is surrounded by the cold. The situation is a battle between healthy qi and the pathogen. It is just like an army not being able to fight its way out of a battle, with but one company breaking

through the besieging enemy forces with the main army still behind. After several battles, if the army manages to break through, it is like a dignified figure. If there is perspiration on the forehead, the situation is just like a company breaking through the besieging army forces; if the perspiration is on the eyebrows, it is just like a few companies breaking through valiantly; if on the cheeks, it is like half the army breaking through slowly. The perspiration on the eyebrows means the illness will be relieved, and the perspiration on the cheeks means there is no more danger.

6 The greater yin person must have millet-like sweating on the forehead, eyebrows and cheeks, and will have a somewhat extended fever before the perspiration stops. This means that the healthy qi is strong and the pathogen is weak. Sweating becomes refreshing for the patient when he perspires little, with tiny drops or none at all. If, shortly after the perspiration stops, the healthy qi is still weak and the pathogen strong, there is no refreshing feeling for the patient.

7 If a greater yin person perspires over the upper back, below the hairline, and does not perspire on the face below the hairline, it is a bad sign. If he sweats over the face, but not around the ears, it is a sign of oncoming death. Generally, if a greater yin person perspires from the posteroauricular area and the hairline of the face to the sternal area, the disease will be relieved; if he has perspiration on the hairline, he will be saved from death; if over the forehead, he will barely escape with his life; if over the eyebrows, he will have just been saved; if over the cheeks, he will be out of danger; if over the lips and jaw, his disease has already been relieved; if over the chest, the disease has been completely relieved. I once observed the following symptoms: when perspiration starts from the forehead to the eyebrows, coldness is not so severe; when perspiration is present from the cheeks to the lips and jaw, coldness is so severe that the patient has chills and a quivering jaw like the wind stirring, and the perspiration directly spreads to both subaxillary areas. It is the same as Zhang Zhongjing's notion that "Extreme coldness will lead to an extreme fever. When coldness is slight, the fever also will be slight." If coldness persists several days in addition to these symptoms, it indicates that the disease is

serious. If only coldness is severe, the disease may be termed as not very serious.

8 The Gyeonggi Province people called the above disease the long-term infectious disease, while the Hamgyeong Province people called it forty day pain or sweatless dry disease. *Jingfang Baidu San*, *Huoxiang Zhengqi San* or *Buzhong Yiqi Tang* was commonly used for this disease, but most of them were inappropriate prescriptions. Only the adoption of Fel Ursi proved fortunate, like a blind man entering the correct door. If, however, the patient was treated by any other prescriptions again, his condition will worsen. There was a saying, "Disease does not kill the patient, and drugs do." Who cannot believe this saying? It is not easy for ordinary doctors to understand the degree of this disease, which is rather difficult to correctly diagnose. If a patient with the above disease has sweating on the eyebrows and cheeks, the disease becomes relieved naturally without administration. Even though the doctor may have given the patient the wrong drugs, there is no sweating on the cheeks, only on the forehead, and coldness as an exterior syndrome is relieved a little. The doctor then regards these drugs as effective, as does the patient, and the drugs become prescription. As a result, the perspiration on the patient's forehead will stop, and he will die. In this disease, we have to judge the degree only according to his perspiration, not according to the degree of coldness. Zhang Zhongjing's notion that the "disease will be relieved naturally" is in actuality a cautious approach, not a false one. However, if the long-term infectious disease has no epidemic pathogens, we can expect that disease will go away on its own. If, however, the epidemic febrile disease has severe epidemic pathogens and the disease is identified, and the prescription evident, it is wrong to wait for the disease to go away on its own, because we are worried that strange symptoms might appear.

9 I have said, "In the greater yin person disease, if coldness causes no perspiration for four days, it indicates a serious condition; if coldness causes no perspiration for five days, the patient is in danger of dying. Fel Ursi powder should be adopted, or *Handa Yeolso Tang* (Decoction for

treating more cold than fever) with five to nine larvae of cicadae (Holotrichia diomphalia Bates) should be taken. If his stool is loose, dried chestnut and Semen Coicis should be adopted; if his stool is dry, Radix Puerariae and Radix et Rhizoma Rhei should be adopted. In case there is perspiration over the forehead and eyebrows, we should wait until the disease is relieved, and then treat the patient with medication; otherwise, a relapse is possible."

10 I once treated the epidemic febrile disease of a greater yin person who had the cold syndrome in the epigastrium. This greater yin person had palpitations, but no perspiration, shortness of breath, a tight cough, and, additionally, sudden diarrhea which continued for dozens of days. This indicates a severe case of the exterior disease. *Taieum Jowi Tang* (Decoction for harmonizing a greater yin person's stomach), with 3.75g of Cortex Ailanthi, was adopted, and the patient took two packs of the prescription every day. The diarrhea stopped after ten days; one month later, he began to sweat on the face every day, and his previous symptoms were relieved. Since several of his relatives suddenly contracted the epidemic febrile disease, he took care of them and stopped taking drugs for several days. He contracted the epidemic febrile disease anew, lost his appetite, and did not eat anything. He took *Taieum Jowi Tang* with Rhizoma Cimicifugae and Radix Scutellariae added, 3.75g each, for ten days, then began to sweat on the face. The epidemic symptoms were slightly relieved, but still he had constipation for two days. Therefore, he took *Galgeun Seunggi Tang* (Decoction for purgation with Radix Puerariae) for five days; within five days, he was able to eat double the amount of thin rice gruel. Most of the epidemic symptoms disappeared, and his disease was cured. He had continuously taken *Taieum Jowi Tang*, adding Rhizoma Cimicifugae and Radix Scutellariae for forty days; his epidemic symptoms almost completely disappeared, and his previous symptoms were cured, as well.

11 A person has "tight cough" whenever he forces himself to cough, but still has difficulty ridding his throat of phlegm. The tight cough of the lesser yin person is called the tight cough associated with the chest, and the

tight cough of the greater yin is the tight cough associated with the jaws.

12 Generally, we can identify the exterior-interior and deficiency-excess syndromes of the patient who has the epidemic febrile disease through examining his previous diseases. A patient, who has suffered primarily from the cold disease, though he contracted the epidemic febrile disease at a later date, will develop cold symptoms. One, who has suffered primarily from the febrile disease, though he contracted the epidemic febrile disease at a later date, will develop febrile syndromes. One whose disease had been primarily mild, and who at a later date contracted an epidemic febrile disease, will see his condition grow serious. One whose disease had been primarily serious, and who at a later date contracted an epidemic febrile disease, will see his condition grow critical.

13 There was a greater yin patient who had a dry throat, and a bluish-whitish face, cold body and occasional diarrhea. His dry throat was induced by Liver heat, and his bluish-whitish colored face, cold body and occasional diarrhea were induced by coldness in the epigastrium. Since this disease is engaged in both the exterior and interior, it was quite a serious case. What was worse, he had contracted the epidemic febrile disease, and it took him twenty days to recover. His stool was smooth or loose during the first third, smooth in the middle third, and dried during the last third; during he had bowel movements two to four times a day. In the beginning, he was taking *Handa Yeolso Tang,* and after recovering he took *Jori Pyewon Tang* (Decoction for regulating Lung vitality) for more than forty days. He barely survived.

14 During the first six days, his stool was sometimes watery or loose, and there was perspiration on the forehead, eyebrows and cheeks. Apart from that, his condition was normal. On the sixth day, he started to take medicine, and on the seventh, he had profuse perspiration all over the face from the forehead to the chin. Afterwards, his face changed into a bluish-whitish color, and he began to stammer. On the eighth and ninth days, he not only stammered, but also he lost his hearing, and the perspiration on the chin moved to his cheeks and eyebrows. He perspired

lightly on the forehead only, from time to time, and became short of breath. On the tenth night, the sweat on the forehead disappeared, his stammering and deafness became worse, and he could not clear his throat of phlegm; he was forced to use his finger to pick out the phlegm. On the eleventh day, his shortness of breath became serious. Suddenly, on the twelfth day, he was able to eat two bowls of rice gruel. At that time, it would have been best to take Fel Ursi powder. Since Fel Ursi was very rare, I thought that he would not live another day; but on that afternoon, his shortness of breath eased slightly, and at the dawn of the thirteenth day, he perspired at the hairline. On the fourteenth and fifteenth days, he could eat two to three bowls of rice gruel and began to perspire on his forehead, eyebrows and cheeks, and the bluish color in his face disappeared. On the sixteenth day, there was perspiration on his chest, a small amount of phlegm was coughed out, and his stammering was relieved. On the twentieth day, he had several bouts of heavy perspirations on his chest and could stand in the room; all the symptoms, except for the deafness, disappeared. Afterwards, he continued to take medicine for forty days, until his deafness and dizziness had disappeared altogether.

2

Discourse on the Greater Yin Person's Interior Febrile Disease Induced from the Liver Affected by Heat*

1 Zhu Gong said, "Symptoms of yang type inflammatory swelling include silky patterns of red spots on the face, sore throat, and hemoptesis with pus, which should be treated with *Gegen Jieji Tang* (Decoction for releasing the flesh with Radix Puerariae) and *Heinu Wan* (Black servant pills). Generally, yang type inflammatory swelling and the deteriorated febrile disease are difficult to treat. Though the patient's spirit and consciousness are poor, if the epigastric region is still warm, open his mouth and let him swallow *Heinu Wan*. Then the patient can be saved immediately."

2 Li Chan said, "Slight chills and fever can be treated with *Gegen Jieji Tang*, and eyeball pain, dry nasal cavity, profuse sweating, constipation, severe thirst and ranting such as that of a madman, should be treated with *Tiaowei Chengqi Tang* (Purgative decoction for harmonizing the stomach). If there is a fever only in the exterior that causes pain in the eye and insomnia, *Jieji Tang* (Decoction for releasing the flesh) should be given. If the heat enters the interior, causing delirium similar to a madman's, *Tiaowei Chengqi Tang* should be given."

---

* 太陰人肝受熱裏熱病論

3 Gong Xin said, "The yang brightness disease with eyeball pain, dry nasal cavity and insomnia can be treated with *Gegen Jieji Tang*."

4 If the three yang diseases worsen, they will become yang type inflammatory swelling. Symptoms include a flushed face with red eyes, and yellowish spots on the body. Sometimes, there is also yellow-reddish diarrhea and a large, pounding pulse. The yang type inflammatory swelling can be treated with *Heinu Wan*.

5 I have said, "The diseases mentioned above should be treated with *Gegen Jieji Tang* and *Heinu Wan*."

6 In the 『*Lingshu*』, we read, "A patient with fever on the inner forearm, a pounding pulse, and the dryness syndrome is pestilent."

7 Wang Shuhe said, "The pulse of pestilence pounds both at the yin and yang locations. If the fever is extreme, the pulse becomes slippery with floating palpation, or scattering and uneven with deep palpation."

8 According to the 『*Maifa*』("Palpation Diagnosis"), the epidemic febrile disease, which has symptoms and signs such as fever, fullness of the abdomen, headache, normal appetite and straight-swift pulse on the second or third day, would cause the patient to die on the eighth day. If the patient has symptoms such as headache, fullness in the abdomen, vomiting and thread-stiff pulse, he will die on the twelfth day. If the patient did not have a headache, aching of the body, red eyes and changes of facial color, but had diarrhea with an uneven pulse that is largely felt by the superficial palpation, and hardness in the epigastrium, he will die on the seventeenth day.

9 Gong Xin said, "If a patient with the epidemic febrile disease has a high fever and a thread-short pulse, he will die, as will a patient with the epidemic febrile disease with severe diarrhea and abdominal pain."

10 "In 1586, when I lived in Daliang, an epidemic febrile disease broke out, and a large number of people died. The symptoms were severe chills with high fever, reddish swelling of the head, face, neck and cheeks, sore

throat and coma. At that time, I made a prescription called *Ersheng Jiuku Wan* (Pills with two wonderful drugs saving from suffering), which was composed of 150g of Radix et Rhizoma Rhei and 75g of Fructus Gleditsiae, and mixed with wheat paste and made into green bean-size pills which were taken 50 to 70 at a time. After just one administration, the patient began to sweat, and eventually recovered. Congenitally healthy patients always recover. Fructus Gleditsiae opens the sweat pores and scatters the exterior qi and Radix et Rhizoma Rhei gets rid of the heat and circulates inside the body."

11 Symptoms brought on by seasonal irregularities include an initially large amount of sputum, fever with discomfort, headache, general soreness, chills with a high fever, neck stiffness and eyeball pain. Appetite and living are normal. When the disease worsens, harshness of voice, red eyes, oral ulcers, buccal inflammations of various sizes, sore throat, coughing with sticky sputum, and sneezing occur.

12 I have said, "In addition to those symptoms mentioned above, if a patient has symptoms such as chills with a high fever, and a feeling of dryness and roughness, he should take *Jogak Daihwang Tang* (Decoction of Fructus Gleditsiae and Radix et Rhizoma Rhei) and *Galgeun Seunggi Tang*. Likewise, if reddish swelling of the head, face and throat appear, he also should take *Jogak Daihwang Tang* and *Galgeun Seunggi Tang*. If the patient has a fever, fullness in the abdomen, diarrhea and a tendency to high fever, it means that he has an interior syndrome and should be treated with *Galgeun Seunggi Tang*. If a symptom such as chills is more severe, it means that the exterior syndrome is quite serious and *Taieum Jowi Tang* added with Rhizoma Cimicifugae and Radix Scutellariae should be adopted."

13 I once treated a greater yin patient who had the epidemic febrile disease induced from the Liver affected by heat. He had been having eye problems for many years, and later contracted the epidemic febrile disease. From the first day, he took *Yeolda Hanso Tang* (Decoction for treating more fever than cold) for three to five days, and his stool became

loose, sometimes to the point of diarrhea. On the sixth day, since he had had no bowel movement, he took *Galgeun Seunggi Tang* continuously for three days and he ate double the amount of rice gruel. He took it continuously for another three days, and then his epidemic febrile disease was mostly relieved. After recovering, he took *Yeolda Hanso Tang*. When his stool was dried, 3.75g of Radix et Rhizoma Rhei was added. When he had severe diarrhea, Radix et Rhizoma Rhei was discontinued. After taking care of his health like this for twenty days, he recovered completely. At the onset, he had nausea, vomiting, unconsciousness and severe pain. Later, his condition improved, and he recovered in twelve days.

14 There was once a ten year old greater yin child suffering from the epidemic febrile disease induced by the interior heat and who could not even eat rice gruel and decoctions. Since his fever was high, he could only drink a small amount of cold water. By the eleventh day, he had had no bowel movement for four days. Trembling with fear, he uttered in delirium, "This room is filled with many worms" or "A rat is dashing into my chest", and crawled around quickly and cried loudly. He sometimes had cold limbs and locked knees induced by the wind stirring syndrome in the case of high fever. At that time, he was given *Galgeun Seunggi Tang* orally and by force. He then began eating double the amount of rice gruel, and the epidemic symptoms were relieved. Fortunately, he survived. Until the fourth or fifth day after onset, the quality of his life, including diet and living conditions, was normal, so there was no difference between himself and a healthy person. Later, however, his condition worsened, and his disease was only relieved after seventeen days.

15 In the 『*Neijing*』[1], we read, "Most physical manifestations, like roughness, fleshlessness, wrinkles and chapness, are related to dryness."*

16 I have said, "When a greater yin person's face is bluish or whitish, he

---

* Note: This statement was taken from the 『*Suwen Xuanji Yuanbingshi*』 ("Profound Ideas and Etiology Based on Plain Questions", 素問玄機原病式), written by Liu Wansu (劉完素, about 1120-1200 A.D.).

generally does not exhibit dryness symptoms. However, if his face is yellowish, reddish or dark, he is generally displaying dryness symptoms. This is caused by the Liver heat and the Lung dryness. I once treated a greater yin person with dryness-heat symptoms such as burnt black colored fingers and gangrenous changes. His left middle finger became burnt black in color, and he lost strength. Within two years, he was bleeding black blood at the palm, and later, on the back of his hands. It ultimately became edematous, and his finger had to be cut off. Within a year, the gangrenous blotches, ranging in size from small to large coins, covered all his body. After three years of this, even in his youth, the patient could neither bear labour work nor walk 12 km per day. After taking 28 packs of *Yeolda Hanso Tang* with 7.5g of Rhizoma et Radix Ligustici and 3.75g of Radix et Rhizoma Rhei, his stool became loose. However, it hardened again a day or two later, so he took twenty packs more. His stool loosened slighly, the blotches on his face improved, and all four limbs grew stronger. I gave him twenty more packs, and his illness was almost cured."

17 In the 『*Lingshu*』, we read, "Two-yang bound is called diabetes. If a patient drinks one liter of water and urinates two liters, he will die."
It was commented, "Two-yang bound means the Heat binding of the stomach and large intestine."

18 In Bianque[2)]'s 『*Nanjing*』[3)], we read, "The pulse with diabetes is tense, forceful and rapid. On the other hand, those who have deep, uneven and weak pulses will die eventually."

19 Zhang Zhongjing said, "Diabetes induces copious urination such as drinking 18 liters causing 18 liters of urine. *Shenqi Wan* (Pill for invigorating Kidney qi) can be adopted."

20 I have said, "The above disease is not the diabetes of a lesser yang person, but the dryness-heat disease of a greater yin person. For this case, we should not adopt *Shenqi Wan*, but rather *Yeolda Hanso Tang* with Rhizoma et Radix Ligustici and Radix et Rhizoma Rhei."

21 I once treated a weak, fifty year old greater yin person who had dryness-heat disease. Since he displayed the symptoms of great thirst, copious urination and constipation, I gave him twenty packs of *Yeolda Hanso Tang* with 7.5g of Rhizoma et Radix Ligustici and 3.75g of Radix et Rhizoma Rhei. It was effective. More than one month later, the patient took five packs of another prescription, and his previous illness recurred. He further took fifty to sixty packs of *Yeolda Hanso Tang* with Rhizoma et Radix Ligustici and Radix et Rhizoma Rhei. He was at death's door throughout this period, and eventually died. I once treated another young greater yin person who had the dryness-heat disease. With three hundred packs of the above prescription, he survived with difficulty for one year, but eventually died. Since he had suffered from the disease for a year, I was not able to determine whether he had also been taking other medications. When the patient was struck with the dryness-heat disease, he generally drank one bowl of water and urinated two bowls of urine. If the disease becomes severe, the patient cannot be cured. Generally, a greater yin person with constipation, copious urination and thirstiness should be treated in the early stages to prevent a more serious condition.

22 The above disease is not a fatal one. One year after its onset and taking medical treatment, the young patient died. His illness was due to his severe Liver heat and Lung dryness, which resulted from his extreme indulgence in luxury and enjoyment. If the young patient had maintained a peaceful mind free of lust, he might have been cured by taking a hundred days' worth of medication; but because he continued harboring burning desires from the first day of his disease to the day he died, he did not survive. A proverb says, "The kindness of the ancestors cannot be fully repaid, while the kindness of respect shall be fully rewarded." Any patient who cultivates and respects his mind, quenches his desires, and maintains a virtuous mind will be cured within a hundred days; within two hundred days, he will be in perfect health. It is true for everything that the kindness of respect shall be indeed rewarded, much more so for diseases.

23 Wei Yilin said, "For the symptoms of yin blood exhaustion, such as deafness, visual difficulty, weakness in the legs, and lower back pains, it

is suitable to take *Heugwon Dan* (Black vitality pills)."

24 Insufficient genuine qi in the young adult male is not an acquired condition, but a congenital weakness. There are so many medications for nourishing and replenishing, but most of them are insufficient to show any desirable effectiveness. None but guarding congenital qi to make water rise and fire fall will promote the autonomous harmony among the five solid organs, and accordingly, the person will be free from disease. *Gongjin Dan* (Pills embracing fortune) is suitable for this case.

25 I have said, "For this case, one should adopt *Heugwon Dan* and *Gongjin Dan*. However, the potency of Radix Angelicae Sinensis and Fructus Corni in those prescriptions is insufficient. To get full strength, use *Gongjin Heugwon Dan* (Modified *Gongjin Dan* for black vitality) and *Nogyong Daibo Tang* (Decoction for major tonification with Cornu Cervi Pantotrichum)."

26 If a greater yin person displays such symptoms as a feeling of fullness in the abdomen after a meal, and weakness in the legs, *Gongjin Heugwon Dan*, *Nogyong Daibo Tang*, *Taieum Jowi Tang* and *Jowi Seungcheong Tang* (Decoction for elevating the clean yang through harmonizing the stomach) should be adopted.

27 A greater yin person may have diarrhea. For diarrhea caused by exterior cold, he should take *Taieum Jowi Tang*, while *Galgeun Naibokja Tang* (Decoction of Radix Puerariae and Semen Raphani) should be adopted in the case of diarrhea caused by exterior-heat.

28 A greater yin person may have a cough. *Taieum Jowi Tang*, *Nogyong Daibo Tang* and *Gongjin Heugwon Dan* should be adopted.

29 A greater yin person may have asthma, a very serious symptom. *Mahwang Jeongcheon Tang* (Decoction for relieving asthma with Herba Ephedrae) should be taken.

30 A greater yin person may have thoracoabdominal pain, a dangerous symptom. *Mahwang Jeongtong Tang* (Decoction for relieving pain with Herba Ephedrae) should be taken.

31 If a greater yin child has frequent diarrhea more than ten times, he certainly suffers from chronic infantile convulsions. He should take *Bopyewon Tang* (Decoction for invigorating Lung vitality) to prevent chronic infantile convulsions.

32 A greater yin person displaying symptoms of abdominal distension and edema–symptoms so fatal that nine out of ten greater yin persons die from it–should take *Geonyul Jejo Tang* (Decoction of dried chestnut and Holotrichia diomphalia Bates). Though treated with medicines, the patient is not successfully cured unless the disease does not recur within three years. The patient should refrain from indulgence in luxury and enjoyment, and calm both his body and mind. For three years, it solely depends on the patient to cultivate his mind and body and take care of himself through willpower. If a greater yin person does not receive medical treatment before he gets edema, he will die in nine out of ten cases. The disease is thus not a disease, but certain death. What should the patient do? In a greater yin person, exertion of the mind and mental stress from repeated failures, dysentery from chronic diarrhea or oliguria from gonorrhea, feelings of fullness in the upper abdomen after a meal, and weakness in the legs are often the cause of edema, a serious and dangerous illness in itself. Thus, we must regard these symptoms as indicative of edema. The patient should quench his lust, and cultivate and respect his mind before medical treatment can prove effective.

33 A greater yin person once had a serious case of spermatorrhea, three or four times a month. One day, suffering from constipation, he was made to take *Yeolda Hanso Tang* with 3.75g of Radix et Rhizoma Rhei. When a patient begins to have bowel movements every day, he should additionally take Os Draconis and a derivative of Radix et Rhizoma Rhei or *Gongjin Heugwon Dan* and *Nogyong Daibo Tang* can be adopted. This illness comes from too much anxiety and thinking.

34 Greater yin person can be fallen by a sudden stroke. If a patient's chest emits a "ge-ge" sound and stares blankly into space, he must be given *Gwache San* (Powder of Pedicellus Melo); if he has convulsions of the four

limbs and drooping eyes, he should take *Wuhwang Cheongsim Hwan* (Bolus for clearing the Heart with Calculcus Bovis). A patient with a dark, yellowish-reddish face generally tends to stare blankly into space, while one with bluish-whitish face tends to have droopy eyelids. If the latter begins to have convulsions of the four limbs, his condition may be termed dangerous; if not, he must quickly be given *Qingxin Wan* (Bolus for clearing the Heart). Ancient *Qingxin Wan* also has dramatic effects: if a patient has a sudden onset of staring eyes, he will die not long afterwards, while one who experiences a sudden onset of droopy eyelids will die in very little time. However, the patient with staring eyes also should begin medical treatment without any delay, or he shall die.

35 *Wuhwang Cheongsim Hwan* is not a common drug and is impossible for every family to acquire it. It is thus advisable to pour powdered Radix Polygalae and Rhizoma Acori Tatarinowii, 3.75g each, into the mouth and blow 0.75g of powdered Fructus Gleditsiae into the nose. When the patient has convulsions of the four limbs and a stiff neck, he is in a dangerous condition. Two men are needed either to hold the wrists of the patient to move the patient's shoulders from left to right, or to hold the patient's ankles to flex and extend the legs. Shaking the greater yin stroke patient's shoulders and legs will do him good, but one should not shake the shoulders and hands of lesser yang stroke patients. Neither should a patient be encouraged to sit up. This is acceptable for a lesser yin stroke patient, but his shoulders should not be shaken; rather, one should slowly massage his limbs.

36 Moschus is suitable to cure stroke and vomiting with diarrhea.

2-1

Four Prescriptions for the Greater Yin Person's Disease from Zhang Zhongjing's『*Shanghanlun*』

1 Decoction of Herba Ephedrae (*Mahuang Tang* 麻黃湯)

- Herba Ephedrae 11.25 g
- Rhizoma Zingiberis Recens 2.25 g
- Semen Armeniacae Amarum 3 slices
- Radix Glycyrrhizae 3.75 g
- Ramulus Cinnamomi 10 pcs.
- Fructus Jujubae 2 pcs.

2 Combination of half *Guizhi Tang* and half *Mahuang Tang* (*Guima Geban Tang* 桂麻各半湯)

- Herba Ephedrae 5.625 g
- Ramulus Cinnamomi 3.75 g
- Rhizoma Zingiberis Recens 3 slices
- Semen Armeniacae Amarum 3.75 g
- Radix Paeoniae Alba 3.75 g
- Radix Glycyrrhizae 2.625 g
- Fructus Jujubae 2 pcs.

3 Purgative decoction for harmonizing the stomach (*Tiaowei Chengqi Tang* 調胃承氣湯)

- Radix et Rhizoma Rhei 15 g
- Radix Glycyrrhizae 3.75 g
- Natrii Sulfas 7.5 g

4 Major decoction of Radix Bupleuri (*Da Chaihu Tang* 大柴胡湯)

· Radix Bupleuri	15 g	· Radix Scutellariae	9.375 g
· Radix Paeoniae Alba	9.375 g	· Radix et Rhizoma Rhei	7.5 g
· Fructus Aurantii Immaturus	5.625 g		

The above prescription treats the transmission of the lesser yang to the yang brightness disease with the symptoms of fever without chills, aversion to heat, constipation, reddish urine, delirium, abdominal distension and tidal fever.

2-2

Nine Prescriptions for the Greater Yin Person's Disease Mentioned in the Writings of Famous Doctors in the Tang, Song and Ming Dynasties

1 Powder of Rhizoma Acori Tatarinowii and Radix Polygalae

(*Shichangpu Yuanzhi San* 石菖蒲遠志散)

· Rhizoma Acori Tatarinowii · Radix Polygalae

Pound the above drugs into a powder and let the patient take 3.75g with liquor three times a day. The patient's eyes and ears will be refreshed.

The original source of this prescription is Sun Simiao's『*Qianjinfang*』.

2 Decoction for harmonizing the middle (*Tiaozhong Tang* 調中湯)

· Radix et Rhizoma Rhei	5.625 g	· Radix Scutellariae	3.75 g
· Radix Platycodi	3.75 g	· Radix Puerariae	3.75 g
· Radix Paeoniae Alba	3.75 g	· Poria (red)	3.75 g
· Rhizoma Ligustici	3.75 g	· Radix Glycyrrhizae	3.75 g
· Rhizoma Atractylodis Macrocephalae			3.75 g

This prescription cures epidemic diseases caused by dryness in the summer, with the symptoms such as dry mouth and choking sensation.

In accordance with the results of recent studies, Rhizoma Atractylodis Macrocephalae, Radix Paeoniae Alba, Poria and Radix Glycyrrhizae should be excluded from this prescription.

3 Black servant pills (*Heinu Wan* 黑奴丸)

· Herba Ephedrae	75 g	· Radix et Rhizoma Rhei	75 g
· Radix Scutellariae	37.5 g	· Cauldron soot	37.5 g
· Natrii Sulfas	37.5 g	· Furnace ash	37.5 g
· Dust (on the girder)	37.5 g	· Smutted ear of barley	37.5 g

Pound the above drugs into a powder and make pills as big as bullets, then take one pill with spring water. After a short bout of shivering and sweating, the patient will recover.

If, through mistaken treatment, a patient with macula caused by yang type inflammatory swelling or with a deteriorated case of acute febrile disease loses consciousness, he can still be treated on the condition that there is warmth in the epigastric region. Administer the above medicine through the mouth. The original source of above two prescriptions is Zhu Gong's 『*Huorenshu*』.

In accordance with the results of recent studies, Natrii Sulfas should be excluded.

4 Pulse-activating powder (*Shengmai San* 生脈散)

· Radix Ophiopogonis	7.5 g	· Radix Ginseng	3.75 g
· Fructus Schizandrae	3.75 g		

If patients drink this in summer instead of water boiled with burned rice, the prescription will give them energy.

In accordance with the results of recent studies, Radix Ginseng should be excluded from this prescription.

5 Cortex Ailanthi Pill (*Chugenpi Wan* 樗根皮丸)

· Cortex Ailanthi

Pound the above drug into a powder and make the pills with liquor and flour paste.

This prescription cures wet dreams. The property of this drug is cool and dry, so it cannot be used alone. The original source of the above two prescriptions is Li Chan's 『*Yixue Rumen*』.

6 Pills with two wonderful drugs saving from suffering

(*Ersheng Jiuku Wan* 二聖救苦丸)

· Radix et Rhizoma Rhei	150 g	· Fructus Gleditsiae	75 g

Pound the above drugs into a powder. Make 50 or 70 pills with flour paste as big as mung beans. One intake causes sweating, which leads to recovery.

The original source of this prescription is Gong Xin's compilation, 『*Wanbing Huichun*』; it cures seasonal epidemic disease.

7 Decoction for releasing the flesh with Radix Puerariae

(*Gegen Jieji Tang* 葛根解肌湯)

· Radix Puerariae	3.75 g	· Rhizoma Cimicifugae	3.75 g
· Radix Scutellariae	3.75 g	· Radix Platycodi	3.75 g
· Radix Bupleuri	3.75 g	· Radix Paeoniae Alba	3.75 g
· Gypsum Fibrosum	3.75 g	· Radix Glycyrrhizae	1.875 g
· Radix Angelicae Dahuricae			3.75 g
· Rhizoma seu Radix Notopterygii			3.75 g

This prescription cures the yang brightness disease with symptoms such as eye pain, dryness in the nasal cavity and insomnia.

In accordance with the results of recent studies, Radix Bupleuri, Radix Paeoniae, Rhizoma seu Radix Notopterygii, Gypsum Fibrosum and Radix Glycyrrhizae must be excluded from this prescription.

8 Bolus for clearing the Heart with Calculus Bovis

(*Niuhuang Qingxin Wan* 牛黃淸心丸)

· Rhizoma Dioscoreae	26.25 g	· Radix Ginseng	9.375 g
· Typhae Pollen	9.375 g	· Cornu Rhinoceri	7.5 g
· Cortex Cinnamomi	6.375 g	· Radix Paeoniae Alba	5.625 g
· Radix Ophiopogonis	5.625 g	· Radix Scutellariae	5.625 g
· Radix Saposhnikoviae	5.625 g	· Radix Bupleuri	4.875 g
· Radix Platycodi	4.875 g	· Poria (white)	4.875 g
· Rhizoma Chuanxiong	4.875 g	· Calculus Bovis	4.5 g
· Cornu Saigae Tataricae	3.75 g	· Borneolum	3.75 g
· Moschus	3.75 g	· Realgar	3 g

· Radix Ampelopsis 2.625 g · Gold sheets 140 pcs.
· Radix Glycyrrhizae (stir-baked) 18.75 g
· Massa Fermentata Medicinalis 9.375 g
· Dried soybean sprouts (stir-baked) 6.375 g
· Colla Corii Asini (stir-baked) 6.375 g
· Rhizoma Atractylodis Macrocephalae 5.625 g
· Cinnabaris (to refine powder with water) 5.625 g
· Semen Armeniacae Amarum 4.875 g
· Rhizoma Zingiberis (stir-baked at high temperature) 2.625 g

Forty of the 140 sheets are used to wrap the pills. Steam twenty pieces of Fructus Jujubae and remove the seeds. Puree the Fructus Jujubae into a paste and mix in there maining pulverized drugs. Add honey and mix thoroughly, from 37.5g of the mixture, make ten pills. Wrap each pill in a thin sheet of gold. Take one pill for each dose with warm water.

This prescription cures stroke, loss of consciousness, accumulation of phlegm, aphagia, wry mouth with distortion of the eye and the paralysis of limbs. The original source of the above two prescriptions is 『*Yijian*』 compiled by Gong Xin.

In accordance with the results of recent studies, Rhizoma Atractylodis Macrocephalae, Radix Ginseng, Radix Glycyrrhizae, Massa Fermentata Medicinalis, Cortex Cinnamomi, Colla Corii Asini, Radix Paeoniae Alba, Radix Angelicae Sinensis, Rhizoma Chuanxiong, Rhizoma Zingiberis, Fructus Jujubae, Radix Bupleuri, Poria, Realgar and Cinnabaris must be excluded from this prescription.

9 Decoction for relieving asthma with Herba Ephedrae

(*Mahuang Dingchuan Tang* 麻黃定喘湯)

· Herba Ephedrae 11.25 g · Radix Scutellariae 3.75 g
· Rhizoma Pinelliae 3.75 g · Cortex Mori 3.75 g
· Fructus Perillae 3.75 g · Flos Farfarae 3.75 g
· Radix Glycyrrhizae 3.75 g
· Semen Armeniacae Amarum 5.625 g
· Semen Ginkgo (remove the cortex, pound and stir-baked it) 21 pcs.

The Huangsege ("Yellow Song") says, "Every disease has its cure." It is most difficult to cure snoring and asthma. There once was a patient who happened upon a medicine, and after taking it, was cured. He then realized the medicine was *Dingchuan Tang* (定喘湯). The original source of this prescription is Gong Xin's compilation, 『*Wanbing Huichun*』. This cures asthma miraculously.

In accordance with the results of recent studies, Rhizoma Pinelliae, Fructus Perillae and Radix Glycyrrhizae should be excluded from this prescription.

2-3

Twenty Four Important Newly Formulated Prescriptions for the Greater Yin Person's Disease

1 Decoction for harmonizing the stomach in a greater yin person

(*Taieum Jowi Tang* : *Taiyin Tiaowei Tang* 太陰調胃湯)

· Semen Coicis	11.25 g	· Chestnut (dried)	11.25 g
· Semen Raphani	7.5 g	· Fructus Schizandrae	3.75 g
· Radix Ophiopogonis	3.75 g	· Radix Platycodi	3.75 g
· Rhizoma Acori Graminei	3.75 g	· Herba Ephedrae	3.75 g

2 Decoction for releasing the flesh with Radix Puerariae

(*Galgeun Haigi Tang* : *Gegen Jieji Tang* 葛根解肌湯)

· Radix Puerariae	11.25 g	· Radix Scutellariae	5.625 g
· Rhizoma Ligustici	5.625 g	· Radix Platycodi	3.75 g
· Radix Angelicae Dahuricae	3.75 g	· Rhizoma Cimicifugae	3.75 g

3 Decoction for elevating the clean yang through harmonizing the stomach

(*Jowi Seungcheong Tang* : *Tiaowei Shengqing Tang* 調胃升清湯)

· Semen Coicis	11.25 g	· Chestnut (dried)	11.25 g
· Semen Raphani	5.625 g	· Herba Ephedrae	3.75 g
· Radix Platycodi	3.75 g	· Radix Ophiopogonis	3.75 g
· Fructus Schizandrae	3.75 g	· Radix Polygalae	3.75 g

· Rhizoma Acori Graminei	3.75 g	· Radix Asparagi	3.75 g
· Semen Ziziphi Spinosae	3.75 g	· Arillus Longan	3.75 g

4 Decoction of Semen Nelumbinis for clearing the Heart

(*Cheongsim Yeonja Tang*: *Qingxin Lianzi Tang* 淸心蓮子湯)

· Semen Nelumbinis	7.5 g	· Rhizoma Dioscoreae	7.5 g
· Radix Ophiopogonis	3.75 g	· Radix Asparagi	3.75 g
· Radix Polygalae	3.75 g	· Arillus Longan	3.75 g
· Semen Platycladi	3.75 g	· Radix Scutellariae	3.75 g
· Semen Ziziphi Spinosae	3.75 g	· Flos Chrysanthemi	1.125 g
· Rhizoma Acori Graminei	3.75 g	· Semen Raphani	3.75 g

5 Decoction for relieving asthma with Herba Ephedrae

(*Mahwang Jeongcheon Tang*: *Mahuang Dingchuan Tang* 麻黃定喘湯)

· Herba Ephedrae	11.25 g	· Radix Scutellariae	3.75 g
· Semen Raphani	3.75 g	· Cortex Mori	3.75 g
· Radix Platycodi	3.75 g	· Radix Ophiopogonis	3.75 g
· Flos Farfarae			3.75 g
· Semen Armeniacae Amarum			5.625 g
· Semen Ginkgo (stir-baked to yellow)			21 pcs.

6 Decoction for relieving pain with Herba Ephedrae

(*Mahwang Jeongtong Tang*: *Mahuang Dingtong Tang* 麻黃定痛湯)

· Semen Coicis	11.25 g	· Herba Ephedrae	7.5 g
· Semen Raphani	7.55 g	· Radix Platycodi	3.75 g
· Rhizoma Acori Graminei	3.75 g	· Radix Ophiopogonis	3.75 g
· Fructus Schizandrae	3.75 g	· Fructus Quisqualis	3.75 g
· Arillus Longan	3.75 g	· Semen Platycladi	3.75 g
· Chestnut (dried)			7 pcs.
· Semen Armeniacae Amarum			3.75 g

7 Decoction for treating more fever than cold

(*Yeolda Hanso Tang* : *Reduo Hanshao Tang* 熱多寒少湯)

- Radix Puerariae 15 g
- Rhizoma Ligustici 7.5 g
- Rhizoma Cimicifugae 3.75 g
- Radix Scutellariae 7.5 g
- Semen Raphani 3.75 g
- Radix Platycodi 3.75 g
- Radix Angelicae Dahuricae 3.75 g

8 Decoction for treating more cold than fever

(*Handa Yeolso Tang* : *Handuo Reshao Tang* 寒多熱少湯)

- Semen Coicis 11.25 g
- Radix Ophiopogonis 3.75 g
- Radix Scutellariae 3.75 g
- Semen Raphani 7.5 g
- Radix Platycodi 3.75 g
- Herba Ephedrae 3.75 g
- Chestnut (dried) 7 pcs.
- Semen Armeniacae Amarum 3.75 g

9 Decoction for purgation with Radix Puerariae

(*Galgeun Seunggi Tang* : *Gegen Chengqi Tang* 葛根承氣湯)

- Radix Puerariae 15 g
- Radix et Rhizoma Rhei 7.5 g
- Radix Angelicae Dahuricae 3.75 g
- Radix Scutellariae 7.5 g
- Rhizoma Cimicifugae 3.75 g
- Radix Platycodi 3.75 g

10 Decoction for regulating Lung vitality

(*Jori Pyewon Tang* : *Tiaoli Feiyuan Tang* 調理肺元湯)

- Radix Ophiopogonis 7.5 g
- Semen Coicis 7.5 g
- Herba Ephedrae 3.75 g
- Radix Platycodi 7.5 g
- Radix Scutellariae 3.75 g
- Semen Raphani 3.75 g

11 Decoction for diaphoresis with Herba Ephedrae

(*Mahwang Balpyo Tang* : *Mahuang Fabiao Tang* 麻黃發表湯)

- Radix Platycodi 11.25 g
- Herba Ephedrae 5.625 g

· Radix Ophiopogonis 3.75 g · Radix Scutellariae 3.75 g
· Semen Armeniacae Amarum 3.75 g

12 Decoction for invigorating Lung vitality

(*Bopyewon Tang*: *Bufeiyuan Tang* 補肺元湯)

· Radix Ophiopogonis 11.25 g · Radix Platycodi 7.5 g
· Fructus Schizandrae 3.75 g

If *3.75g* each of Rhizoma Dioscoreae, Semen Coicis and Semen Raphani are added to the above, the results will be more effective.

13 Decoction for major tonification with Cornu Cervi Pantotrichum

(*Nogyong Daibo Tang*: *Lurong Dabu Tang* 鹿茸大補湯)

· Radix Ophiopogonis 5.625 g · Semen Coicis 5.625 g
· Rhizoma Dioscoreae 3.75 g · Radix Asparagi 3.75 g
· Fructus Schizandrae 3.75 g · Herba Ephedrae 3.75 g
· Semen Armeniacae Amarum 3.75 g
· Cornu Cervi Pantotrichum 7.5g, 11.25g or 15 g

This prescription cures weak patients displaying exterior symptoms and cold syndromes.

14 Modified *Gongchen Dan* for black vitality

(*Gongjin Heugwon Dan*: *Gongchen Heiyuan Dan* 拱辰黑元丹)

· Rhizoma Dioscoreae 150 g · Radix Asparagi 150 g
· Moschus 18.75 g
· Holotrichia diomphalia Bates 37.5~75 g
· Cornu Cervi Pantotrichum 150g, 187.5g or 225 g

Boil the flesh of Fructus Mume and puree into a soft paste. Together with the other pulverized drugs, make the pills as big as the seed of an empress tree. Take 50~70 pills for each dose with warm water or liquor. This cures the weak patient who has interior symptom.

15 Decoction of Fructus Gleditsiae and Radix et Rhizoma Rhei

(*Jogak Daihwang Tang* : *Zaojiao Dahuang Tang* 皂角大黃湯)

· Rhizoma Cimicifugae	11.75 g	· Radix Puerariae	11.75 g
· Radix et Rhizoma Rhei	3.75 g	· Fructus Gleditsiae	3.75 g

Do not use this medicine over three or four packs. Since 11.25g of Rhizoma Cimicifugae, Radix et Rhizoma Rhei and Fructus Gleditsiae are included, the potency of this drug is extremely strong.

16 Decoction of Radix Puerariae and Herba Spirodelae

(*Galgeun Bupyeong Tang* : *Gegen Fuping Tang* 葛根浮萍湯)

· Radix Puerariae	11.75 g	· Semen Raphani	7.5 g
· Radix Scutellariae	7.5 g	· Herba Spirodelae	3.75 g
· Radix et Rhizoma Rhei			3.75 g
· Holotrichia diomphalia Bates			10 pcs.

This prescription cures edema and the interior symptoms with more fever than chills.

17 Decoction of dried chestnut and Holotrichia diomphalia Bates

(*Geonyul Jejo Tang* : *Ganli Qicao Tang* 乾栗蠐螬湯)

· Chestnut (dried)	100 pcs.
· Holotrichia diomphalia Bates	100 pcs.

Take these as a decoction or stir-bake them with an adjuvant. Pound ten dried chestnuts and ten Holotrichia diomphalia Bates into a powder. Take the above medicine with the decoction of dried chestnuts.

This prescription cures edema and the exterior symptoms with more chills than fever.

18 Decoction of dried chestnut and Cortex Ailanthi

(*Geonyul Jeogeunpi Tang* : *Ganli Chugenpi Tang* 乾栗樗根皮湯)

· Chestnut (dried)	37.5 g	· Cortex Ailanthi	11.25~18.75 g

This prescription cures dysentery. Take this as a decoction or pills. In the pill form, it is taken only with 18.5g of Cortex Ailanthi.

19 Melo Pedicellus powder (*Gwache San*: *Guadi San* 瓜蒂散)

· Melo Pedicellus (stir-baked to yellow)

Pound the above drug into a powder of 1.125 or 1.875g. Take it with warm water or take a quickly prepared decoction of dried Melo Pedicellus, 3.75g.

This prescription cures stroke. Patients with congested sounds emanating from the chest and blankly staring into space absolutely require this medicine. This medicine must be used on patients who have this disease and display symptoms like it, but it must not be used on those who have another disease or exhibit different symptoms. It most certainly cannot be used on patients with abdominal and chest pains, or cough and asthma due to cold. It is also forbidden to use it on patients with indigestion. In these cases, other medicines have to be used.

Stroke patients with a pale complexion and the exterior deficiency syndrome of the cold type require *Wungdam San (Xiongdan San)*, *Wuhwang Cheongsim Hwan (Niuhuang Qingxin Wan)* and *Seokchangpo Wonji San (Shichangpu Yuanzhi San)*, but not *Gwache San*.

20 Fel Ursi powder (*Wungdam San* : *Xiongdan San* 熊膽散)

· Fel Ursi 1.125~1.875 g

This prescription should be taken with warm water.

21 Moschus powder (*Sahyang San* : *Shexiang San* 麝香散)

· Moschus 1.125~1.875 g

This prescription should be taken with warm water or warm liquor.

22 Powder of Rhizoma Acori Graminei and Radix Polygalae

(*Seokchangpo Wonji San*: *Shichangpu Yuanzhi San* 石菖蒲遠志散)

· Radix Polygalae (powder)	37.5 g
· Spina Gleditsiae (powder)	1.125 g
· Rhizoma Acori Graminei (powder)	3.75 g

This prescription should be taken with warm water. Another way is to take the powder of Radix Polygalae and Rhizoma Acori Graminei with warm water and breathe the powder of Spina Gleditsiae into the nasal cavity.

23 Powder of Radix Ophiopogonis and Radix Polygalae

(*Maigmundong Wonji San*: *Maimendong Yuanzhi San* 麥門冬遠志散)

· Radix Ophiopogonis	11.25 g	· Radix Polygalae	3.75 g
· Rhizoma Acori Graminei	3.75 g	· Fructus Schizandrae	1.875 g

24 Bolus for clearing the Heart with Calculus Bovis

(*Wuhwang Cheongsim Hwan*: *Niuhuang Qingxin Yuan* 牛黃淸心元)

· Rhizoma Dioscoreae	26.25 g	· Cornu Rhinoceri	7.5 g
· Radix Ophiopogonis	5.625 g	· Radix Scutellariae	5.625 g
· Radix Platycodi	4.875 g	· Calculus Bovis	4.5 g
· Cornu Saigae Tataricae	3.75 g	· Borneolum	3.75 g
· Radix Ampelopsis	2.625 g	· Moschus	3.75 g
· Gold			70 sheets
· Pollen Typhae (stir-baked)			9.375 g
· Dried soybean sprouts (stir-baked)			6.375 g
· Semen Armeniacae Amarum			4.875 g

Twenty sheets of gold are used to wrap the pills. Make a soft extract of twenty Fructus Mume, steamed and pared. Pound the above drugs into a powder, knead it with the soft extract of the Fructus Mume and, from 37.5g of the mixture, make twenty pills wrapped in thin sheets of gold. Take one pill for each dose with warm water.

The drugs for the greater yin person are Semen Armeniacae Amarum (remove the twinned seed and the husk), Radix Ophiopogonis, Radix Polygalae (remove the core), Semen Ginkgo (remove the horn), chestnut (remove the horn), Radix et Rhizoma Rhei (steamed with liquor or crude),

Cornu Cervi Pantotrichum (stir-baked with vinegar), Spina Gleditsiae (stir-baked with vinegar), Semen Ziziphi Spinosae (stir-baked), Semen Armeniacae Amarum (stir-baked) and Semen Ginkgo (stir-baked).

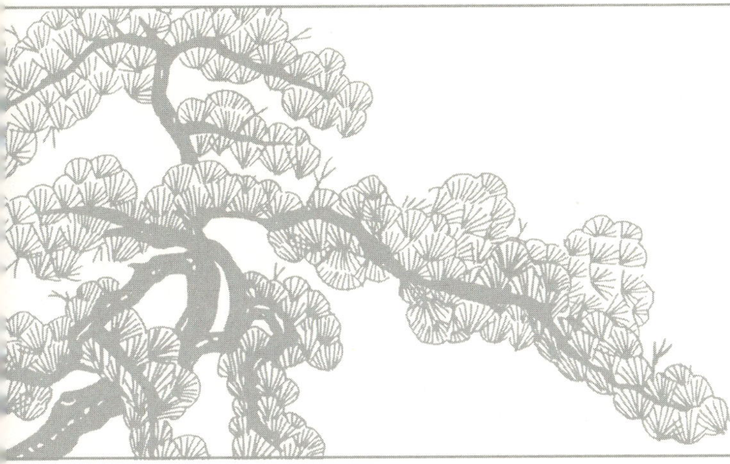

PART / V

1

Discourse on the Taiyang (Greater Yang) Person's Lumbar Vertebrae Disease Induced by Exopathogen*

1 In the 『*Neijing*』, we read, "Moderate and uneven *chi* (cubit) pulses are the manifestations of *jieyi* (generalized fatigue and lassitude)."

As a comment on this sentence, "Since a *chi* pulse manifests itself in the yin portion, it is dominated by the Liver and Kidney. Since a moderate pulse manifests itself as heat affects the middle-*jiao*, and an uneven pulse manifests itself as blood exhaustion, this condition is called generalized fatigue and lassitude. Since the symptoms of generalized fatigue and lassitude are neither chilly nor febrile, or weak nor strong, it cannot be identified exactly and is called generalized fatigue and lassitude."

2 In the 『*Lingshu*』, it is said, "If a disease in the spinal cord develops, the patient's cord deteriorates, then his shins ache and his body is generally fatigued and cannot go." "Cannot go." means that the patient is unable to walk.

3 I have said, "The above symptoms belong to the quite serious lumbar vertebrae disease of the greater yang person. The patient should refrain from feeling deep sorrow and anger, and secure peace of his mind; then the disease can be cured. For this disease, *Ogapi Jangcheok Tang* (Decoction for

* 太陽人外感腰脊病論

strengthening spine with Cortex Acanthopanacis) should be adopted."

4 The patient with generalized fatigue and lassitude is perfectly healthy in the upper part of the body, but experiences fatigue in the lower part of the body, so that he is unable to walk. Yet, his feet do not have the symptoms of palsy or swelling with pain, and his feet are not so weak. Since his physical condition is neither weak nor strong, neither cold nor heat, the disease belongs to the lumbar vertebrae disease. The generalized fatigue and lassitude patient does not have the symptoms of severe chills with fever and aching of the body. If a greater yang patient displays the symptoms of severe chills with fever and aching of the body, it is because his lumbar vertebrae are rich in exterior qi. The disease can easily be cured, and the patient made healthy again.

2

Discourse on the Greater Yang Person's Small Intestine Disease Induced by Endopathogen*

1 Zhu Zhenheng said, "*Yege* (Dysphagia) and *fanwei* (regurgitation of food from the stomach) are induced by the exhaustion of blood and fluid. This exhaustion causes a dry esophagus. If the upper part of the esophagus near the throat grows dry, the patient will most likely only be able to drink, not eat. If he is able to swallow food at all, it will only be in small amounts. This symptom is called *ye*. If the lower part of the esophagus near the stomach grows dry, the patient will be able to ingest food, but the food will not reach or stay in the stomach and be regurgitated. This symptom is called *ge* or regurgitation of food from the stomach. The patient also has constipation with dried fecal masses like goat's dung. Though their terms are different, their pathogenic factor is the same." Zhu Zhenheng also said, "Dysphagia of the upper-*jiao* shows pain in the epigastric region after food is taken. The patient regurgitates the food promptly, and the pain disappears. For dysphagia of the middle-*jiao*, though the food can be swallowed, it cannot enter the stomach and vomiting is delayed. Dysphagia of the lower-*jiao* shows vomiting in the afternoon what was taken in the morning, and vomiting in the morning of what was taken in the previous afternoon. Patients with deficiency of both qi and blood may foam at the mouth; and those who foam heavily at

---

* 太陽人内觸小腸病論

the mouth will die. A patient with dried fecal masses like goat's dung is hard to cure. He who does not take light food is also hard to cure."

2 Zhang Jihfeng[1)] said, "*Ye* may stem from mental problems. Inward contemplation and self-cultivation can cure it."

3 In Gong Xin's 『(*Gujin*) *Yijian*』, we read, "Regurgitation of food from the stomach, *ge* and *ye* have the same pathogenic factor. The symptoms of dysphagia do not belong to a deficiency or an excess, cold or heat; but it is one of the diseases related to spiritual qi."

4 I have said, "This is the most serious case among the small intestine diseases in greater yang persons. Only patients who avoid anger and eat plain food can be cured. We should apply *Mihudeung Sikjang Tang* (Decoction for planting intestine with Caulis Actinidiae Chinensis)."

5 The difficulty some people experience in swallowing food is called *ye*, while the difficulty some people experience in keeping food down is called *ge*. When a patient regurgitates in the afternoon what was taken in the morning, or regurgitates in the morning what was taken in the previous afternoon, his condition is called regurgitation of food from the stomach. However, when a patient regurgitates in the afternoon what was taken in the morning and regurgitates in the morning what was taken in the previous afternoon, not all the food comes up. When a patient spontaneously regurgitates in the morning what was taken in the previous afternoon, his illness is an obstruction located in the upper part of the stomach. Those symptoms are called regurgitation of food from the stomach or dysphagia. Generally, dysphagia is dysphagia in the esophageal region, and regurgitation of food from the stomach is dysphagia in the gastric region. In other words, they are the same disease. Inevitably, the patient with dysphagia does not have symptoms such as abdominal pain, borborygmus, diarrhea and dysentery. If the greater yang person has symptoms of abdominal pain, borborygmus, diarrhea and dysentery, it means that his interior qi of the small intestine is rich, making the disease easy to cure.

6 Though both generalized fatigue and lassitude, and the dysphagia are serious symptoms, their relative seriousness can be identified. Generalized fatigue and lassitude without dysphagia is a mild type of generalized fatigue and lassitude. Dysphagia without dysphagia is mild type of dysphagia. A combination of generalized fatigue and lassitude and dysphagia represents a serious and dangerous condition; but among serious and dangerous conditions, there is also a relative seriousness. Since the quality of life of a greater yang patient with generalized fatigue and lassitude and dysphagia seems normal until he is practically at death's door, we are apt to treat him as a common case. Therefore, once his condition reaches the serious stage, it becomes very hard to cure him. Since I am possessed of a greater yang constitution, I once had this disease. I vomited foamy saliva from the mouth for six to seven years, and afterwards continuously paid attention to my health for several decades in order to avoid dying young. I thus report my case in order to alert all greater yang patients with the same disease. The advisable treatment, in one sentence, is "Just avoid anger."

7 The greater yang person originally has a strong will and weak integrity. Since the strong will induces the qi of the esophagus to flow upward, and that qi which exhales and disperses becomes too great and overflows, and since weak integrity induces the qi of the small intestine to be stuck in the middle-*jiao*, and that qi which inhales and concentrates becomes exhausted and deficient, diseases such as dysphagia and regurgitation of food from the stomach are generated.

8 Someone once asked me, "Zhu Zhenheng said, 'Dysphagia and regurgitation of food from the stomach are induced by the exhaustion of blood and fluid which causes a dry esophagus, and such a patient is unable to swallow food.' What is your opinion on the subject?" I answered, "When food enters the stomach, the Spleen works with the stomach; when the food is sent to the large intestine, the Kidney works with the large intestine. So the Spleen and the Kidney are the storerooms, which promote the coming and going of food, and supplement and drain by turns. When the air and the fluid are exhaled from the epigastrium, the

Lung works with it, and when the air and the fluid are inhaled by the small intestine, the Liver works with it. So the Lung and the Liver are the gates that promote the respiration of air and fluid, and act back and forth by turns. Therefore, if the power of the lesser yang person's large intestine, which expels the yin cold qi of food, is insufficient, the yang hot qi of food inside the stomach will inevitably prosper. If the power of the greater yang person's small intestine, which absorbs the yin cool qi of air and fluid, is insufficient, the yang warm qi of air and fluid in the epigastrium will inevitably prosper. If the yang warm qi of air and fluid in the epigastrium is too prosperous, the blood in the epigastric part will dry up. This is quite natural; however, the causes of the above diseases are not limited to dryness, but also include a strong, upwardly exhaling qi and weak, inhaling qi in the middle-*jiao*. The result is an inability to swallow food and vomiting"

9 Someone once asked me, "How do you know that the dysphagia and regurgitation of food from the stomach mentioned by Zhu Zhenheng do not belong to the disease of the lesser yin, lesser yang, or greater yin person, and how did you conclude that they were, in fact, diseases of the greater yang person? Also, how do you know that the dysphagia mentioned in the 『*Neijing*』 does not belong to the disease of the lesser yin, lesser yang or greater yin person, and how did you conclude that it was, in fact, a disease of the greater yang person? Your conclusions are difficult to believe; please explain your position." I answered, "The vomiting of a lesser yang person must be induced by severe heat. The vomiting of a lesser yin person must be induced by severe cold. The vomiting of a greater yin person certainly brings about the release from the disease. However, dysphagia and regurgitation of food from the stomach are not manifest in cold or heat, deficiency or excess. Is it not, therefore, logical to conclude that those are the diseases of the greater yang person? The generalized fatigue and lassitude is the disease in which the patient's upper body is normally healthy, while his lower body suffers from fatigue. His shins ache, and he cannot walk. If a lesser yin, lesser yang or greater yin person has this disease; it must be in combination

with other symptoms. There is no reason to have just fatigue without cold or heat, or deficiency or excess."

10 Someone once asked me, "You have mentioned that the treatment for a greater yang person's generalized fatigue and lassitude was to refrain from feeling deep sorrow and sudden anger, and to secure peace of mind. You also mentioned that the treatment of a greater yang person's dysphagia was to avoid anger and eat plain food. I understand that generalized fatigue and lassitude is more serious than dysphagia in a greater yang person. Does this mean that, in a greater yang person, the disease induced by sorrow is more serious than the disease induced by anger?" I answered, "No. On the contrary, since dysphagia is far more serious than generalized fatigue and lassitude in a greater yang person, the damage caused by anger is more serious than that by sorrow in a greater yang person. Deepening sorrow in a greater yang person injures the exterior qi, and exploding anger injures the interior qi. Since the generalized fatigue and lassitude is an exterior disease, I advise patients to refrain from feeling deep sorrow and anger at the same time." I was asked again, "Then the angry nature of a lesser yang person injures the qi of the mouth and the bladder, and his sorrow injures the qi of the Kidney and the large intestine. The joyous nature of a lesser yin person injures the qi of the eyes and the paravertebral musculature of the back, and pleasure injures the qi of the Spleen and stomach. A greater yin person's feelings of pleasure injure the qi of the ears and the nape of the neck, and joy emotion injures the qi of the Lung and the epigastrium. Is that correct?" I replied, "Yes."

11 The stool of greater yang people should be first, smooth, and, second, large in its shape and quantity. Their urine should be first, copious, and next, frequent. Their complexion should be pale, not dark. Their flesh should be thin, not fatty. There should be no hard mass in the pit of the stomach. If the mass is small, it can be easily extinguished; if it is large, the disease will become serious, and the mass will prove difficult to reduce.

2-1

Ten Recommended Herbs for the Greater Yang Person's Disease (Mentioned in the "Materia Medica") Based on My Experiences, and Two Herbs Based on the Experiences of Li Chan and Gong Xin

1 In the "Materia Medica", we read that Cortex Acanthopanacis cures the arthralgia of the lower limbs, contraction of the near joints, flaccidity and lameness. There once was a crippled three year old child, who, after taking this herb, was able to walk again.

- Pine knots cure flaccidity of the lower limbs.
- Fructus Chaenomelis stops vomiting. To drink its decoction or its freshly squeezed juice is best.
- Grape roots stop hiccups. To drink the decoction in high concentration is best.
- Fructus Actinidiae cures regurgitation of food from the stomach due to the blockage of heat. Drink the sap. The vine's sap is a great lubricant, and controls the blockage of the stomach, which induces vomiting. It is very good to drink its decoction.
- Rhizoma Phragmitis cures retching and five kinds of dysphagia with dysphoria. Take a 1.804 liter decoction of Rhizoma Phragmitis 187.5g at a draught. The patient shall recover by the time he has ingested 5.6 liters.
- Shells (Solen gouldii) cure regurgitation and vomiting.
- Crucian cures regurgitation.
- Water shieleds (Bracenia Schreberi) is cooked with crucian and made into a soup. This cures regurgitation and the inability to swallow, and stops vomiting.
- Buckwheat reinforces the intestine and stomach, and invigorates the primordial qi.

2 Li Chan said that bran (on the pestle) cures dysphagia, the inability to swallow and obstructed throats. Pound the above drug into a powder and take it with rice gruel.

3 Gong Xin said that shells cure regurgitation.

2-2

Two Newly Formulated Prescriptions Applicable to the Greater Yang Person's Disease

1 Decoction for strengthening spine with Cortex Acanthopanacis

(*Ogapi Jangcheok Tang* : *Wujiapi Zhuangji Tang* 五加皮壯脊湯)

· Cortex Acanthopanacis	15 g	· Fructus Chaenomelis	7.5 g
· Green pine knot	7.5 g	· Grape root	3.75 g
· Rhizoma Phragmitis	3.75 g	· Semen Pruni	3.75 g
· Buckwheat	half of a spoon		

If no green pine knots can be found, the newborn sprout of a pine can be used instead. This prescription cures the exterior syndrome.

2 Decoction for planting intestine with Caulis Actinidiae Chinensis

(*Mihudeung Sikjang Tang* : *Mihouteng Zhichang Tang* 獼猴藤植腸湯)

· Caulis Actinidiae Chinensis	15 g	· Fructus Chaenomelis	7.5 g
· Grape root	7.5 g	· Rhizoma Phragmitis	3.75 g
· Semen Pruni	3.75 g	· Cortex Acanthopanacis	3.75 g
· Bran (on the pestle)	half of a spoon	· Pine flower	3.75 g

If there is no Caulis Actinidiae Chinensis, its vine can be used instead.

This prescription cures the interior syndrome.

Generally, fruits and vegetables have a clear and plain taste, so they belong to the medicinal ingredient for the Liver. Shells also have a medicine value for the Liver; specifically, they invigorate it.

I have said, "People lack experience with these drugs because they have little experience treating these diseases. Greater yang people are so few in number that descriptions of greater yang people's diseases and of the drugs used for treatment are rare. *Ogapi Jangcheok Tang* and *Mihudeung Sikjang Tang* are simple and not at all satisfactory. If, however, a greater yang person contracts a disease, and we are able to create a new prescription based on the principles of those two drugs, why should we worry about the scarcity of available prescriptions?"

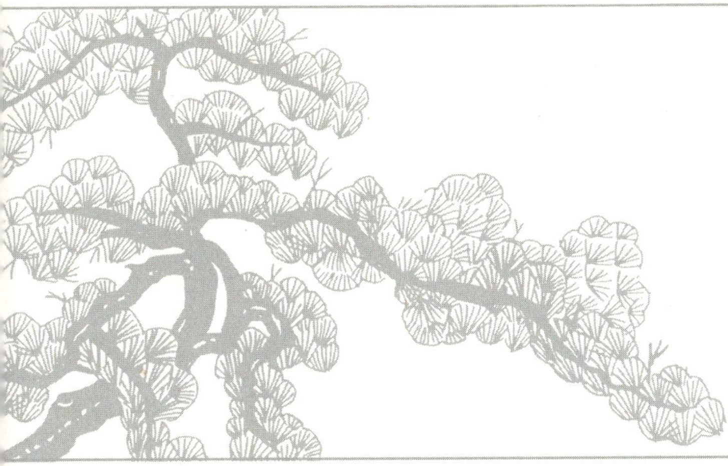

PART / VI

1

Discourse on General Health Maintenance*

1 The period from the age of 1 to 16 is called childhood; from 17 to 32, young adulthood; from 33 to 48, prime of adulthood; and from 49 to 64, old age.

2 Children, like new spring buds, long for knowledge and information, and love and respect others. Young adults esteem bravery and daring, and flourish and shoot up swiftly, like the young trees of summer. Adults enjoy making friends and allowing life to ripen, like the fruits of autumn. The elderly prefer orderliness, and can keep secrets, like the roots of winter.

3 The child who likes to study is the most admired among children; the young adult who respects the aged is the most admired among young adults; the adult who can love others broadly is the most admired among adults; and the elderly person who protects and encourages the righteous is the most admired among old people. He who has genuine abilities and, moreover, a good heart is the real hero. There are, however, people who are possessed of genuine abilities, but lack a good heart.

---

* 廣濟說

4 Before the age of seven or eight, the child may become ill when constrained by the four emotions–joy, anger, sorrow and pleasure–due to a lack of information and knowledge. The affectionate mother should take care of such a child. Before the age of 24 or 25, the young adult may become ill when he is constrained by the four emotions–joy, anger, sorrow and pleasure–due to a lack of bravery and daring. The wise father and able brother should take care of him. Concerning a man before the age of 38 or 39, he should be helped by a sensible younger brother and his good friends. Concerning a man before the age of 56 or 57, he should be encouraged by his dutiful sons and grandsons.

5 The good man, who is admirable, attracts good people to his house, while the bad man, who is disreputable, attracts bad people to his house. When many good people gather together, their qi is activated. When many bad people gather together, their qi is aroused. A house where bad men have gathered to engage in drink, sensual pleasures, and the pursuit of wealth and power can easily make dutiful sons and wives ill.

6 In a house where people hunger for power, factions are created, and it is these factions that destroy the house. In a house where people hunger for wealth, sons become haughty and stupid, and it is they who eventually destroy the house.

7 In a house where all work ends in vain, illness remains constant, and good and evil are struggling with each other, collapse is certain. In such circumstances, only the wise and affectionate father and dutiful son have the means to solve this problem.

8 Overindulgence in luxury can decrease one's life span. Laziness can decrease one's life span. Prejudice can decrease one's life span. Greediness can decrease one's life span. The overindulgent man will surely abandon himself to sensual pleasures. The lazy man will surely give himself up to drinking. The prejudiced man will surely fight for power. The greedy man will surely die for the pursuit of money.

9 Simplicity allows one to live one's natural life span. Diligence allows one

to live one's natural life span. Self-control allows one to live one's natural life span. Integrity allows one to live one's natural life span. The simple man avoids sensual pleasures. The diligent man avoids drinking. The deliberate man avoids pursuing power. The man with integrity avoids pursuing wealth.

10 Overindulgence makes one's living quarters dreary. Overdrinking makes one's behavior clumsy. Fighting for power makes one's mind anguished. Pursuing wealth creates disorder in appointed roles.

11 When a man respects the gentle woman, sensual pleasure can be enjoyed in the right way. When a man loves his good friends, drinking together can lead to virtue. When a man respects the wise man, his pursuit of power can lead to the proper course of action. When a man cares for the poor, his wealth is put to proper use.

12 These four pursuits-overdrinking, sensual pleasures, wealth and power-from ancient times were compared to the constraints of four walls, and to a jail. Not only a man's longevity or a family's fortune, but also the maintenance of society, depends upon refraining from these four vices. Therefore, if we allow society to fall into the trap of these four vices, we will revert to the troubled eras of Yao, Shun, and the Southern States of Zhou and Shao.

13 Generally, a man has to pursue simplicity, diligence, self-control and integrity. If someone has these four, he automatically can enjoy his full life span. If he is possessed of simplicity, diligence and self-control, or integrity, self-control and diligence, his life span will be shorter than who has all four qualities. More examples of people are those who are both overindulgent in luxury and yet diligent, or self-controlled and yet greedy, or simple and yet lazy, or prejudiced and yet honest. If they are cautious, then they may enjoy a long life. If they are neglectful, however, they will die young.

14 Generally, a cautious man will live long, a neglectful man will die young, a diligent man will live long, and a greedy man will die young. If a

hungry man, upon receiving food, eats it hastily, the qi of his intestines will be disturbed. When a poor man suddenly gets money, his life will be disturbed. Even though a man is hungry, if he is content, the qi of his intestines will be in order. Even though a man is poor, if he is content, his inner strength will be preserved. If one can bear hunger and not refrain from eating greedily, it is laudable. If one can bear the cold, and not indulge in too many warm clothes, it is laudable. If one uses one's physical strength for labors, and does not live in idleness, it is laudable. If one can gain through diligence, and not wait for windfall, it is laudable.

15 The man who lives in the mountains without integrity will die young. The man who lives in the city without simplicity will die young. The man living in the countryside without diligence will die young. The intellectual man without self-control will also die young.

16 The man living in the mountains must have integrity; if he has integrity, he will live long and prosper. The man living in the city must have simplicity; if he has simplicity, he will live long and prosper. The man living in the countryside must be diligent; if he is diligent, he will live long and prosper. The intellectual man must have self-control; if he has self-control, he will live long and prosper.

17 If a man living in the mountains has integrity, not only will he live long and prosper, but he will also be the most distinguished man in that area. If a man living in the city has simplicity, not only will he live long and prosper, but he will also be the most distinguished man in the city. If a man who lives in the countryside has diligence, not only will he live long and prosper, but he will also be the most distinguished man in that area. If an intellectual man has self-control, not only will he live long and prosper, but he will also be the most distinguished man among intellectuals.

18 Someone once asked me, "The farmer cultivates his land with his physical strength, so he must be diligent. Why do you say he is not diligent? Likewise, the intellectual studies very hard, and is self-controlled. Why do you say he is not self-controlled?" I answered, "The farmer is always anxious that he cannot cultivate one hundred Mau. If he

were truly diligent, there would be no need for him to be anxious. Thus, compared to the intellectual, the farmer is actually idle. The intellectual, however, studies hard and becomes arrogant in his learning; whereas the farmer is ignorant of book learning, and must always remain cautious. Thus, compared to the farmer, the intellectual lacks self-control. If, however, the farmer learns how to study from the intellectual, and the intellectual learns how to perform physical labors from the farmer, their abilities and characters will develop, and their organic qi strengthen."

19 The overindulgent man looks down on ordinary life and makes light of domestic life. He is surrounded by luxury, and does not understand the difficulties of earning a living. He lacks the proper skills for acquiring property. He is always overindulgent in sensual pleasures, and never feels any regret to the end of his life.

20 A lazy man is very crude and refuses to work diligently. He spends his time dreaming idly. He is generally unwilling to work hard, and so takes to drink; rarely are lazy men not also drunkards. When we see such drunken men, we are able to understand just how crude the lazy man's mind is.

21 It is said that overdrinking and overindulging in sexual pleasures kill men. As alcohol poisoning dries out the intestines, so does sexual overindulgence dry up the essence of a body. People who say this, however, fail to understand completely. Drunkards, in fact, loathe physical labors, and their worries are as great as mountains. He who is blinded by lust experiences anxieties that cut him like a knife. Such overindulgence in drinking and sexual pleasure break a man's mental vitality, while alcohol poisoning and sexual exhaustion attack his body. Together, they can kill a man.

22 The sensualist will certainly be attracted to the lewd woman, and likewise, the lewd woman will be attracted to the sensualist. The foolish man will certainly be attracted to the jealous woman, and the jealous woman will likewise be attracted to the foolish man. According to the law of nature, the lewd woman is a proper partner for the sensual man, and the foolish man is also a proper partner for the jealous woman. Generally,

women both lewd and jealous are well suited to vulgar, not noble, men. Among the seven valid reasons for divorce, lewd and jealous behavior is the worst. Most people, however, do not understand the meaning of jealousy. They think jealousy refers to the hatred of a wife for her husband's many concubines, but for a noble man to have a son is the most important thing. Thus, his wife should not be jealous or hateful towards her husband's concubines. However, since the cause of turmoil in a family is often due to there being many concubines, a wife who is jealous and hateful of the bad behavior of these concubines displaces wisdom. So how can we say that these two kinds of jealousy are the same? In the 『*Shijing*』 ("Classic of Poetry"), we read the following verse: The peach tree beams so red; Its leaves are lush and green. The maiden's getting wed; On household she'll be keen. 'On household she'll be keen' means that women love wisdom, follow virtue, and are keen on their household duties. Not being keen on household means being jealous of the wise and the able, and not being keen on household duties. Generally, if the husband is foolish, and the wife is jealous of the wise and able, illness will continuously plague the household, death will follow, sons will become fools, and property will be lost.

23 Being jealous of the wise and the able is the worst thing in the world. Loving wisdom and following virtue is the best thing in the world. He, who harbors no jealousy of the wise and the able, though he may perform some bad acts, is actually not such a bad person. He, who harbors no love of wisdom and does not follow virtue, though he may perform some good actions, is actually not such a good person. It is considered that all the diseases in the world come from being jealous of the wise and the able, and the cure for all the diseases in the world depends on having respect for wisdom and following virtue. Therefore, being jealous of the wise and the able is the most prevalent disease in the world, and respecting the wise and following virtue is the greatest medicine in the world.

2

Discourse on Identifying the Four Constitutions*

1 In a town of 10,000 people, half will be of the greater yin type. Three thousand will be of the lesser yang type, and two thousand of the lesser yin type. Only three to ten or more people will be of the greater yang type.

2 The greater yang person has a developed nape for the rising posture and a slender waist for the standing posture. The lesser yang person has a developed chest for the self-embracing posture and small hips for the sitting posture. The greater yin person has a thick waist for the standing posture and a weak nape for the rising posture. The lesser yin person has developed hips for the sitting posture and a weak chest for the self-embracing posture.

3 The greater yang person is skilled at communicating and has a talent for social acquaintances. The lesser yang person has a warrior mentality and a talent for appointed roles. The greater yin person is skilled at accomplishments and has a talent for living quarters. The lesser yin person is skilled at good conduct and has a talent for clanships.

4 The greater yang person's body is easily recognizable, but because they are very rare, they are the most difficult to identify. Greater yang people's

* 四象人辨證論

napes are developed, and they communicate well. They have a determined character, but have dysphagia, regurgitation of food from the stomach and generalized fatigue and lassitude, so they are easy to identify. Until their illness becomes serious, they appear to be normal. The elderly lesser yin person also may have generalized fatigue and lassitude, so we should not confuse him with the greater yang person.

5 The body of the greater yang female is big and strong, but since she has a small Liver, narrow waist, and her uterus function is weak, she can seldom give birth. We can easily see this to be true by noticing the greater yang mare and cow–though their bodies are big and strong, they too seldom are able to give birth.

6 The lesser yang person has a developed upper body and weak lower body, his chest is well developed, and his feet are light. He is quick, sharp and brave. Since lesser yang people are numerous, they are the most easily identified among the four types.

7 Since some lesser yang people, like lesser yin people, are small and smart in appearance, we must carefully observe their symptoms, such as chills and fever, and not confuse them with the lesser yin types.

8 Greater yin and lesser yin persons are similar in body shape and thus are difficult to distinguish, but if we diagnose the symptoms carefully, we can distinguish them clearly. When the greater yin person spontaneously sweats, he is healthy, but if the lesser yin person has spontaneous sweating, he is seriously ill. If the skin of the greater yin person is too solid and hard, he will have a serious illness. If the skin of the lesser yin person is very solid, he will be healthy. The greater yin person tends to have severe palpitations and chest pains, and the lesser yin person tends to exhibit restless involuntary movement of the limbs. The corners of a greater yin person's eyes tend to turn upward, and he often experiences eye pain. The lesser yin type does not have the same characteristics. The lesser yin type generally breathes smoothly, but sometimes sighs deeply. The greater yin type, on the other hand, does not sigh deeply. If the two get malaria with chills, the greater yin is able to drink cold water, but the

lesser yin cannot. The greater yin's pulse is long and tight, while the lesser yin's is smooth and weak. The greater yin's flesh is solid, while the lesser yin's is tender. The greater yin is gentle in appearance and inarticulate in speech, but persistent and well behaved. The lesser yin's appearance is neat, his speech natural, and his behavior shrewd.

9 Lesser yin persons are generally short, but some of them may be six to seven feet tall. As for the greater yins, they are usually tall, but some of them are five feet or shorter.

10 The greater yin person always has a fearful mind. If he achieves peace of mind, he will also achieve stability and harmony. If he is too fearful, his mind will worsen, and he will experience severe palpitations. Severe palpitations are a serious problem for the greater yin person.

11 The lesser yang person always suffers from anxiety. If he achieves peace of mind, he will also achieve stability and harmony. If he is too anxious, his mind will be bound. If his anxiety becomes extreme, he will become seriously ill and experience amnesia, a serious problem for the lesser yang person.

12 The lesser yin type always has a nervous mind. If his nervous mind becomes stable, then his Spleen qi will be activated. The greater yang person always has a rash personality. If he can slow down his pace, his Liver blood will become regulated.

13 The lesser yin person has problems with his pharynx and larynx. Those problems are serious and chronic. We should not let these problems go untreated, but administer *Shengui Bawu Tang* (Decoction of eight precious ingredients with Radix Ginseng and Ramulus Cinnamomi), roe liver or gold snake liquor.

14 Some greater yang people may have constipation for eight or nine days. This indicates nothing too serious, and so is nothing to worry too much about. However, we still must not ignore it. We can treat it with *Mihudeung Ogapi Tang* (Decoction of Caulis Actinidiae Chinensis and Cortex Acanthopanacis).

15 If the greater yang person passes a lot of urine, he is very healthy. If the greater yin person sweats a lot, he is very healthy. If the lesser yang person's bowel movements are smooth, he is very healthy. If the lesser yin person's digestion is good, he is very healthy.

16 When the greater yang person gets dysphagia, the upper-*jiao* of the epigastrium feels like a harsh wind is passing through. When the greater yin person gets dysentery, the middle-*jiao* of the small intestine feels obstructed, as if by dense fog. When the lesser yang person gets constipation, then his diaphragm will surely feel like fire. When the lesser yin person has continuous diarrheas, the hypogastric region surely feels as cold as ice. If we know the person's type and the patterns of his symptoms, there will be no uncertainty in prescribing the proper medicine.

17 We must identify the person's constitution very carefully by observing his appearance. If we fail after several attempts, we can identify his type clearly by referring to the patterns of symptoms. Only after ascertaining the patient's nature can we prescribe medicine. We must not even prescribe a single pack of medicine carelessly, for a single pack may kill a seriously ill patient.

18 Hua Tuo said, "The key to a healthy life lies in engaging in moderate labors, and avoiding excessive fatigue." An elderly man once said, "People may eat twice a day, but should not eat four or five times a day. People should not continue to eat after meals. If you follow those instructions, you will have a long life."

19 I have added, "I would like to say that the greater yin person always calms his fearful mind by looking outside himself. The lesser yang person always calms his anxious mind by looking within. The greater yang person slows down his rash mind by taking one step back. The lesser yin person can calm his nervous mind by moving one step forward. In this way, all four types may live a long life."

20 Again, I have said, "The greater yang type should be careful not to be angry or sorrowful. The lesser yang type should be careful not to become

sorrowful or angry. The greater yin type should be careful not to be excessively joyful or pleased. The lesser yin type should be careful not to be excessively pleased or joyful. In this way, all four types may live a long life."

21 The great King Shun was willing to learn farming, pottery and fishing from others. Confucius said, "Among three men walking together, there will surely be at least one teacher." Accordingly, we can say that the sage studies widely, learns carefully from many people, integrates his knowledge, and thus becomes great. Each constitution has its own strong point in intelligence and talents. Therefore, in each field–the arts of writing, calligraphy, archery, equestrianism, singing, dancing, etiquette, *baduk* (Go) and *janggi* (Korean chess)–there are differences in techniques, as well. All these various techniques are harmonized together and used to form society.

22 The 『*Lingshu*』 also suggested constitution ideas according to the four types and the five phases, but it only referred to the body's outer appearance, and neglected the principles of the internal organs. People in those ancient times recognized that there were four types, but they could not identify them in detail.

Identifying the Four Constitutions

	Greater Yang (Taiyang)	Lesser Yang (Soyang)	Greater Yin (Taieum)	Lesser Yin (Soeum)
Population	very rare	30 %	50 %	20 %
General figure	developed nape of the neck slender waist	developed chest small hips	thick waist weak nape of the neck	developed hips weak chest
Face	large & thin shiny eyes wide	small thin lips narrow jaws protruding	rounded looks serious	smart
Skin	soft	dry & thin	solid	tender
Walking	very rare	unstable	heavy & gentle	stable
Characters	creative positive progressive charismatic heroic rash mind	unstable easily gets bored outside-oriented sacrificing righteous easily acceptable hot tempered anxious mind	gentle commercial endurable humorous looks foolish coward fearful mind	neat negative mild inside-oriented intelligent systematic selfish jealous narrow-minded nervous mind
Healthy sign	urination	bowel movement	perspiration	digestion
Pulse		rapid & floating	long & tight	smooth & weak

3
Epilogue*

For almost a year, I devoted myself solely to the writing of this book, working day and night, without interruption, from July 13, 1893 to April 13, 1894. I have described lesser yang and lesser yin persons in detail, but was not able to do the same for greater yin and greater yang people, due to both a lack of experience and exhaustion from writing this book.

In the 『*Liji*』[1] ("Record of Rites"), we read, "If you cannot understand what you read, then you must think for yourself." If you are able to understand the theories underlying the greater yin and greater yang types through your own efforts, then my own rough explanations need not be consulted. If there is but one potter in a town of ten thousand people, he will not be able to meet the needs of the entire town; and if there is only one doctor in a village of one hundred families, he will not be able to meet the medical needs of the village. Likewise, if we can spread the ideas of medical science and see to it that every family understands medical science, and that every person understands disease, then all will have good health and a long life.

(On April 13, 1894, Lee Je-ma finished this work at Namsan in Seoul. The next year, he returned to his hometown, Hamheung city. From 1895 to 1900, he revised his writings and modified the manuscript from the "Discourse on

---

* 跋文

Nature and Order" to the discourses on the greater yin person. He did not have the chance to modify the last three discourses, and published them unrevised.)

東醫壽世保元 全文

1

性命論*

1 天機有四一曰地方二曰人倫三曰世會四曰天時

2 人事有四一曰居處二曰黨與三曰交遇四曰事務

3 耳聽天時目視世會鼻嗅人倫口味地方

4 天時極蕩也世會極大也人倫極廣也地方極邈也

5 肺達事務脾合交遇肝立黨與腎定居處

6 事務克修也交遇克成也黨與克整也居處克治也

7 頷有籌策臆有經綸臍有行檢腹有度量

8 籌策不可驕也經綸不可矜也行檢不可伐也度量不可夸也

9 頭有識見肩有威儀腰有材幹臀有方略

10 識見必無奪也威儀必無侈也材幹必無懶也方略必無竊也

11 耳目鼻口觀於天也肺脾肝腎立於人也頷臆臍腹行其知也頭肩腰臀行其行也

12 天時大同也事務各立也世會大同也交遇各立也人倫大同也黨與各立也地方大同也居處各立也

13 籌策博通也識見獨行也經綸博通也威儀獨行也行檢博通也材幹獨行也度量博通也方略獨行也

14 大同者天也各立者人也博通者性也獨行者命也

15 耳好善聲目好善色鼻好善臭口好善味

16 善聲順耳也善色順目也善臭順鼻也善味順口也

---

* Part I–1 Discourse on Nature and Order

17 肺惡惡聲脾惡惡色肝惡惡臭腎惡惡味

18 惡聲逆肺也惡色逆脾也惡臭逆肝也惡味逆腎也

19 頷有驕心臆有矜心臍有伐心腹有夸心

20 驕心驕意也矜心矜慮也伐心伐操也夸心夸志也

21 頭有擅心肩有侈心腰有懶心臀有慾心

22 擅心奪利也侈心自尊也懶心自卑也慾心竊物也

23 人之耳目鼻口好善無雙也人之肺脾肝腎惡惡無雙也人之頷臆臍腹邪心無雙也人之頭肩腰臀怠心無雙也

24 堯舜之行仁在於五千年前而至于今天下之稱善者皆曰堯舜則人之好善果無雙也桀紂之行暴在於四千年前而至于今天下之稱惡者皆曰桀紂則人之惡惡果無雙也以孔子之聖三千之徒受教而惟顔子三月不違仁其餘日月至焉而心悅誠服者只有七十二人則人之邪心果無雙也以文王之德百年而後崩未洽於天下武王周公繼之然後大行而管叔蔡叔猶以至親作亂則人之怠行果無雙也

25 耳目鼻口人皆可以爲堯舜頷臆臍腹人皆自不爲堯舜肺脾肝腎人皆可以爲堯舜頭肩腰臀人皆自不爲堯舜

26 人之耳目鼻口好善之心以衆人耳目鼻口論之而堯舜未爲加一鞭也人之肺脾肝腎惡惡之心以堯舜肺脾肝腎論之而衆人未爲少一鞭也人皆可以爲堯舜者以此人之頷臆臍腹之中誣世之心每每隱伏也存其心養其性然後人皆可以爲堯舜之知也人之頭肩腰臀之下罔民之心種種暗藏也修其身立其命然後人皆可以爲堯舜之行也人皆自不爲堯舜者以此

27 耳目鼻口之情行路之人大同於協義故好善也好善之實極公也極公則亦極無私也肺脾肝腎之情同室之人各立於擅利故惡惡也惡惡之實極無私也極無私則亦極公也頷臆臍腹之中自有不息之知如切如磋而驕矜伐夸之私心卒然敗之則自棄其知而不能博通也頭肩腰臀之下自有不息之行赫兮咺兮而奪侈懶竊之慾心卒然陷之則自棄其行而不能正行也

28 耳目鼻口人皆知也頷臆臍腹人皆愚也肺脾肝腎人皆賢也頭肩腰臀人皆不肖也

29 人之耳目鼻口天也天知也人之肺脾肝腎人也人賢也我之頷臆臍腹我自爲心而未免愚也我之免愚在我也我之頭肩腰臀我自爲身而未免不肖也我之免不肖在我也

30 天生萬民性以慧覺萬民之生也有慧覺則生無慧覺則死慧覺者德之所由生也

31 天生萬民命以資業萬民之生也有資業則生無資業則死資業者道之所由生也

32 仁義禮智忠孝友悌諸般百善皆出於慧覺士農工商田宅邦國諸般百用皆出於資業

33 慧覺欲其兼人而有教也資業欲其廉己而有功也慧覺私小者雖有其傑巧如曹操而不可爲教也資業橫濫者雖有其雄猛如秦王而不可爲功也

34 好人之善而我亦知善者至性之德也惡人之惡而我必不行惡者正命之道

也知行積則道德也道德成則仁聖也道德非他知行也性命非他知行也

35 或曰擧知而論性可也而擧行而論命何義耶曰命者命數也善行則命數自美也惡行則命數自惡也不待卜筮而可知也詩云永言配命自求多福卽此義也

36 或曰吾子之言曰耳聽天時目視世會鼻嗅人倫口味地方耳之聽天時目之視世會則可也而鼻何以嗅人倫口何以味地方乎曰處於人倫察人外表黙探各人才行之賢不肖者此非嗅耶處於地方均嘗各處人民生活之地利者此非味耶

37 存其心者責其心也心體之明暗雖若自然而責之者清不責者濁馬之心覺黠於牛者馬之責心黠於牛也鷹之氣勢猛於鴟者鷹之責氣猛於鴟也心體之清濁氣宇之强弱在於牛馬鴟鷹者以理推之而猶然况於人乎或相倍蓰或相千萬者豈其生而輒得茫然不思居然自至而然哉

2

四端論*

1 人稟臟理有四不同肺大而肝小者名曰太陽人肝大而肺小者名曰太陰人脾大而腎小者名曰少陽人腎大而脾小者名曰少陰人

2 人趨心慾有四不同棄禮而放縱者名曰鄙人棄義而偸逸者名曰懦人棄智而飾私者名曰薄人棄仁而極慾者名曰貪人

3 五臟之心中央之太極也五臟之肺脾肝腎四維之四象也中央之太極聖人之太極高出於衆人之太極也四維之四象聖人之四象旁通於衆人之四象也

4 太少陰陽之臟局短長四不同中有一大同天理之變化也聖人與衆人一同也鄙薄貪懦之心地淸濁四不同中有萬不同人慾之闊狹也聖人與衆人萬殊也

5 太少陰陽之短長變化一同之中有四偏聖人所以希天也鄙薄貪懦之淸濁闊狹萬殊之中有一同衆人所以希聖也

6 聖人之臟四端也衆人之臟亦四端也以聖人一四端之臟處於衆人萬四端之中聖人者衆人之所樂也聖人之心無慾也衆人之心有慾也以聖人一無慾之心處於衆人萬有慾之中衆人者聖人之所憂也

7 然則天下衆人之臟理亦皆聖人之臟理而才能亦皆聖人之才能也以肺脾肝腎聖人之才能而自言曰我無才能云者豈才能之罪哉心之罪也

8 浩然之氣出於肺脾肝腎也浩然之理出於心也仁義禮智四臟之氣擴而充之則浩然之氣出於此也鄙薄貪懦一心之慾明而辨之則浩然之理出於此也

9 聖人之心無慾云者非淸淨寂滅如老佛之無慾也聖人之心深憂天下之不治故非但無慾也亦未暇及於一己之慾也深憂天下之不治而未暇及於一

---

* Part I-2 Discourse on the Four Principles

己之慾者必學不厭而教不倦也學不厭而教不倦者卽聖人之無慾也毫有一己之慾則非堯舜之心也暫無天下之憂則非孔孟之心也

10 太陽人哀性遠散而怒情促急哀性遠散則氣注肺而肺益盛怒情促急則氣激肝而肝益削太陽之臟局所以成形於肺大肝小也少陽人怒性宏抱而哀情促急怒性宏抱則氣注脾而脾益盛哀情促急則氣激腎而腎益削少陽之臟局所以成形於脾大腎小也太陰人喜性廣張而樂情促急喜性廣張則氣注肝而肝益盛樂情促急則氣激肺而肺益削太陰之臟局所以成形於肝大肺小也少陰人樂性深確而喜情促急樂性深確則氣注腎而腎益盛喜情促急則氣激脾而脾益削少陰之臟局所以成形於腎大脾小也

11 肺氣直而伸脾氣栗而包肝氣寬而緩腎氣溫而畜

12 肺以呼肝以吸肝肺者呼吸氣液之門戶也脾以納腎以出腎脾者出納水穀之府庫也

13 哀氣直升怒氣橫升喜氣放降樂氣陷降

14 哀怒之氣上升喜樂之氣下降上升之氣過多則下焦傷下降之氣過多則上焦傷

15 哀怒之氣順動則發越而上騰喜樂之氣順動則緩安而下墜哀怒之氣陽也順動則順而上升喜樂之氣陰也順動則順而下降

16 哀怒之氣逆動則暴發而竝於上也喜樂之氣逆動則浪發而竝於下也上升之氣逆動而竝於上則肝腎傷下降之氣逆動而竝於下則脾肺傷

17 頻起怒而頻伏怒則腰脇頻迫而頻蕩也腰脇者肝之所住着處也腰脇迫蕩不定則肝其不傷乎乍發喜而乍收喜則胸腋乍闊而乍狹也胸腋者脾之所住着處也胸腋闊狹不定則脾其不傷乎忽動哀而忽止哀則脊曲忽屈而忽伸也脊曲者腎之所住着處也脊曲屈伸不定則腎其不傷乎屢得樂而屢失樂則背霍暴揚而暴抑也背霍者肺之所住着處也背霍抑揚不定則肺其不傷乎

18 太陽人有暴怒深哀不可不戒少陽人有暴哀深怒不可不戒太陰人有浪樂深喜不可不戒少陰人有浪喜深樂不可不戒

19 皐陶曰都在知人在安民禹曰吁咸若時惟帝其難之知人則哲能官人安民則惠黎民懷之能哲而惠何憂乎觀菟何遷乎有苗何畏乎巧言令色孔壬

20 三復大禹之訓而欽仰之曰帝堯之喜怒哀樂每每中節者以其難於知人也大禹之喜怒哀樂每每中節者以其不敢輕易於知人也天下喜怒哀樂之暴動浪動者都出於行身不誠而知人不明也知人帝堯之所難而大禹之所吁也則其誰沾沾自喜乎蓋亦益反其誠而必不可輕易取舍人也

21 雖好善之心偏急而好善則好善必不明也雖惡惡之心偏急而惡惡則惡惡必不周也天下事宜與好人做也不與好人做則喜樂必煩也天下事不宜與不好人做也與不好人做則哀怒益煩也

22 哀怒相成喜樂相資哀性極則怒情動怒性極則哀情動樂性極則喜情動喜性極則樂情動太陽人哀極不濟則忿怒激外少陽人怒極不勝則悲哀動中少陰人樂極不成則喜好不定太陰人喜極不服則侈樂無厭如此而動者無異於以刀割臟一次大動十年難復此死生壽夭之機關也不可不知也

23 太少陰陽之臟局短長陰陽之變化也天稟之已定固無可論天稟已定之外又有短長而不全其天稟者則人事之修不修而命之傾也不可不愼也

24 太陽人怒以一人之怒而怒千萬人其怒無術於千萬人則必難堪千萬人也少陰人喜以一人之喜而喜千萬人其喜無術於千萬人則必難堪千萬人也少陽人哀以一人之哀而哀千萬人其哀無術於千萬人則必難堪千萬人也太陰人樂以一人之樂而樂千萬人其樂無術於千萬人則必難堪千萬人也

25 太陽少陽人但恒戒哀怒之過度而不可强做喜樂虛動不及也若强做喜樂而煩數之則喜樂不出於眞情而哀怒益偏也太陰少陰人但恒戒喜樂之過度而不可强做哀怒虛動不及也若强做哀怒而煩數之則哀怒不出於眞情而喜樂益偏也

26 喜怒哀樂之未發謂之中發而皆中節謂之和喜怒哀樂未發而恒戒者此非漸近於中者乎喜怒哀樂已發而自反者此非漸近於節者乎

3

擴充論*

1 太陽人哀性遠散而怒情促急哀性遠散者太陽之耳察於天時而哀衆人之相欺也哀性非他聽也怒情促急者太陽之脾行於交遇而怒別人之侮己也怒情非他怒也少陽人怒性宏抱而哀情促急怒性宏抱者少陽之目察於世會而怒衆人之相侮也怒性非他視也哀情促急者少陽之肺行於事務而哀別人之欺己也哀情非他哀也太陰人喜性廣張而樂情促急喜性廣張者太陰之鼻察於人倫而喜衆人之相助也喜性非他嗅也樂情促急者太陰之腎行於居處而樂別人之保己也樂情非他樂也少陰人樂性深確而喜情促急樂性深確者少陰之口察於地方而樂衆人之相保也樂性非他味也喜情促急者少陰之肝行於黨與而喜別人之助己也喜情非他喜也

2 太陽之耳能廣博於天時而太陽之鼻不能廣博於人倫太陰之鼻能廣博於人倫而太陰之耳不能廣博於天時少陽之目能廣博於世會而少陽之口不能廣博於地方少陰之口能廣博於地方而少陰之目不能廣博於世會

3 太陽之脾能勇統於交遇而太陽之肝不能雅立於黨與少陰之肝能雅立於黨與而少陰之脾不能勇統於交遇少陽之肺能敏達於事務而少陽之腎不能恒定於居處太陰之腎能恒定於居處而太陰之肺不能敏達於事務

4 太陽之聽能廣博於天時故太陽之神充足於頭腦而歸肺者大也太陽之嗅不能廣博於人倫故太陽之血不充足於腰脊而歸肝者小也太陰之嗅能廣博於人倫故太陰之血充足於腰脊而歸肝者大也太陰之聽不能廣博於天時故太陰之神不充足於頭腦而歸肺者小也少陽之視能廣博於世會故少陽之氣充足於背膂而歸脾者大也少陽之味不能廣博於地方故少陽之精不充足於膀胱而歸腎者小也少陰之味能廣博於地方故少陰之精充足於膀胱而歸腎者大也少陰之視不能廣博於世會故少陰之氣不充足於背膂而歸脾者小也

5 太陽之怒能勇統於交遇故交遇不侮也太陽之喜不能雅立於黨與故黨與侮也是故太陽之暴怒不在於交遇而必在於黨與也少陰之喜能雅立於黨

---

* Part I-3 Discourse on the Establishment and Supplement

與故黨與助也少陰之怒不能勇統於交遇故交遇不助也是故少陰之浪喜不在於黨與而必在於交遇也少陽之哀能敏達於事務故事務不欺也少陽之樂不能恒定於居處故居處欺也是故少陽之暴哀不在於事務而必在於居處也太陰之樂能恒定於居處故居處保也太陰之哀不能敏達於事務故事務不保也是故太陰之浪樂不在於居處而必在於事務也

6 太陽之交遇可以怒治之而黨與不可以怒治之也若遷怒於黨與則無益於黨與而肝傷也少陰之黨與可以喜治之而交遇不可以喜治之也若遷喜於交遇則無益於交遇而脾傷也少陽之事務可以哀治之而居處不可以哀治之也若遷哀於居處則無益於居處而腎傷也太陰之居處可以樂治之而事務不可以樂治之也若遷樂於事務則無益於事務而肺傷也

7 太陽之性氣恒欲進而不欲退少陽之性氣恒欲擧而不欲措太陰之性氣恒欲靜而不欲動少陰之性氣恒欲處而不欲出

8 太陽之進量可而進也自反其材而不莊不能進也少陽之擧量可而擧也自反其力而不固不能擧也太陰之靜量可而靜也自反其知而不周不能靜也少陰之處量可而處也自反其謀而不弘不能處也

9 太陽之情氣恒欲爲雄而不欲爲雌少陰之情氣恒欲爲雌而不欲爲雄少陽之情氣恒欲外勝而不欲内守太陰之情氣恒欲内守而不欲外勝

10 太陽之人雖好爲雄亦或宜雌若全好爲雄則放縱之心必過也少陰之人雖好爲雌亦或宜雄若全好爲雌則偸逸之心必過也少陽之人雖好外勝亦宜内守若全好外勝則偏私之心必過也太陰之人雖好内守亦宜外勝若全好内守則物慾之心必過也

11 太陽人雖至愚其性便便然猶延納也雖至不肖人之善惡亦知之也少陽人雖至愚其性恢恢然猶式度也雖至不肖人之知愚亦知之也太陰人雖至愚其性卓卓然猶教誘也雖至不肖人之勤惰亦知之也少陰人雖至愚其性坦坦然猶撫循也雖至不肖人之能否亦知之也

12 太陽人謹於交遇故恒有交遇生疎人慮患之怒心此心出於秉彝之敬心也莫非至善而輕於黨與故每爲親熟黨與人所陷而偏怒傷臟以其擇交之心不廣故也

13 少陰人謹於黨與故恒有黨與親熟人擇交之喜心此心出於秉彝之敬心也莫非至善而輕於交遇故每爲生疎交遇人所誣而偏喜傷臟以其慮患之心不周故也

14 少陽人重於事務故恒有出外興事務之哀心此心出於秉彝之敬心也莫非至善而不謹於居處故每爲主内做居處人所陷而偏哀傷臟以其重外而輕内故也

15 太陰人重於居處故恒有主内做居處之樂心此心出於秉彝之敬心也莫非至善而不謹於事務故每爲出外興事務人所誣而偏樂傷臟以其重内而輕外故也

16 太陰之頷宜戒驕心太陰之頷若無驕心絶世之籌策必在於此也少陰之臆宜戒矜心少陰之臆若無矜心絶世之經綸必在於此也太陽之臍宜戒伐心太陽之臍若無伐心絶世之行檢必在於此也少陽之腹宜戒夸心少陽之腹若無夸心絶世之度量必在於此也

17 少陰之頭宜戒奪心少陰之頭若無奪心大人之識見必在於此也太陰之肩宜戒侈心太陰之肩若無侈心大人之威儀必在於此也少陽之腰宜戒懶心

少陽之腰若無懶心大人之才幹必在於此也太陽之臂宜戒竊心太陽之臂若無竊心大人之方略必在於此也

4

臟腑論*

1 肺部位在膻下背上胃脘部位在頷下胸上故背上胸上以上謂之上焦脾部位在膂胃部位在膈故膂膈之間謂之中上焦肝部位在腰小腸部位在臍故腰臍之間謂之中下焦腎部位在腰脊下大腸部位在臍腹下故脊下臍下以下謂之下焦

2 水穀自胃脘而入于胃自胃而入于小腸自小腸而入于大腸自大腸而出于肛門者水穀之都數停畜於胃而薰蒸爲熱氣消導於小腸而平淡爲凉氣熱氣之輕清者上升於胃脘而爲溫氣凉氣之質重者下降於大腸而爲寒氣

3 胃脘通於口鼻故水穀之氣上升也大腸通於肛門故水穀之氣下降也胃之體廣大而包容故水穀之氣停畜也小腸之體狹窄而屈曲故水穀之氣消導也

4 水穀溫氣自胃脘而化津入于舌下爲津海津海者津之所舍也津海之清氣出于耳而爲神入于頭腦而爲膩海膩海者神之所舍也膩海之膩汁清者內歸于肺濁滓外歸于皮毛故胃脘與舌耳頭腦皮毛皆肺之黨也

5 水穀熱氣自胃而化膏入于膻間兩乳爲膏海膏海者膏之所舍也膏海之清氣出于目而爲氣入于背膂而爲膜海膜海者氣之所舍也膜海之膜汁清者內歸于脾濁滓外歸于筋故胃與兩乳目背膂筋皆脾之黨也

6 水穀凉氣自小腸而化油入于臍爲油海油海者油之所舍也油海之清氣出于鼻而爲血入于腰脊而爲血海血海者血之所舍也血海之血汁清者內歸于肝濁滓外歸于肉故小腸與臍鼻腰脊肉皆肝之黨也

7 水穀寒氣自大腸而化液入于前陰毛際之內爲液海液海者液之所舍也液海之清氣出于口而爲精入于膀胱而爲精海精海者精之所舍也精海之精汁清者內歸于腎濁滓外歸于骨故大腸與前陰口膀胱骨皆腎之黨也

8 耳以廣博天時之聽力提出津海之清氣充滿於上焦爲神而注之頭腦爲膩

---

* Part I-4 Discourse on Viscera and Bowels

積累爲膩海目以廣博世會之視力提出膏海之淸氣充滿於中上焦爲氣而注之背膂爲膜積累爲膜海鼻以廣博人倫之嗅力提出油海之淸氣充滿於中下焦爲血而注之腰脊爲凝血積累爲血海口以廣博地方之味力提出液海之淸氣充滿於下焦爲精而注之膀胱爲凝精積累爲精海

9 肺以鍊達事務之哀力吸得膩海之淸汁入于肺以滋肺元而內以擁護津海鼓動其氣凝聚其津脾以鍊達交遇之怒力吸得膜海之淸汁入于脾以滋脾元而內以擁護膏海鼓動其氣凝聚其膏肝以鍊達黨與之喜力吸得血海之淸汁入于肝以滋肝元而內以擁護油海鼓動其氣凝聚其油腎以鍊達居處之樂力吸得精海之淸汁入于腎以滋腎元而內以擁護液海鼓動其氣凝聚其液

10 津海之濁滓則胃脘以上升之力取其濁滓而以補益胃脘膏海之濁滓則胃以停畜之力取其濁滓而以補益胃油海之濁滓則小腸以消導之力取其濁滓而以補益小腸液海之濁滓則大腸以下降之力取其濁滓而以補益大腸

11 膩海之濁滓則頭以直伸之力鍛鍊之而成皮毛膜海之濁滓則手以能收之力鍛鍊之而成筋血海之濁滓則腰以寬放之力鍛鍊之而成肉精海之濁滓則足以屈强之力鍛鍊之而成骨

12 是故耳必遠聽目必大視鼻必廣嗅口必深味耳目鼻口之用深遠廣大則精神氣血生也淺近狹小則精神氣血耗也肺必善學脾必善問肝必善思腎必善辨肺脾肝腎之用正直中和則津液膏油充也偏倚過不及則津液膏油爍也

13 膩海藏神膜海藏靈血海藏魂精海藏魄

14 津海藏意膏海藏慮油海藏操液海藏志

15 頭腦之膩海肺之根本也背膂之膜海脾之根本也腰脊之血海肝之根本也膀胱之精海腎之根本也

16 舌之津海耳之根本也乳之膏海目之根本也臍之油海鼻之根本也前陰之液海口之根本也

17 心爲一身之主宰負隅背心正向膻中光明瑩徹耳目鼻口無所不察肺脾肝腎無所不忖頷臆臍腹無所不誠頭手腰足無所不敬

5

醫源論*

1 書曰若藥不瞑眩厥疾不瘳商高宗時已有瞑眩藥驗而高宗至於稱歎則醫藥經驗其來已久於神農黃帝之時其說可信於眞也而本草素問出於神農黃帝之手其說不可信於眞也何以言之神農黃帝時文字無應後世文字澆漓例法故也衰周秦以來扁鵲有名而張仲景具備得之始爲成家著書醫道始興張仲景以後南北朝隋唐醫繼之而至于宋朱肱具備得之著活人書醫道中興朱肱以後元醫李杲王好古朱震亨危亦林繼之而至于明李梴龔信具備得之許浚具備傳之著東醫寶鑑醫道復興蓋自神農黃帝以後秦漢以前病證藥理張仲景傳之魏晉以後隋唐以前病症藥理朱肱傳之宋元以後明以前病證藥理李梴龔信許浚傳之若以醫家勸勞功業論之則當以張仲景朱肱許浚爲首而李梴龔信次之

2 本草自神農黃帝以來數千年世間流來經驗而神農時有本草殷時有湯液本草唐時有孟詵食療本草陳藏器本草拾遺宋時有龐安常本草補遺日華子本草元時有王好古湯液本草

3 少陰人病證藥理張仲景庶幾乎昭詳發明而宋元明諸醫盡乎昭詳發明少陽人病證藥理張仲景半乎昭詳發明而宋元明諸醫庶幾乎昭詳發明太陰人病證藥理張仲景略得影子而宋元明諸醫太半乎昭詳發明太陽人病證藥理朱震亨略得影子而本草略有藥理

4 余生於醫藥經驗五六千載後因前人之述偶得四象人臟腑性理著得一書名曰壽世保元原書中張仲景所論太陽病少陽病陽明病太陰病少陰病厥陰病以病證名目而論之也余所論太陽人少陽人太陰人少陰人以人物名目而論之也二者不可混看又不可厭煩然後可以探其根株而採其枝葉也若夫脈法者執證之一端也其理在於浮沈遲數而不必究其奇妙之致也三陰三陽者辨證之同異也其理在於腹背表裏而不必究其經絡之變也

5 古人以六經陰陽論病故張仲景著傷寒論亦以六經陰陽該病證而以頭痛

* Part I–5 Discourse on the Origin of Eastern Medicine

身疼發熱惡寒脈浮者謂之太陽病證以口苦咽乾目眩耳聾胸脇滿寒熱往來頭痛發熱脈弦細者謂之少陽病證以不惡寒反惡熱汗自出大便秘者謂之陽明病證以腹滿時痛口不燥心不煩而自利者謂之太陰病證以脈微細但欲寐口燥心煩而自利者謂之少陰病證以初無腹痛自利等證而傷寒六七日脈微緩手足厥冷舌卷囊縮者謂之厥陰病證六條病證中三陰病證皆少陰人病證也少陽病證卽少陽人病證也太陽病證陽明病證則少陽人少陰人太陰人病證均有之而少陰人病證居多也古昔以來醫藥法方流行世間經歷累驗者仲景採摭而著述之蓋古之醫師不知心之愛惡所欲喜怒哀樂偏着者爲病而但知脾胃水穀風寒暑濕觸犯者爲病故其論病論藥全局都自少陰人脾胃水穀中出來而少陽人胃熱證藥間或有焉至於太陰人太陽人病情則全昧也

6 岐伯曰傷寒一日巨陽受之故頭項痛腰脊强二日陽明受之陽明主肉其脈挾鼻絡於目故身熱目疼而鼻乾不得臥也三日少陽受之少陽主膽其脈循脇絡於耳故胸脇痛而耳聾三陽經絡皆受其病而未入於臟故可汗而已四日太陰受之太陰脈布胃中絡於嗌故腹滿而嗌乾五日少陰受之少陰脈貫腎絡於肺繫舌本故口燥舌乾而渴六日厥陰受之厥陰脈循陰器而絡於肝故煩滿而囊縮三陰三陽五臟六腑皆受病榮衛不行五臟不通則死矣

7 兩感於寒者必不免於死兩感於寒者一日巨陽少陰俱病則頭痛口乾而煩滿二日陽明太陰俱病腹滿身熱不飮食譫語三日少陽厥陰俱病耳聾囊縮而厥水漿不入口不知人六日死其死皆以六七日之間其愈皆以十日已上

8 論曰靈樞素問假托黃帝異怪幻惑無足稱道方術好事者之言容或如是不必深責也然此書亦是古人之經驗而五臟六腑經絡針法病證修養之辨多有所啓發則實是醫家格致之宗主而苗脈之所自出也不可全數其虛誕之罪而廢其啓發之功也蓋此書亦古之聰慧博物之言方士淵源修養之述也其理有可考而其說不可盡信

9 岐伯所論巨陽少陽少陰經病皆少陽人病也陽明太陰經病皆太陰人病也厥陰經病少陰人病也

1

少陰人腎受熱表熱病論*

1 張仲景傷寒論曰發熱惡寒脈浮者屬表卽太陽證也

2 太陽傷風脈陽浮而陰弱陽浮者熱自發陰弱者汗自出嗇嗇惡寒淅淅惡風翕翕發熱鼻鳴乾嘔桂枝湯主之

3 危亦林得效方曰四時瘟疫當用香蘇散

4 龔信醫鑑曰傷寒頭痛身疼不分表裏證當用藿香正氣散

5 論曰張仲景所論太陽傷風發熱惡寒者卽少陰人腎受熱表熱病也此證發熱惡寒而無汗者當用桂枝湯川芎桂枝湯香蘇散芎歸香蘇散藿香正氣散發熱惡寒而有汗者此亡陽初證也必不可輕易視之先用黃芪桂枝湯補中益氣湯升陽益氣湯三日連服而汗不止病不愈則當用桂枝附子湯人蔘桂枝附子湯升陽益氣附子湯

6 張仲景曰太陽病脈浮緊發熱無汗而衄者自愈也

7 太陽病六七日表證因在脈微而沈反不結胸其人如狂者以熱在下焦小腹當滿小便自利者下血乃愈抵當湯主之

8 太陽證身黃發狂小腹硬滿小便自利者血證宜抵當湯傷寒小腹滿應小便不利今反利者以有血也

9 太陽病不解熱結膀胱其人如狂血自下者自愈但小腹急結者宜攻之宜桃仁承氣湯

10 太陽病外證未除而數下之遂下利不止心下痞硬表裏不解人蔘桂枝湯主之

11 論曰此證其人如狂者腎陽困熱也小腹硬滿者大腸怕寒也二證俱見當先其急腎陽困熱則當用川芎桂枝湯黃芪桂枝湯八物君子湯升補之大腸怕

---

* Part II-1 Discourse on the Lesser Yin Person's Exterior Febrile Disease Induced From the Kidney Affected by Heat

寒則當用藿香正氣散香砂養胃湯和解之若外熱包裏冷而毒氣重結於内或將有養虎遺患之弊則當用巴豆丹下利一二度因以藿香正氣散八物君子湯和解而峻補之

12 張仲景所論下焦血證卽少陰人脾局陽氣爲寒邪所掩抑而腎局陽氣爲邪所拒不能直升連接於脾局鬱縮膀胱之證也其人如狂者其人亂言也如見鬼狀者恍惚譫語也太陽病表證因在者身熱煩惱而惡寒之證間有之也太陽病外證除者身熱煩惱而惡寒之證都無之也此證益氣而升陽則得其上策也破血而解熱則出於下計也太陽病外證未除而數下之逐下利不止云云者亦可見古人之於此證用承氣湯則下利不止故遂變其方而用抵當桃仁湯耳太陽病外證未除則陽氣其力雖有鬱抑猶能振寒而與寒邪相爭於表也若外證盡除則陽氣其力不能振寒而遂爲窮困縮伏之勢也攻下之藥何甚好藥而必待陽氣窮困縮伏之時而應用耶人蔘桂枝湯不亦晩乎

13 張仲景曰婦人傷寒發熱經水適來適斷晝日明了夜則譫語如見鬼狀此爲熱入血室無犯胃氣及上二焦必自愈

14 陽明病口燥嗽水不欲嚥此必衄不可下

15 陽明病不能食攻其熱必噦傷寒嘔多雖有陽明不可攻胃家實不大便若表未解及有半表者先以桂枝柴胡和解乃可下也

16 論曰右諸證當用藿香正氣散香砂養胃湯八物君子湯

17 張仲景曰陽明之爲病胃家實也問曰緣何得陽明病答曰太陽病發汗若下若利小便者此亡津液胃中乾燥因轉屬陽明不更衣内實大便難者此名陽明病也

18 傷寒轉屬陽明其人濈然微汗出也

19 傷寒若吐若下後不解不大便五六日至十餘日日晡所發潮熱不惡寒狂言如見鬼狀若劇者發則不識人循衣摸床惕而不安微喘直視脈弦者生脈濇者死

20 論曰秦漢時醫方治法大便秘燥者有大黃治法無巴豆治法故張仲景亦用大黃大承氣湯治少陰人太陽病轉屬陽明其人濈然微汗出胃中燥煩實不大便五六日至十餘日日晡發潮熱不惡寒狂言如見鬼狀之時而用之則神效若劇者發則不識人循衣摸床惕而不安微喘直視用之於此則脈弦者生脈濇者死蓋此方治少陰人太陽病轉屬陽明不大便五六日日晡發潮熱者可用而其他則不可用也仲景知此方有可用不可用之時候故亦能昭詳少陰人太陽陽明病證候也蓋仲景一心精力都在於深得大承氣湯可用時候故不可用之時候亦昭詳知之也仲景太陽陽明病藥方中惟桂枝湯人蔘桂枝湯得其彷佛而大承氣湯則置人死生於茫無津涯之中必求大承氣湯可用之時候而待其不大便五六日日晡發潮熱狂言時是豈美法也哉蓋少陰人病候自汗不出則脾不弱也大便秘燥則胃實也少陰人太陽陽明病自汗不出脾不弱者輕病也大便雖硬用藥則易愈也故大黃枳實厚朴芒硝之藥亦能成功於此時而劇者猶有半生半死若用八物君子湯升陽益氣湯與巴豆丹則雖劇者亦無脈弦者生脈濇者死之理也又太陽病表證因在時何不早用溫補升陽之藥與巴豆預圖其病而必待陽明病日晡發潮熱狂言時用承氣湯使人半生半死耶

21 許叔微本事方曰一人病傷寒大便不利日晡發潮熱手循衣縫兩手撮空直視喘急諸醫皆走此誠惡候仲景雖有證而無法但云脈弦者生脈濇者死謾且救之與小承氣湯一服而大便利諸疾漸退脈且微弦半月愈

22 王好古海藏書曰一人傷寒發狂欲走脈虛數用柴胡湯反劇以蔘芪歸朮陳皮甘草煎湯一服狂定再服安睡而愈

23 醫學綱目曰嘗治循衣摸床者數人皆用大補氣血之劑惟一人兼瞤振脈代遂於補劑中略加桂亦振止脈和而愈

24 成無己明理論曰潮熱屬陽明必於日晡時發者乃爲潮熱也陽明之爲病胃家實也胃實則譫語手足濈然汗出者此大便已硬也譫語有潮熱承氣湯下之熱不潮者勿服

25 朱震亨丹溪心法曰傷寒壞證昏沈垂死一切危急之證好人蔘一兩水煎一服而盡汗自鼻梁上出涓涓如水

26 論曰右論皆以張仲景大承氣湯始作俑而可用不可用時候難知故紛瘩多惑而始知張仲景之不可信也張仲景大承氣湯元是殺人之藥而非活人之藥則大承氣湯不必擧論此胃家實病不更衣發狂證當用巴豆全粒或用獨蔘八物君子湯或先用巴豆後用八物君子湯以壓之

27 張仲景曰陽明病外證身熱汗自出不惡寒反惡熱

28 傷寒陽明病自汗出小便數則津液內竭大便必難其脾爲約麻仁丸主之

29 陽明病自汗出小便自利者此爲津液內竭大便雖硬不可攻之宜用蜜導法通之

30 陽明病發熱汗多者急下之宜大承氣湯

31 李梴醫學入門曰汗多不止謂之亡陽如心痞胸煩面青膚瞤者難治色黃手足溫者可治凡汗漏不止眞陽脫亡故謂之亡陽其身必冷多成痺寒四肢拘急桂枝附子湯主之

32 嘗治少陰人十一歲兒汗多亡陽病此兒勞心焦思素證有時以泄瀉爲憂而每飯時汗流滿面矣忽一日頭痛發熱汗自出大便秘燥以此兒素證泄瀉爲憂故頭痛身熱便秘汗出之熱證以其反於泄瀉寒證而曾不關心尋常治之以黃芪桂枝白芍藥等屬發表矣至于四五日頭痛發熱不愈六日平明察其證候則大便燥結已四五日小便赤澁二三匙而一晝夜間小便度數不過二三次不惡寒而發熱汗出度數則一晝夜間二三四次不均而人中則或有時有汗或有時無汗汗流滿面滿體其證可惡始覺汗多亡陽證候眞是危證也急用巴豆一粒仍煎黃芪桂枝附子湯用附子一錢連服二貼以壓之至于未刻大便通小便稍淸而稍多其翌日卽得病七日也以小兒附子太過之慮故以黃芪桂枝附子湯一貼分兩日服矣兩日後其兒亡陽證又作不惡寒發熱汗多而小便赤澁大便秘結如前面色帶青間有乾咳病勢比前太甚其日卽得病九日也時則巳時末刻也急用巴豆一粒仍煎人蔘桂枝附子湯用人蔘五錢附子二錢連二貼以壓之至于日晡大便始通小便稍多而色赤則一也又用人蔘桂枝附子湯人蔘五錢附子二錢一貼服矣至于二更夜其兒側臥而頭不能擧自吐痰一二匙而乾咳仍止其翌日又用人蔘桂枝附子湯人蔘五錢附子二錢三貼食粥二三匙每用藥後則身淸凉無汗小便稍多而大便必通又翌日用此方二貼食粥半碗又翌日用此方二貼食粥半碗有餘身淸凉自起坐房室中此日卽得病十二日也此三日內身淸凉無汗大便通小便淸而多者連用附子二錢日二三貼之故也至于十三日又起步門庭而擧頭不能仰面懲前小兒附子太過之慮用黃芪桂枝附子湯用附子一錢每日二貼服至于七八日頭面稍得仰擧而面部浮腫又每日二貼服至于七八日頭面又得仰擧而面部浮腫亦減其後用此方每日二貼服自得病初至於病解前後一月餘用附子凡八兩矣

33 張仲景曰陽明病有三病太陽陽明者脾約是也正陽陽明者胃家實是也少陽陽明者發汗利小便胃中燥煩實大便難是也

34 論曰張仲景所論陽明三病一曰脾約者自汗出小便利之證也二曰胃家實者不更衣大便難之證也三曰發汗利小便胃中燥煩實者此亦胃家實也其實非三病也二病而已仲景意脾約云者津液漸竭脾之潤氣漸約之謂也胃家實云者津液已竭胃之全局燥實之謂也中古戰國秦漢之時醫家單方經驗其苓已久汗吐下三法始爲盛行太陽病表證因在者或以麻黃湯發汗或以猪苓湯利小便或以承氣湯下之承氣湯下之則下利不止之證作矣麻黃湯猪　湯發汗利小便則胃中燥煩實大便難之證作矣仲景有見於此故以脾約之自汗出自利小便者脾之潤氣漸約亦將爲胃燥實之張本矣然脾約自脾約也胃家實自胃家實也寧有其病先自脾約而後至於胃家實之理耶

35 胃家實脾約二病如陰證之太陰少陰病虛實證狀顯然不同自太陽病表證因在時已爲兩路分岐元不相合太陽病表證因在而其人如狂者鬱狂之初證也陽明病胃家實不更衣者鬱狂之中證也陽明病潮熱狂言微喘直視者鬱狂之末證也太陽病發熱惡寒汗自出者亡陽之初證也陽明病不惡寒反惡熱汗自出者亡陽之中證也陽明病發熱汗多者亡陽之末證也蓋鬱狂證都是身熱自汗不出也亡陽證都是身熱自汗出也

36 陰證口中和而有腹痛泄瀉者太陰病也口中不和而有腹痛泄瀉者少陰病也陽證自汗不出而有頭痛身熱者太陽陽明病鬱狂證也自汗出而頭痛身熱者太陽陽明病亡陽證也陰證之太陰病陽證之鬱狂病有輕證重證也陰證之少陰病陽證之亡陽病有險證危證也亡陽少陰病自初痛已爲險證繼而爲危證也

37 亡陽病證非但觀於汗也必觀於小便多少也若小便清利而自汗出則脾約病也此險證也小便赤澁而自汗出則陽明病發熱汗多也此危證也然少陽人裏熱證太陰人表熱證亦有汗多而小便赤澁者宜察之不可誤藥

38 胃家實病其始焉汗不出不惡寒但惡熱而其病垂危則濈然微汗出潮熱也濈然微汗出潮熱者表寒振發之力永竭故也胃竭之候也脾約病其始焉身熱汗自出不惡寒而若其病垂危則發熱汗多而惡寒也發熱汗多而惡寒者裏熱撑支之勢已窮故也脾絶之候也

39 張仲景曰厥陰證手足厥冷小腹痛煩滿囊縮脈微欲絶宜當歸四逆湯

40 凡厥者陰陽氣不相順接便爲厥厥者手足逆冷是也

41 傷寒六七日尺寸脈微緩者厥陰受病也其證小腹煩滿而囊縮宜用承氣湯下之

42 六七日脈至皆大煩而口噤不能言躁擾者必欲解也

43 朱肱活人書曰厥者手足逆冷是也手足指頭微寒者謂之清此疾爲輕陰厥者初得病便四肢厥冷脈沈微而不數足多攣

44 傷寒六七日煩滿囊縮尺寸俱微緩者足厥陰經受病也其脈微浮爲欲愈不浮爲難愈脈浮緩者必囊不縮外證必發熱惡寒爲欲愈宜桂麻各半湯若尺寸俱沈短者必囊縮毒氣入腹宜承氣湯下之速用承氣湯可保五生一死六七日脈微浮者否極泰來水升火降寒熱作而大汗解矣

45 諸手足厥冷皆屬厥陰不可汗下然有須汗須下者謂手足雖逆冷時有溫時手足掌心必煖非正厥逆當消息之

46 李梴曰舌卷厥逆冷過肘膝小腹絞痛三味蔘萸湯四順湯主之囊縮手足乍冷乍溫煩滿者大承氣湯主之

47 論曰張仲景所論厥陰病初無腹痛下利等證而六七日猝然而厥手足逐冷則此非陰證之類也乃少陰人太陽傷風惡寒發熱汗自出之證正邪相持日久當解不解而變爲此證也此證當謂之太陽病厥陰證也此證不必用當歸四逆湯桂麻各半湯而當用蔘萸湯人蔘吳茱萸湯獨蔘八物湯不當用大承氣湯而當用巴豆

48 凡少陰人外感病六七日不得汗解而死者皆死於厥陰也四五日觀其病勢用黃芪桂枝湯八物君子湯三四五貼豫防可也

49 朱肱曰厥陰病消渴氣上衝心心中疼熱飢不欲食食則吐蛔

50 龔信曰傷寒有吐蛔者雖有大熱忌下涼藥犯之必死蓋胃中有寒則蛔不安所而上膈大凶之兆也急用理中湯

51 論曰此證當用理中湯日三四服又連日服或理中湯加陳皮官桂白何首烏

52 重病危證藥不三四服則藥力不壯也又不連日服則病加於少愈也或病愈而不決也連日服者或日再服或日一服或日三服或二三日連日服或五六日連日服或數十日連日服觀其病勢圖之

2

少陰人胃受寒裏寒病論*

1 張仲景曰太陰之證腹滿而吐食不下自利益甚時腹自痛

2 腹滿時痛吐利不渴者爲太陰宜四逆湯理中湯腹滿不減減不足言宜大承氣湯

3 傷寒自利不渴者屬太陰以其臟有寒故也當溫之宜用四逆湯

4 太陰證腹痛自利不渴宜理中湯理中丸四順理中湯丸亦主之

5 論曰右證當用理中湯四順理中湯四逆湯而古方草刱藥力不具備此證當用白何烏理中湯白何烏附子理中湯腹滿不減減不足言者有痼冷積滯也當用巴豆而不當用大承氣湯

6 張仲景曰病發於陰而反下之因作痞傷寒嘔而發熱者若心下滿而不痛此爲痞半夏瀉心湯主之胃虛氣逆者亦主之

7 下後下利日數十行穀不化腹雷鳴心下痞硬乾嘔心煩此乃結熱乃胃中虛客氣上逆故也甘草瀉心湯主之

8 太陰證下利清穀若發汗則必脹滿發汗後腹脹滿宜用厚朴半夏湯

9 汗解後胃不和心下痞硬脇下有水氣腹中雷鳴下利者生薑瀉心湯主之

10 傷寒下利心下痞硬服瀉心湯後以他藥下之利不止與理中湯利益甚赤石脂禹餘粮湯主之

11 論曰病發於陰而反下之云者病發於胃弱當用藿香正氣散而反用大黃下之之謂也麻黃大黃自是太陰人藥非少陰人藥則少陰人病無論表裏麻黃大黃汗下元非可論少陰人病下利清穀者積滯自解也太陰證下利清穀者當用藿香正氣散香砂養胃湯薑朮寬中湯溫胃而降陰少陰證下利清穀者當用官桂附子理中湯健脾而降陰

---

* Part II-2 Discourse on the Lesser Yin Person's Interior Cold Disease Induced From the Stomach Affected by Cold

12 藿香正氣散香砂六君子湯寬中湯蘇合元皆張仲景瀉心湯之變劑也此所謂青於藍者出於藍噫青雖自青若非其藍青何得青

13 張仲景曰傷寒陰毒之病面青身痛如被杖五日可治七日不治

14 李梴曰三陰病深必變爲陰毒其證四肢厥冷吐利不渴靜踡而臥甚則咽痛鄭聲加以頭痛頭汗眼睛內痛不欲見光面脣指甲青黑身如被杖又此證面青白黑四肢厥冷多睡

15 論曰右證當用人蔘桂皮湯人蔘附子理中湯

16 張仲景曰傷寒直中陰經初來無頭痛無身熱無渴怕寒踡臥沈重欲眠脣青厥冷脈微而欲絶或脈伏宜四逆湯四逆者四肢逆冷也

17 論曰嘗治少陰人直中陰經乾藿亂關格之病時屬中伏節候少陰人一人面部氣色或青或白如彈丸圈四五點成團起居如常而坐於房室中倚壁一身委靡無力而但欲寐問其這間原委則曰數日前下利清水一二行仍爲便閉至今爲兩晝夜別無他故云問所飮食則曰食麥飯云急用巴豆如意丹一半時刻其汗自人中穴出而達于面上下利一二度時當日暮觀其下利則清水中雜穢物而出終夜下利十餘行翌日平明至日暮又十餘行下利而清穀麥粒皆如黃豆大其病爲食滯故連三日絶不穀食日所食但進好熟冷一二碗至第三日平明病人面色則無不顯明而一身皆冷頭頸墜下去地二三寸而不能仰擧病證更重計出無聊仔細點檢病人一身則手足膀胱腰腹皆如氷冷臍下全腹堅硬如石而胸腹上中脘熱氣熏騰炙手可熱最爲可觀至第五日平朝一發吐清沫而清沫中雜米穀一朶而出自此病勢大減因進米飮聯服數碗其翌日因爲粥食此病在窮村故未暇溫胃和解之藥其後又有少陰人一人日下利數次而仍下清水全腹浮腫初用桂附藿陳理中湯倍加人蔘官桂各二錢附子二錢或一錢日四服數日後則日三服至十餘日遂下利清穀連三日三四十行而浮腫大減又少陰人小兒一人下利青水面色青黯氣陷如睡用獨蔘湯加生薑二錢陳皮砂仁各一錢日三四服數日後下利十餘行大汗解蓋少陰人藿亂關格病得人中汗者始免危也食滯大下者次免危也自然能吐者快免危也禁進粥食但進好熟冷或米飮者扶正抑邪之良方也宿滯之彌留者得好熟冷乘熱溫進則消化無異於飮食雖絶食二三四日不必爲慮

18 張仲景曰少陰病脈微細但欲寐

19 傷寒欲吐不吐心煩但欲寐五六日自利而渴者屬少陰小便色白宜四逆湯

20 少陰病身體痛手足寒骨節痛脈沈者附子湯主之

21 下利腹脹滿身體疼痛先溫其裏乃攻其表溫裏宜四逆湯攻表宜桂枝湯

22 論曰右證當用官桂附子理中湯

23 張仲景曰少陰病始得之反發熱脈沈者麻黃附子細辛湯主之

24 少陰病一二日口中和背惡寒宜附子湯

25 少陰病二三日用麻黃附子甘草湯微發之以二三日無證故微發汗也無證謂無吐利厥證也

26 下利脈沈而遲其人面小赤身有微汗下利清穀必鬱冒汗出而解病人必微厥所以然者其面戴陽下虛故也

27 少陰病脈細沈數病爲在裏不可發汗少陰病但厥無汗而强發之必動其血

或從口鼻或從目出是爲下厥上渴難治

28 論曰張仲景所論太陰病少陰病俱是少陰人胃氣虛弱泄瀉之證而太陰病泄瀉重證中平證也少陰病泄瀉危證中險證也人但見泄瀉同是一證而易於尋常做圖少陰病泄瀉尋常做圖則必不免死蓋太陰病泄瀉大腸之泄瀉也少陰病泄瀉胃中之泄瀉也太陰病泄瀉溫氣逐冷氣之泄瀉也少陰病泄瀉冷氣逼溫氣之泄瀉也

29 少陰病欲自愈則面小赤身有微汗必鬱冒汗出而解故古人有見於此少陰病但厥無汗者亦以麻黃强發汗欲其自愈而反動其血從口鼻出故於是乎始爲戒懼凡少陰病不敢輕易用麻黃而少陰病始得之一二日二三日初證以麻黃附子甘草湯微發之也然麻黃爲少陰病害藥則雖二三日初證必不可用麻黃發之也此證當用官桂附子理中湯或以桂枝易官桂

30 少陰病初證因爲險證繼而爲危證此病初證早不辨證而措置則危境也凡腹痛自利無口渴口中和者爲太陰病腹痛自利而有口渴口中不和者爲少陰病少陰病有身體痛骨節痛表證此則表裏俱病而大腸寒氣必勝胃中溫氣而上升也太陰病無身體痛骨節痛表證此則裏病表不病而胃中溫氣猶勝大腸寒氣而下降也

31 張仲景曰少陰病自利純青水心下痛口燥乾者宜大承氣湯

32 朱肱曰少陰病口燥咽乾而渴宜急下之非若陽明宜下而可緩也

33 李杲東垣書曰少陰證口中辨口中和者當溫口中乾燥者當下少陰證下利辨色不青者當溫色青者當下

34 李梴曰舌乾口燥或下利清水譫語便閉宜小承氣湯脣青四肢厥冷指甲青黑宜薑附湯

35 論曰下利青水者欲下之則當用巴豆欲溫之則當用官桂附子理中湯下利青水仍爲便閉者先用巴豆後用薑朮寬中湯

36 嘗見少陰人十歲兒思慮耗氣每有憂愁一二日則必腹痛泄瀉一二日用白何烏理中湯二三四貼或甚則附子理中湯一二貼則泄瀉必愈矣忽一日此兒心有憂愁氣度不平數日故豫治次用白何烏理中湯二貼則泄瀉因作下利青水連用六貼青水不止急用附子理中湯六貼青水變爲黑水又二貼黑水泄瀉亦愈又二三貼調理以此觀之則下利青水者病人有藿亂關格而後成此證也此證當用巴豆破積滯痼冷自是無疑此兒十歲冬十二月有下利青水病十一歲春二月又得亡陽病

37 朱肱曰躁無暫定而厥者爲藏厥

38 李梴曰藏厥者發躁無休息時發熱七八日脈微膚冷而躁或吐或瀉無時暫安者乃厥陰眞藏氣絶故曰藏厥仲景無治法而四逆湯冷飮救之又少陰病厥而吐利發躁者亦不治而三味蔘萸湯救之

39 論曰少陰人喜好不定而計窮力屈則心煩躁也少陰病傷寒欲吐不吐心煩但欲寐者此非計窮力屈者之病乎蓋喜好者所慾也何故至於計窮力屈而得此少陰病乎何不早用君子寬平心乎然初證傷寒欲吐不吐心煩但欲寐者早用藥則猶可免死也其病至於躁無暫定而厥則勢在極危也豈不可憐乎此證當用蔘萸湯四逆湯官桂附子理中湯吳茱萸附子理中湯

40 朱肱曰病人身冷脈沈細而疾煩躁而不飮水者陰盛隔陽也若飮水者非此證也厥陰病渴欲飮水者小小與之愈

41 成無己曰煩謂心中鬱煩也躁謂氣外熱躁也但煩不躁及先煩後躁者皆可治但躁不煩及先躁後煩者皆不可治先躁後煩謂怫怫然更作躁悶此陰盛隔陽也雖大躁欲於泥水中臥但水不得入口是也此氣欲絶而爭譬如燈將滅而暴明

42 李梴曰傷寒陰盛隔陽其證身冷反躁欲投井中脣青面黑渴欲飮水復吐大便自利黑水六脈沈細而疾或無脈陰盛隔陽大虛證也宜霹靂散又曰厥逆煩躁者不治

43 論曰此證當用官桂附子理中湯吳茱萸附子理中湯或用霹靂散

44 藏厥與陰盛隔陽病情大同小異俱在極危如存一髮措手難及若論此病之可治上策莫如此證未成之前早用官桂附子理中湯吳茱萸附子理中湯

45 凡觀少陰人病泄瀉初證者當觀於心煩與不煩也心煩則口渴而口中不和也心不煩則口不渴而口中和也觀少陰人病危證者當觀於躁之有定無定也欲觀躁之有定無定則必占心之範圍有定無定也心之範圍綽綽者心之有定而躁之有定也心之範圍耿耿者心之無定而躁之無定也心雖耿耿忽忽猶有一半時刻綽綽卓卓則其病可治可治者用薑附而可效也

46 凡少陰人泄瀉日三度重於一二度也四五度重於二三度也而日四度泄瀉則太重也泄瀉一日輕於二日也二日輕於三四日也而連三日泄瀉則太重也少陰人平人一月間或泄瀉二三次則不可謂輕病人也一日間乾便三四度則不可謂輕病人也下利清穀者雖日數十行口中必不燥乾而冷氣外解也下利清水者腹中必有青水也若下利黃水則非清水而又必雜穢物也

47 張仲景曰傷寒七八日身黃如梔子色小便不利腹微滿屬太陰宜茵蔯蒿湯傷寒但頭汗出餘無汗劑頸而還小便不利身必發黃

48 李梴曰天行疫癘亦能發黃謂之瘟黃殺人最急宜瘴疸丸

49 論曰右證當用茵蔯橘皮湯茵蔯附子湯茵蔯四逆湯瘴疸丸或用巴豆丹

50 醫學綱目曰但結胸無大熱者此爲水結但頭汗出名曰水結胸小半夏湯主之

51 龔信曰寒實結胸無熱證者宜三物白散

52 論曰右證當用桂枝半夏生薑湯赤白何烏寬中湯三物白散或用巴豆丹

53 少陽人病心下結硬者名曰結胸病其病可治也少陰人病心下結硬者名曰藏結病其病不治也醫學綱目醫鑑所論水結胸寒實結胸證藥俱是少陰人太陰病而與張仲景茵蔯蒿湯證相類則此病想必非眞結硬於心下而卽痞滿於心下者也張仲景瀉心湯證傷寒下利心下痞硬汗解後心下痞硬云者亦皆痞滿於心下或臍上近處結硬也而非眞結硬於心下者也若少陰人病而心下右邊結硬則不治

54 張仲景曰病有結胸有藏結其狀如何曰按之痛寸脈浮關脈沈名曰結胸也何謂藏結曰如結胸狀飮食如故時時下利寸脈浮關脈細小沈緊名曰藏結舌上白胎滑者難治病人胸中素有痞連在臍傍引入小腹入陰筋者此名藏結死

55 朱肱曰藏結狀如結胸飮食如故時時下利而舌上白胎歌曰飮食如常時下利更加舌上白胎時連臍腹痛引陰筋此疾元來死不醫

56 論曰嘗見少陰人一人心下右邊結硬百藥無效與巴豆如意丹反劇搖頭動

風有頃而止數月後死其後又有少陰人一人有此證者用巴豆丹面上身上有汗而獨上脣人中穴左右邊無汗此人一周年後亦死凡少陰人心下結硬有此證者目睹四五人或半年或一年針灸醫藥無不周至而個個無回生之望此卽藏結病而少陰人病也

57 張仲景曰黃疸之病當以十八日爲期十日以上宜差反劇爲難治發於陰部其人必嘔發於陽部其人振寒而發熱

58 諸疸小便黃赤色者爲濕熱當作濕熱治小便色白不可除熱者無熱也若有虛寒證當作虛勞治

59 腹脹滿面萎黃躁不得睡

60 黃家日晡時當發熱反惡寒此爲女勞得之膀胱急小腹滿一身盡黃額上黑足下熱因作黑疸腹脹如水狀大便黑或時溏此女勞之病非水也腹滿者難治

61 朱肱曰陰黃煩躁喘嘔不渴宜用茵蔯橘皮湯一人傷寒發黃脈微弱身冷次第用藥至茵蔯四逆湯大效一人傷寒發黃脈沈細遲無力次第用藥至茵蔯附子湯大效

62 醫學綱目曰濕家之黃色暗不明一身不痛熱家之黃如橘子一身盡痛

63 王好古曰凡病當汗而不汗當利小便而不利亦生黃

64 朱震亨曰黃疸因食積者下其食積其餘但利小便小便利白其黃自退

65 李梴曰黃疸十日以上入腹喘滿煩渴面黑者死

66 王叔和脈經曰黃家寸口脈近掌無脈口鼻冷黑色並不可治

67 論曰陰黃卽少陰人病也當用朱氏茵蔯橘皮湯茵蔯四逆湯女勞之黃熱家之黃利小便之黃想或非少陰人病而余所經驗未嘗一遇黃疸而治之故未得仔細裏許然痞滿黃疸浮腫同出一證而有輕重若欲利小便則乾薑良薑陳皮青皮香附子益智仁能利少陰人小便荊芥防風羌活獨活茯苓澤瀉能利少陽人小便

3

少陰人泛論*

1 論曰發熱惡寒者爲太陽病發熱不惡寒者爲陽明病太陽陽明之發熱形證一也而惡寒不惡寒之間相去遠甚而陽氣之進退强弱泰山之比岡陵也自利而不渴者爲太陰病自利而渴者爲少陰病太陰少陰之自利形證一也而渴不渴之間相去遠甚而冷氣之聚散輕重雲夢之比瀦澤也是故藿香正氣散香砂養胃湯之證勢平地駿馬之病勢也獨蔘八物湯桂附理中湯之證勢太行短笻之病勢也若使一天下少陰人稟賦者自知其病之陽明少陰證如太行之險路得之可畏救之不易攝身療病戒懼謹愼之道有若大路然而不迷則其庶幾乎

2 太陽病汗出熱氣卻寒氣之汗出也陽明病汗出寒氣犯熱氣之汗出也太陰病下利溫氣逐冷氣之下利也少陰病下利冷氣逼溫氣之下利也

3 少陰人病有二吉證人中汗一吉證也能飮水一吉證也

4 少陰人病有二急證發熱汗多一急證也下利淸水一急證也

5 少陰人病有六大證一曰少陰病二曰陽明病三曰太陰病陰毒證也四曰太陽病厥陰證也五曰太陰病黃疸證也六曰太陽病胃家實證也

6 發熱汗出則病必解也而發熱汗出而病益甚者陽明病也通滯下利則病必解也而通滯下利而病益甚者少陰病也陽明少陰以邪犯正之病不可不急用藥也惡寒汗出則病必盡解也而惡寒汗出而其病半解半不解者厥陰之漸也腹痛下利則病必盡解也而腹痛下利而其病半解半不解者陰毒之漸也厥陰陰毒正邪相傾之病不可不預用藥也發熱一汗而病卽解者太陽之輕病也食滯一下而病卽解者太陰之輕病也太陽太陰之輕病不用藥而亦自愈也發熱三日不得汗解者太陽之尤病也食滯三日不能化下者太陰之尤病也太陽太陰之尤病已不可謂輕證而用藥二三貼亦自愈也發熱六日不得汗解食滯六日不能化下者太陽太陰之胃家實黃疸病也太陽太陰之胃家實黃疸正邪壅錮之病不可不大用藥也

* Part II-3 General Remarks on the Lesser Yin Person

7 太陽太陰之病六七日或成危證或成重證而十日内必有險證陽明少陰之病自始發已爲重證而二三日内亦致險證是故陽明少陰之病不可不察於始發也太陽太陰之病不可不察於四五日間也

8 太陽太陰之病病勢緩而能曠日持久故變證多也陽明少陰之病病勢急而不能曠日持久故變證少也蓋陽明少陰病過一日而至二日則不可不用藥也太陽太陰病過四日而至五日則不可不用藥也太陽太陰之厥陰陰毒皆六七日之死境也尤不可不謹也

9 陽明太陽之危者獨蔘八物湯補中益氣湯可以解之而病勢危時若非日三四服而又連日服則難解也少陰太陰之危者獨蔘附子理中湯桂附藿陳理中湯可以解之而病勢危時若非日三四服而又連日服則難解也病勢極危時日四服病勢半危時日三服病勢不減則日二服病勢少減則二日三服而一日則一服一日則二服病勢大減則日一服病勢又大減則間二三四五日一服蓋有病者可以服藥無病者不可以服藥重病可以重藥輕病不可以重藥若輕病好用重藥無病者好服藥臟氣脆弱益招病矣

10 膏粱雖則助味常食則損味羊裘雖則禦寒常着則攝寒膏粱羊裘猶不可以常食常着況藥乎若論常服藥之有害則反爲百倍於全不服藥之無利也蓋有病者明知其證則必不可不服藥無病者雖明知其證必不可服藥歷觀於世之服鴉片煙水銀山參鹿茸者屢服則無不促壽者以此占之則可知矣

11 少陰人吐血當用獨蔘八物湯咽喉痛當用獨蔘官桂理中湯

12 嘗見少陰人飮食倍常口味甚甘不過一月其人浮腫而死少陰人食消卽浮腫之屬而危證也不可不急治當用芎歸葱蘇理中湯

13 嘗見少陰人浮腫獐肝一部切片作膾一服盡連用五部其病卽效又有少陰人服獐肝一部眼力倍常眞氣湧出少陽人虛勞病服獐肝一部其人吐血而死

14 嘗見少陰人浮腫有醫教以服海鹽自然汁日半匙四五日服浮腫大減一月服永爲完健病不再發

15 嘗見少陰人咽喉痛經年不愈有醫教以服金蛇酒卽效金蛇酒卽金色黃章蛇釀酒者也

16 嘗見少陰人痢疾有醫教以服項赤蛇煎湯卽效項赤蛇去頭斷尾納二疊紬囊中藥缸内別設横木懸空掛之用水五碗煎取一碗服二疊紬囊懸空掛煎者恐犯蛇骨故也蛇骨有毒

17 嘗見少陰人痢疾有醫教以大蒜三顆清蜜半匙同煎三日服卽效

18 嘗見少陰人乳傍近脇有漏瘡歷七八月瘡口不合惡汁常流有醫教以山參熊膽末各一分傅之卽效又少陰人一人滿身有瘡以人蔘末塗傅卽效

19 嘗見少陰人乳傍近脇發内癰有醫教以火針取膿醫曰内癰外證惡寒發熱似傷寒而有痛處也察其痛處明知有膿則不可不用火針

20 嘗見少陰人背癰有醫教以火刀裂瘡醫曰火刀裂瘡宜早也若疑訝而緩不及事則全背堅硬悔之無及

21 嘗見少陰人半身不遂病有醫教以服鐵液水得效

22 嘗見少陰人小兒腹瘧病有醫教以瘧病將發之早朝用火煅金頂砒極細末六厘生甘草湯調下卽效醫曰砒藥必金頂砒然後可用而又火煅然後可用

也必不可過六厘而又不可不及六厘也過六厘則藥毒太過也不及六厘則瘧不愈也此藥屢試屢驗而有一服愈後瘧又再發者又用之則其病益甚而危蓋此藥可以一服不可再服云聽醫言而究其理則一服愈而瘧不再發者皆少陰人兒也一服愈而瘧又再發者皆非少陰人兒也惟少陰人兒腹瘧病難治者用此藥尋常瘧不必用此不祥之藥少陰人尋常間日瘧惡寒時用川芎桂枝湯二三貼則亦無不愈又腹中實滿而大便硬瘧發者亦可用巴豆

23 百藥莫非善藥而惟少陰人信砒藥太陰人瓜蒂藥最爲惡藥也何哉少陰人信砒藥百病用之皆殆而秖有治瘧之一能者亦有名無實不無危慮萬不如桂枝人蔘白芍藥三四服之治瘧則此非天下萬害無用之藥乎太陰人瓜蒂藥百病用之皆殆而秖有治痰涎壅塞之一能者亦有名無實不無危慮萬不如桔梗麥門冬五味子三四服之治痰涎壅塞則此非天下萬害無用之藥乎此二藥外治可用內服不可用

24 嘗見少陰人中氣病舌卷不語有醫針合谷穴而其效如神其他諸病之藥不能速效者針能速效者有之蓋針穴亦有太少陰陽四象人應用之穴而必有升降緩束之妙繫是不可不察敬俟後之謹厚而好活人者

3-1

張仲景傷寒論中少陰人病經驗設方藥二十三方*

1 桂枝湯桂枝三錢白芍藥二錢甘草一錢薑三片棗二枚

2 理中湯人蔘白朮乾薑各二錢甘草灸一錢

3 薑附湯乾薑炮兩附子竝炮一枚剉取五錢水煎服附子生用名曰白通湯

4 四順理中湯人蔘白朮乾薑甘草灸各二錢

5 人蔘桂枝湯甘草灸桂枝各一錢八分白朮人蔘乾薑各一錢五分

6 四逆湯甘草灸六錢乾薑炮五錢生附子一枚剉分二貼水煎服

7 厚朴半夏湯厚朴三錢人蔘半夏各一錢五分甘草七分五厘薑七片

8 半夏散半夏製甘草灸桂枝各二錢

9 赤石脂禹餘粮湯赤石脂禹餘粮各二錢五分

10 附子湯白朮四錢白芍藥白茯苓各三錢附子炮人蔘各二錢

11 麻黃附子細辛湯麻黃細辛各二錢附子炮一錢

12 麻黃附子甘草湯麻黃甘草各三錢附子炮一錢

13 當歸四逆湯白芍藥當歸各二錢桂枝一錢五分細辛通草甘草各一錢

14 半夏瀉心湯半夏製二錢人蔘甘草黃芩各一錢五分乾薑一錢黃連五分薑三片棗二枚

15 生薑瀉心湯生薑半夏各二錢人蔘乾薑各一錢五分黃連甘草各一錢黃芩五分棗三枚

16 甘草瀉心湯甘草二錢乾薑黃芩各一錢五分半夏製人蔘各一錢棗三枚

---

* Part II-3-1 Twenty Three Prescriptions for the Lesser Yin Person's Disease form Zhang Zhongjing's 『*Shanghanlun*』

17 茵蔯蒿湯茵蔯一兩大黃五錢梔子二錢先煎茵蔯減半納二味煎又減半服日二小便當利色正赤腹漸減黃從小便去也

18 抵當湯水蛭虻蟲竝炒去足翅桃仁留尖各十枚大黃蒸三錢

19 桃仁承氣湯大黃三錢桂心芒硝各二錢甘草一錢桃仁留尖十枚

20 麻仁丸大黃蒸四兩枳實厚朴赤芍藥各二兩麻子仁一兩五錢杏仁一兩二錢五分爲末蜜丸梧子大空心溫湯下五十丸

21 蜜導法老人虛人不可用藥者用蜜熬入皂角末少許捻作錠子納肛門卽通

22 大承氣湯大黃四錢厚朴枳實芒硝各二錢水二大盞先煎枳朴至一盞乃下大黃煎至七分去滓入芒硝再一沸溫服

23 小承氣湯大黃四錢厚朴枳實各一錢五分剉作一貼水煎服

3-2

宋元明三代醫家著述中少陰人病經驗行用要藥十三方巴豆藥六方*

1 十全大補湯人蔘白朮白芍藥甘草灸黃芪肉桂當歸川芎白茯苓熟地黃各一錢薑三片棗二枚此方出於王好古海藏書中治虛勞今考更定此方當去白茯苓熟地黃當用砂仁陳皮

2 補中益氣湯黃芪一錢五分甘草灸人蔘白朮各一錢當歸陳皮各七分升麻柴胡各三分薑三片棗二枚此方出於李杲東垣書中治勞倦虛弱身熱而煩自汗倦怠今考更定此方黃芪當用三錢而當去升麻柴胡當用藿香紫蘇葉

3 香砂六君子湯香附子白朮白茯苓半夏陳皮厚朴白豆蔲各一錢人蔘甘草木香縮砂益智仁各五分薑三片棗二枚此方出於龔信醫鑑書中治不思飮食食不下食後倒飽今考更定此方當去白茯苓當用白何首烏

4 木香順氣散烏藥香附子靑皮陳皮厚朴枳殼半夏各一錢木香縮砂各五分桂皮乾薑甘草灸各三分薑三片棗二枚此方出於龔信萬病回春書中治中氣病中氣者與人相爭暴怒氣逆而暈倒也先以薑湯救之甦後用此藥

5 蘇合香元白朮木香沈香麝香丁香安息香白檀香訶子皮香附子華撥犀角朱砂各二兩朱砂半爲衣蘇合油入安息香膏內乳香龍腦各一兩右細末用安息香膏竝煉蜜搜和千搗每一兩分作四十丸每取二三丸井華水或溫水下此方出於局方治一切氣疾中氣上氣氣逆氣鬱氣痛許叔微本事方曰凡人暴喜傷陽暴怒傷陰憂愁怫意氣多厥逆當用此藥若槩作中風治多致殺人危亦林得效方曰中風脈浮身溫口多痰涎中氣脈沈身涼口無痰涎今考更定此方當去麝香犀角朱砂龍腦乳香當用藿香茴香桂皮五靈脂玄胡索

6 藿香正氣散藿香一錢五分紫蘇葉一錢厚朴大腹皮白朮陳皮半夏甘草桔梗白芷白茯苓各五分薑三片棗二枚此方出於龔信醫鑑書中治傷寒今考更定此方當去桔梗白芷白茯苓當用桂皮乾薑益智仁

---

* Part II-3-2 Thirteen Prescriptions and Six Other Prescriptions Containing Semen Crotonis for the Lesser Yin Person's Disease Mentioned in the Writings of Famous Doctors in the Song, Yuan and Ming Dynasties

7 香蘇散香附子三錢紫蘇葉二錢五分陳皮一錢五分蒼朮甘草各一錢薑三片蔥白二莖此方出於危亦林得效方書中治四時瘟疫局方曰昔有一老人授此方與一人令其合施城中大疫服此皆愈

8 桂枝附子湯附子炮桂枝各三錢白芍藥二錢甘草灸一錢薑三片棗二枚此方出於李梴醫學入門書中治汗漏不止四肢拘急難以屈伸

9 茵蔯四逆湯茵蔯一兩附子乾薑竝炮甘草灸各一錢治陰黃病冷汗不止

10 茵蔯附子湯茵蔯一兩附子炮甘草灸各一錢治陰黃病身冷

11 茵蔯橘皮湯茵蔯一兩陳皮白朮半夏生薑各一錢治陰黃病喘嘔不渴
右三方出於朱肱活人書中

12 三味蔘萸湯吳茱萸三錢人蔘二錢薑四片棗二枚治厥陰證嘔吐涎沫少陰證厥冷煩躁陽明證食穀欲嘔皆妙

13 霹靂散附子一枚炮過以冷灰培半時取出切半枚細剉入臘茶一錢水一盞煎至六分去渣入熟蜜半匙放冷服之須臾躁止得睡汗出差治陰盛隔陽證
右二方出於李梴醫學入門書中

14 溫白元川烏炮二兩五錢吳茱萸桔梗柴胡石菖蒲紫菀黃連乾薑炮肉桂川椒炒赤茯苓皂角灸厚朴人蔘巴豆霜各五錢右爲末煉蜜和丸梧子大薑湯下三丸或五丸至七丸此方出於局方治積聚癥癖黃疸鼓脹十種水氣九種心痛八種痞塞五種淋疾遠年瘧疾龔信醫鑑曰婦人腹中積聚有似懷孕羸瘦困弊或歌哭如邪祟服此藥自愈久病服之則皆瀉出蟲蛇惡膿之物

15 瘴疸丸茵蔯梔子大黃芒硝各一兩杏仁六錢常山鱉甲巴豆霜各四錢豆豉二錢右爲末蒸餠和丸梧子大每三丸或五丸溫水送下此方出於危亦林得效方書中一名茵蔯丸治時行瘟疫及瘴瘧黃疸濕熱病

16 三稜消積丸三稜蓬朮神麴各七錢巴豆和皮入米同炒黑去米青皮陳皮茴香各五錢丁香皮益智仁各三錢右爲末醋糊和丸梧子大薑湯下三四十丸此方出於李杲東垣書中治生冷物不消滿悶

17 秘方化滯丸三稜蓬朮竝煨各四錢八分半夏麴木香丁香青皮陳皮竝去白黃連各二錢五分巴豆肉醋浸一宿熬乾六錢右爲末以烏梅末入麵少許煮作糊和丸黍尖大每服五七丸至十丸欲通利則以熱湯下欲磨積則陳皮湯下欲止泄則飮冷水此方出於朱震亨丹溪心法書中理一切氣化一切積久堅沈痼磨之自消暴積乍留導之立法奪造化有通塞之功調陰陽有補瀉之妙

18 三物白散桔梗貝母各三錢巴豆去皮心熬研如脂一錢右爲末和勻白湯和服半錢弱人減半或吐或利不利進熱粥一碗利不止進冷粥一碗

19 如意丹川烏炮八錢檳榔人蔘柴胡吳茱萸川椒白茯苓白薑黃連紫菀厚朴肉桂當歸桔梗皂角石菖蒲各五錢巴豆霜二錢五分右爲末煉蜜和丸梧子大朱砂爲衣每五丸或七丸溫水下專治瘟疫及一切鬼祟右二方出於李梴醫學入門書中
論曰右巴豆六方卽古人之各自置方各自經驗而此六方同是一巴豆之力則所用亦無異而同歸於一也蓋巴豆少陰人病之必不可不用而又不可輕用必不可浪用而又不可疑用之藥故聯錄六方備述經驗昭明其理者欲其用之必中而不敢輕忽也

3-3

新定少陰人病應用要藥二十四方*

1 黃芪桂枝附子湯桂枝黃芪各三錢白芍藥二錢當歸甘草炙各一錢附子炮一錢或二錢薑三片棗二枚

2 人蔘桂枝附子湯人蔘四錢桂枝三錢白芍藥黃芪各二錢當歸甘草炙各一錢附子炮一錢或二錢薑三片棗二枚

3 升陽益氣附子湯人蔘桂枝白芍藥黃芪各二錢白何首烏官桂當歸甘草炙各一錢附子炮一錢或二錢薑三片棗二枚

4 人蔘官桂附子湯人蔘五錢或一兩官桂黃芪各三錢白芍藥二錢當歸甘草炙各一錢附子炮二錢或二錢五分薑三片棗二枚右四方皆亡陽危病藥也亡陽病人小便白而多危有餘地則用附子一錢日再服小便赤而少危無餘地則用附子二錢日二三服病在將危用一錢病在免危用一錢病在調理亦一錢日再服

5 升陽益氣湯人蔘桂枝黃芪白芍藥各二錢白何首烏官桂當歸甘草炙各一錢薑三片棗二枚

6 補中益氣湯人蔘黃芪各三錢甘草炙白朮當歸陳皮各一錢藿香蘇葉各三分或五分薑三片棗二枚

7 黃芪桂枝湯桂枝三錢白芍藥黃芪各二錢白何首烏當歸甘草炙各一錢薑三片棗二枚

8 川芎桂枝湯桂枝三錢白芍藥二錢川芎蒼朮陳皮甘草炙各一錢薑三片棗二枚

9 芎歸香蘇散香附子二錢紫蘇葉川芎當歸蒼朮陳皮甘草炙各一錢葱白五莖薑三片棗二枚

10 藿香正氣散藿香一錢五分紫蘇葉一錢蒼朮白朮半夏陳皮青皮大腹皮桂

---

* Part II-3-3 Twenty Four Newly Created Prescriptions for the Lesser Yin Person's Disease

皮乾薑益智仁甘草炙各五分薑三片棗二枚

11 八物君子湯人蔘二錢黃芪白朮白芍藥當歸川芎陳皮甘草炙各一錢薑三片棗二枚本方以白何首烏易人蔘則名曰白何首烏君子湯本方用蔘芪各一錢加白何首烏官桂各一錢則名曰十全大補湯本方用人蔘一兩黃芪一錢則名曰獨蔘八物湯

12 香附子八物湯香附子當歸白芍藥各二錢白朮白何首烏川芎陳皮甘草炙各一錢薑三片棗二枚嘗治婦人思慮傷脾咽乾舌燥隱隱有頭痛神效

13 桂枝半夏生薑湯生薑三錢桂枝半夏各二錢白芍藥白朮陳皮甘草炙各一錢治虛寒嘔吐水結胸等證

14 香砂養胃湯人蔘白朮白芍藥甘草炙半夏香附子陳皮乾薑山査肉砂仁白豆蔻各一錢薑三片棗二枚

15 赤白何烏寬中湯白何首烏赤何首烏良薑乾薑青皮陳皮香附子益智仁各一錢棗二枚治四體倦怠小便不快陽道不興將有浮腫之漸者用之本方加厚朴枳實木香大腹皮各五分則又有通氣脈之功力雖浮腫已成者安心靜慮一百日而日再服則自無不效之理本方以人蔘易赤何首烏則名曰人蔘白何烏寬中湯以當歸易赤何首烏則名曰當歸白何烏寬中湯古方有乾薑良薑青皮陳皮等分作湯丸名曰寬中湯嘗治少陰人小便不快陽道不興四體倦怠無力者用之必效百發百中又寬中丸本方加五靈脂益智仁各一錢則治腹痛神效

16 蒜蜜湯白何首烏白朮白芍藥桂枝茵蔯益母草赤石脂罌粟殼各一錢薑三片棗二枚大蒜五根清蜜半匙治痢疾

17 鷄蔘膏人蔘一兩桂皮一錢鷄一首濃煎服或以胡椒清蜜助滋味無妨此方自古有方治瘧疾痢疾神效嘗治久瘧先用巴豆通利大便後數三日連用鷄蔘膏快效桂皮或以桂心代用

18 巴豆丹巴豆一粒去殼取粒溫水呑下全粒或半粒仍煎湯藥以煎藥時刻巴豆獨行腸胃間太半用力然後服湯藥則湯藥可以與巴豆同行通快腸胃升提其氣也再煎湯藥大便通後又連服之巴豆全粒下利半粒化積

19 人蔘陳皮湯人蔘一兩生薑砂仁陳皮各一錢棗二枚本方以炮乾薑易生薑又加桂皮一錢則尤有溫胃逐冷之力以本方嘗治未周年小兒陰毒慢風連服數日病快愈矣病愈後更不服藥再發不治

20 人蔘吳茱萸湯人蔘一兩吳茱萸生薑各三錢白芍藥當歸官桂各一錢

21 官桂附子理中湯人蔘三錢白朮乾薑炮官桂各二錢白芍藥陳皮甘草炙各一錢附子炮一錢或二錢

22 吳茱萸附子理中湯人蔘白朮乾薑炮官桂各二錢白芍藥陳皮甘草炙吳茱萸小茴香破故紙各一錢附子炮一錢或二錢

23 白何烏附子理中湯白何首烏白朮炒白芍藥微炒桂枝乾薑炮各二錢陳皮甘草炙附子炮各一錢

24 白何烏理中湯白何首烏白朮白芍藥桂枝乾薑炮各二錢陳皮甘草炙各一錢有人蔘則用人蔘無人蔘則用白何首烏白何首烏與人蔘性味相近而清越之力不及溫補之力過之不無異同之處險病危證人蔘二錢以上不可全恃白何首烏代用古方經驗不多藥材生踈故也然此一味必不可遺棄於補

藥中而古方何人飲用白何首烏五錢治瘧病右少陰人藥諸種附子炮用甘草灸用乾薑炮用或生用黃芪灸用或生用窮巷僻村病起倉卒雖單方猶百勝於束手無策陽明病雖單黃芪桂皮人蔘芍藥亦可用少陰病雖單附子芍藥人蔘甘草亦可用太陽病雖單蘇葉蔥白黃芪桂枝亦可用太陰病雖單白朮乾薑陳皮藿香亦可用爲先用單方而一邊求得全方則必無救病失機之理然當用全方中所有之藥不當用全方中所無

1

少陽人脾受寒表寒病論*

1 張仲景曰太陽病脈浮緊發熱惡寒身痛不汗出而煩躁者大青龍湯主之

2 論曰發熱惡寒脈浮緊身痛不汗出而煩躁者卽少陽人脾受寒表寒病也此證不當用大青龍湯當用荊防敗毒散

3 張仲景曰少陽之爲病口苦咽乾目眩

4 眩而口苦舌乾者屬少陽

5 口苦耳聾胸滿者少陽傷風證也

6 口苦咽乾目眩耳聾胸脇滿或往來寒熱而嘔屬少陽忌吐下宜小柴胡湯和之

7 論曰此證不當用小柴胡湯當用荊防敗毒散荊防導赤散荊防瀉白散

8 張仲景所論少陽病口苦咽乾胸脇滿或往來寒熱之證卽少陽人腎局陰氣爲熱邪所陷而脾局陰氣爲熱邪所壅不能下降連接於腎局而凝聚膂間膠固囚滯之病也此證嘔者外寒包裏熱而挾痰上逆也寒熱往來者脾局陰氣欲降未降而或降故寒熱或往或來也口苦咽乾目眩耳聾者陰氣囚滯膂間欲降未降故但寒無熱而至於耳聾也口苦咽乾目眩者例證也耳聾者重證也胸脇滿者結胸之漸也脇滿者猶輕也胸滿者重證也古人之於此證用汗吐下三法則其病輒生譫語壞證病益危險故仲景變通之而用小柴胡湯清痰燥痰溫冷相雜平均和解欲其病不轉變而自愈此法以汗吐下三法論之則可謂近善而巧矣然此小柴胡湯亦非平均和解病不轉變之藥則從古斯今得此病者眞是寒心矣耳聾胸滿傷風之病豈可以小柴胡湯擬之乎噫後來龔信所製荊防敗毒散豈非少陽人表寒病三神山不死藥乎此證清裏熱而降表陰則痰飮自散而結胸之證預防不成也清痰而燥痰則無益於陰降痰散延拖結胸將成而或別生奇證也

9 朱肱曰凡發汗腰以上雖淋漓而腰以下至足微潤則病終不解

---

* Part Ⅲ-1 Discourse on the Lesser Yang Person's Exterior Cold Disease Induced form the Spleen Affected by Cold

10 論曰少陽人病無論表裏病手足掌心有汗則病解手足掌心不汗則雖全體皆汗而病不解

11 少陽人傷寒病有再痛三痛發汗而愈者此病非再三感風寒而再痛發汗三痛發汗也少陽人頭痛腦强寒熱往來耳聾胸滿尤甚之病元來如此表邪深結至於三痛然後方解也無論初痛再痛三痛用荊防敗毒散或荊防導赤散荊防瀉白散每日二貼式至病解而用之病解後又用十餘貼如此則自無後病而完健

12 張仲景曰少陽證濈濈汗出心下痞硬滿引脅下痛乾嘔短氣不惡寒表解裏未和也宜十棗湯若合下不下令人脹滿遍身浮腫

13 傷寒表未解醫反下之膈内拒痛手不可近心下滿而硬痛此爲結胸宜大陷胸湯

14 渴欲飮水水入卽吐名曰水逆五苓散主之

15 杜壬曰裏未和者蓋痰與燥氣壅於中焦故頭痛乾嘔汗出痰隔也非十棗湯不治

16 龔信曰心下硬痛手不可近燥渴譫語大便實脈沈實有力爲大結胸大陷胸湯下之反加煩躁者死小結胸正在心下按之則痛宜小陷胸湯

17 論曰右張仲景所論三證皆結胸病而膈内拒痛手不可近燥渴譫語者結胸之最尤甚證也飮水水入卽吐心下痞硬滿乾嘔短氣者次證也凡結胸病皆藥湯入口輒還吐惟甘遂末入口口涎含下因以溫水嗽口而下則藥不還吐嘗治結胸用甘遂散溫水調下五次輒還吐至六次不還吐而下利一度其翌日又水還吐又用甘遂一次快通利而病愈凡結胸無非險證當先用甘遂仍煎荊防導赤散以壓之乾嘔短氣而藥不還吐者不用甘遂但用荊防導赤散加茯苓澤瀉各一錢二三服又連日服而亦病愈燥渴譫語者尤極險證也急用甘遂仍煎地黃白虎湯三四貼以壓之又連日服地黃白虎湯張仲景曰傷寒表未解醫反下之云者以大承氣湯下之之謂也非十棗陷胸下之之謂也然十棗陷胸不如單用甘遂或用甘遂天一丸結胸甘遂末例用三分大結胸用五分龔信所論燥渴譫語煩躁死者若十棗湯下後因以譫語證治之連用白虎湯則煩躁者必無不治之理

18 甘遂表寒病破水結之藥也石膏裏熱病通大便之藥也表病可用甘遂而不可用石膏裡病可用石膏而不可用甘遂然揚手擲足引飮泄瀉證用石膏痺風膝寒大便不通證用甘遂

19 少陰人傷寒病有小腹硬滿之證少陽人傷寒病有心下結胸之證此二證俱是表氣陰陽虛弱正邪相爭累日不決之中裡氣亦秘澁不和而變生此證也

20 李子建傷寒十勸論曰傷寒腹痛亦有熱證不可輕服溫煖藥又曰傷寒自利當觀陰陽證不可例服溫煖及止瀉藥

21 朱震亨曰傷寒陽證身熱脈數煩渴引飮大便自利宜柴苓湯

22 盤龍山老人論曰少陽人身熱頭痛泄瀉當用猪苓車前子湯荊防瀉白散身寒腹痛泄瀉當用滑石苦參湯荊防地黃湯此病名謂之亡陰病

23 少陽人身熱頭痛泄瀉一二日或三四日而泄瀉無故自止身熱頭痛不愈大便反秘者此危證也距譫語不遠

24 泄瀉後大便一晝夜間艱辛一次滑利或三四五次小小滑利身熱頭痛因存者此便秘之兆也譫語前有此證則譫語當在數日譫語後有此證則動風必

在咫尺

25 少陽人忽然有吐者必生奇證也當用荊防敗毒散以觀動靜而身熱頭痛泄瀉者用石膏無疑身寒腹痛泄瀉者用黃連苦參無疑

26 嘗見少陽人兒生未一周年忽先一吐而後泄瀉身熱頭痛揚手擲足轉輾其身引飮泄瀉四五六次無度數者用荊防瀉白散日三貼兩日六貼然後泄瀉方止身熱頭痛清淨又五六貼而安

27 少陽人身熱頭痛揚手擲足引飮者此險證也雖泄瀉必用石膏無論泄瀉有無當用荊防瀉白散加黃連瓜蔞各一錢或地黃白虎湯

28 凡少陽人有身熱頭痛則已非輕證而兼有泄瀉則危險證也必用荊防瀉白散日二三服又連日服身熱頭痛清淨然後可免危險

29 少陽人身寒腹痛泄瀉一晝夜間三四五次者當用滑石苦參湯身寒腹痛二三晝夜間無泄瀉或艱辛一次泄瀉者當用滑石苦參湯或用熟地黃苦參湯

30 嘗見少陽人恒有腹痛患苦者用六味地黃湯六十貼而病愈又見少陽人十餘年腹痛患苦一次起痛則或五六個月或三四個月一二個月叫苦者每起痛臨時急用滑石苦參湯十餘貼不痛時平心靜慮恒戒哀心怒心如此延拖一周年而病愈又見少陽人少年兒恒有滯證痞滿間有腹痛腰痛又有口眼喎斜初證者用獨活地黃湯一百日內二百貼服使之平心靜慮恒戒哀心怒心一百日而身健病愈

31 古醫有言頭無冷痛腹無熱痛此言非也何謂然耶少陰人元來冷勝則其頭痛亦自非熱痛而卽冷痛也少陽人元來熱勝則其腹痛亦自非冷痛而卽熱痛也古醫又言汗多亡陽下多亡陰此言是也何謂然耶少陰人雖則冷勝然陰盛格陽敗陽外遁則煩熱而汗多也此之謂亡陽病也少陽人雖則熱勝然陽盛格陰敗陰內遁則畏寒而泄下也此之謂亡陰病也亡陽亡陰病非用藥必死也不急治必死也

32 亡陽者陽不上升而反爲下降則亡陽也亡陰者陰不下降而反爲上升則亡陰也陰盛格陽於上則陽爲陰抑不能上升於胸膈下陷大腸而外遁膀胱故背表煩熱而汗出也煩熱而汗出者非陽盛也此所謂內冰外炭陽將亡之兆也陽盛格陰於下則陰爲陽壅不能下降於膀胱上逆背膂而內遁膈裡故腸胃畏寒而泄下也畏寒而泄下者非陰盛也此所謂內炭外冰陰將亡之兆也

33 少陰人病一日發汗陽氣上升人中穴先汗則病必愈也而二日三日汗不止病不愈則陽不上升而亡陽無疑也少陽人病一日滑利陰氣下降手足掌心先汗則病必愈也而二日三日泄不止病不愈則陰不下降而亡陰無疑也凡亡陽亡陰證明知醫理者得病前可以預執證也得病一二日明白易見也至于三日則雖愚者執證亦明若觀火矣用藥必無過二三日矣四日則晩矣五日則臨危也

34 少陰人平居裡煩汗多者得病則必成亡陽也少陽人平居表寒下多者得病則必成亡陰也亡陽亡陰人平居預治補陰補陽可也不可至於亡陽亡陰得病臨危然後救病也

35 少陰人病愈之汗人中先汗而一次發汗胸膈壯快而活潑亡陽之汗人中或汗或不汗屢次發汗胸膈悶躁而下陷也少陽人病愈之泄手足掌心先汗而一次滑泄表氣清寧而精神爽明亡陰之泄手足掌心不汗屢次泄利表氣溯寒而精神鬱冒

36 少陰人胃家實病少陽人結胸病正邪陰陽相敵而相格故日久而後危證始

見也少陰人亡陽病少陽人亡陰病正邪陰陽不敵而相格故初證已爲險證繼而因爲危證矣譬如用兵合戰交鋒初一日合戰正兵爲邪兵所敗折正兵幾許兵數二日又戰又敗又折幾許數三日又戰又敗又折幾許數以三日交鋒觀之則將愈益戰而愈益敗愈益折矣若四日復戰五日復戰則正兵之全軍覆沒可知矣所以用藥必無過三日也

37 盤龍山老人者李翁所居地有盤龍山故李翁自謂盤龍山老人也此書中論曰二者無非盤龍山老人之論而此章特擧盤龍山老人者蓋亡陽亡陰最是險病而人必尋常視之易於例治故別以盤龍山老人提擧驚呼而警覺之也

38 亡陰證古醫別無經驗用藥頭話而李子建朱震亨書中若干論及之然自無明的快驗蓋此病從古以來殺人孟浪甚速未暇經驗獵得裡許故也

39 張仲景曰太陽病不解轉入少陽者脇下硬滿乾嘔不能食往來寒熱者尚未吐下脈沈緊者與小柴胡湯若已吐下發汗譫語柴胡證證罷此爲壞證依壞法治之

40 傷寒脈弦細頭痛發熱者屬少陽不可發汗發汗則譫語

41 嘗治少陽人傷寒發狂譫語證時則乙亥年淸明節候也少陽人一人得傷寒寒多熱少之病四五日後午未辰刻喘促短氣伊時經驗未熟但知少陽人應用藥六味湯最好之理故不敢用他藥而紙用六味湯一貼病人喘促卽時頓定又數日後病人發狂譫語喘促又發又用六味湯一貼則喘促雖少定而不如前日之頓定矣病人發狂連三日午後喘促又發又用六味湯喘促略不少定有頃舌卷動風口噤不語於是而始知六味湯之無能爲也急煎白虎湯一貼以竹管吹入病人鼻中下咽而察其動靜則舌卷口噤之證不解而病人腹中微鳴仍以兩爐煎藥荏苒灌鼻數三貼後病人腹中大鳴放氣出焉三人扶持病人竹管吹鼻灌藥而病人氣力益屈强三人扶持之力幾不能支當矣又荏苒灌鼻自未申時至亥子時凡用石膏八兩末境病人腹中大脹角弓反張之證出焉角弓反張後少頃得汗而睡翌日平明病人又服白虎湯一貼日出後滑便一次而病快愈愈後有眼病用石膏黃柏末各一錢日再服七八日後眼病亦愈伊時未知大便驗法故不察大便之秘閉幾日然想必此病人先自表寒病得病後有大便秘閉而發此證矣

42 其後又有少陽人一人得傷寒熱多寒少之病有人敎服雉肉湯仍成陽毒發斑余敎服白虎湯連三貼而其人只服半貼數日後譫語而病重病家㥦急顚倒往觀則病人外證昏憒已有動風之漸而耳聾譫語舌上白胎藥囊秖有石膏一斤滑石一兩而無他藥故急煎石膏一兩滑石一錢頓服而其翌日又服石膏一兩滑石一錢此兩日則大便皆不過一晝夜至于第三日病家以過用石膏歸咎故一日不用石膏矣至于第四日病家㥦急顚倒往觀則病人大便秘閉兩夜一晝而語韻不分明牙關緊急水飮不入急煎石膏二兩艱辛下咽而半吐半下咽少頃牙關開而語韻則不分明如前又連用石膏一兩其翌日則以午後動風藥不下咽之慮故預爲午前用藥以備動風而又五六日用之前後用石膏凡十四兩而末境發狂數日語韻宏壯而病愈數月然後方出門庭

43 其後又有少陽人一人初得頭痛身熱表寒病八九日其間用黃連瓜蔞羌活防風等屬病勢少愈而永不快袪矣仍爲發狂三日病家以尋常例證視之而秖用黃連瓜蔞等屬又譫語數日始用地黃白虎湯一貼其翌日午後動風急煎地黃白虎湯連三貼救急而艱辛下咽其翌日則白虎湯加石膏一兩午前用之以備動風而連三日用之病人自起坐立能大小便病勢比前快蘇快壯矣不幸病加於少愈慮不周於完治此人竟不救恨不午前秖用白虎湯二貼

以備動風而午後全不用藥以繼之也以此三人病觀之則發狂譫語證白虎湯非但午前用藥以備動風而已矣日用五六貼七八貼十餘貼以晝繼夜則好矣不必待譫語後而用藥發狂時當用藥可也不必待發狂後而用藥發狂前早察發狂之漸可也

44 其後又有一少陽人十七歲女兒素證間有悖氣食滯腹痛矣忽一日頭痛寒熱食滯有醫用蘇合元三箇薑湯調下仍爲泄瀉日數十行十餘日不止引飮不眠間有譫語證時則己亥年冬十一月二十三日也卽夜用生地黃石膏各六兩知母三兩其夜泄瀉度數減半其翌日用荊防地黃湯加石膏四錢二貼連服安睡而能通小便荊防地黃湯二貼藥力十倍於知母白虎湯可知矣於是每日用此藥四貼晝二貼連服夜二貼連服數日用之泄瀉永止頭部兩鬢有汗而病兒譫語證變爲發狂證病家驚惑二晝夜疑不用藥病勢遂危頭汗不出小便秘結口噙冰片不省人事爻象可惡矣勢無奈何以不得已之計一夜間用荊防地黃湯加石膏一兩連十貼灌口其夜小便通三碗狂證不止然知人看面稍有知覺其翌日又用六貼連五日日用四五六貼發狂始止夜間或霎時就睡然不能久睡便覺又日用三四貼連五日頭頂兩鬢有汗而能半時刻就睡稍進粥飮少許其後每日荊防地黃湯加石膏一錢日二貼用之大便過一日則加四錢至于十二月二十三日始得免危能起立房室中一朔內凡用石膏四十五兩新年正月十五日能行步一里地而來見我其後又連用荊防地黃湯加石膏一錢至于新年三月

45 論曰少陽人病以火熱爲證故變動甚速初證不可輕易視之也凡少陽人表病有頭痛裡病有便秘則已爲重病也重病不當用之藥一二三貼誤投則必殺人險病危證當用之藥一二三貼不及則亦不救命

2

少陽人胃受熱裏熱病論*

1 張仲景曰太陽病八九日如瘧狀發熱惡寒熱多寒小脈微而惡寒者此陰陽俱虛不可更發汗更下更吐面色反有熱色者未欲解也不能得小汗出身必痒宜桂麻各半湯

2 太陽病似瘧發熱惡寒熱多寒小脈微弱者此亡陽也身不痒不可發汗宜桂婢各半湯

3 論曰此證大便不過一晝夜而通者當用荊防瀉白散大便過一晝夜而不通者當用地黃白虎湯

4 張仲景曰陽明證小便不利脈浮而渴猪苓湯主之

5 三陽合病頭痛面垢譫語遺尿中外俱熱自汗煩渴腹痛身重白虎湯主之

6 論曰陽明證者但熱無寒之謂也三陽合病者太陽少陽陽明證俱有之謂也此證當用猪苓湯白虎湯然古方猪苓湯不如新方猪苓車前子湯之俱備古方白虎湯不如新方地黃白虎湯之全美矣若陽明證小便不利者兼大便秘燥則當用地黃白虎湯

7 朱肱曰陽厥者初得病必身熱頭痛外有陽證至四五日方發厥厥至半日却身熱蓋熱氣深方能發厥若微厥却發熱者熱甚故也其脈雖伏按之滑者爲裏熱或飮水或揚手擲足或煩躁不得眠大便秘小便赤外證多昏憒用白虎湯

8 論曰少陽人裏熱病地黃白虎湯爲聖藥而用之者必觀於大便之通不通也大便一晝夜有餘而不通則可用也二晝夜不通則必用也凡少陽人大便一晝夜不通則胃熱已結也二晝夜不通則熱重也三晝夜不通則危險也一晝夜八九辰刻二晝夜恰好用之無至三晝夜之危險若譫語證便秘則不可過一晝夜

---

* Part Ⅲ-2 Discourse on the Lesser Yang Person's Interior Febrile Disease Induced from the Stomach Affected by Heat

9 少陽人胃受熱則大便燥也脾受寒則泄瀉也故亡陰證泄瀉二三日而大便秘一晝夜則淸陰將亡而危境也胃熱證大便三晝夜不通而汗出則淸陽將竭而危境也

10 少陽人大便不通病用白虎湯三四服當日大便不通者將爲融會貫通大吉之兆也不必疑惑而翌日又服二三貼則必無不通

11 少陽人表裏病結解必觀於大便而少陽人大便頭燥尾滑體大而疏通者平時無病者之大便也其次大滑便一二次快滑泄廣多而止者有病者之病快解之大便也其次一二次尋常滑便者有病者病勢不加之大便也其次或過一晝夜有餘不通或一晝夜間三四五次小小滑利者將溢之候也非好便也宜預防

12 少陰人裡寒病臍腹冷證受病之初已有腹鳴泄瀉之機驗而其機甚顯則其病執證易見而用藥可早也少陽人裡熱病胸隔熱證受病之初雖有胸煩悶燥之機驗而其機不甚顯則執證難見而用藥太晚也若使少陽人病胸煩悶燥之驗顯然露出使人可覺則其病已險而難爲措手矣凡少陽人表病有頭痛則自是表病明白易見之初證也若復引飮小便赤則可畏也泄瀉揚手擲足則大畏也少陽人裡病大便過一晝夜有餘而不通則自是裡病明白易見之初證也若復大便過三晝夜不通則危險矣背癰腦疽脣譫纏喉風咽喉等病受病之日已爲危險證也陽毒發斑流注丹毒黃疸等病受病之日已爲險證也面目口鼻牙齒之病成病之日皆爲重證也凡少陽人表病有頭痛證則必用荊防敗毒散裡病有大便過一晝夜不通證則用白虎湯

13 王好古曰渴病有三曰消渴曰消中曰消腎熱氣上騰胸中煩躁舌赤唇紅此渴引飮常多小便數而少病屬上焦謂之消渴熱蓄於中消穀善飢飮食倍常不生肌肉此渴亦不甚煩小便數而甛病屬中焦謂之消中熱伏於下腿膝枯細骨節痠疼飮水不多隨卽尿下小便多而濁病屬下焦謂之消腎又有五石過度之人眞氣旣盡石勢獨留陽道興强不交精泄謂之强中消渴輕也消中甚焉消腎尤甚焉若强中則其斃可立而待也

14 朱震亨曰上消者舌上赤裂大渴引飮白虎湯主之中消者善食而瘦自汗大便硬小便數黃連猪肚丸主之下消者煩躁引飮小便如膏腿膝枯細六味地黃湯主之

15 醫學綱目曰渴而多飮爲上消消穀善飢爲中消渴而尿數有膏油爲下消

16 危亦林曰因耽嗜色慾或服丹石眞氣旣脫熱邪獨盛飮食如湯消雪肌膚日削小便如膏油陽强興盛不交精泄三消之中最爲難治

17 論曰消渴者病人胸次不能寬遠闊達而陋固膠小所見者淺所欲者速計策霍突意思艱乏則大腸淸陽上升之氣自不快足日月耗困而生此病也胃局淸陽上升而不快足於頭面四肢則成上消病大腸局淸陽上升而不快足於胃局則成中消病上消自爲重證而中消倍重於上消中消自爲險證而下消倍險於中消上消宜用凉膈散火湯中消宜用忍冬藤地骨皮湯下消宜用熟地黃苦參湯尤宜寬闊其心不宜膠小其心寬濶則所欲必緩淸陽上達膠小則所欲必速淸陽下耗

18 平心靜思則陽氣上升輕淸而充足於頭面四肢也此元氣也淸陽也勞心焦思則陽氣下陷重濁而鬱熱於頭面四肢也此火氣也耗陽也

19 危亦林曰消渴須防發癰疽忍冬藤不拘多少根莖花葉皆可服

20 李杲曰消渴之疾能食者末傳必發腦疽背瘡不能食者必傳中滿鼓脹

21 東醫醫方類聚曰消嬰之病變成發癰疽或成水病或雙目失明

22 論曰癰疽眼病皆是中消之變證也中消自爲險證則上消當早治也中消必急治也下消則瀕死

23 王好古曰一童子自　至童盜汗七年諸藥不效服凉膈散三日病已

24 論曰少陽人大腸淸陽快足於胃充溢於頭面四肢則汗必不出也少陽人汗者自是陽弱也而服凉膈散病已則此病卽上消而其病輕也

25 東醫醫方類聚曰夫渴者數飮水其人必頭面眩背寒而嘔因虛故也

26 龔信曰凡陰虛證每日午後惡寒發熱至晚亦得微汗而解誤作瘧治多致不救

27 孫思邈千金方書曰消渴宜愼者有三一飮酒二房勞三醎食及麵能愼此三者雖不服藥亦可自愈

28 論曰上消中消裏陽升氣雖則虛損表陰降氣猶恃完壯故其病雖險猶能歲月支撑者以此也若夫陰虛午熱飮水背寒而嘔者表裡陰陽俱爲虛損所以爲病尤險與下消略相輕重然能善攝身心服藥則十之六七尙可生也不善攝身心服藥則百之百必死也此證當用獨活地黃湯十二味地黃湯

29 易之需九三爻辭曰需于泥致寇至象曰需于泥災在外也自我致寇敬愼不敗也以此意而倣之曰陰虛午熱背寒而嘔其病雖險然死尙在外也能齋戒其心恭敬其身又服好藥不死也

3

少陽人泛論*

1 少陽人病中風吐血嘔吐腹痛食滯痞滿五證同出一屬而自有輕重浮腫喘促結胸痢疾寒熱往來胸脇滿五證同出一屬而自有輕重

2 少陽人中風半身不遂一臂不遂未如何之疾也重者必死輕者猶生間以服藥安而復之待其自愈而不可期必治法之疾也

3 少陽人吐血者必蕩滌剛愎偏急與人並驅爭塗之淡食服藥修養如釋道一百日則可以少愈二百日則可以大愈一周年則可以快愈三周年則可保其壽凡吐血調養失道則必再發再發則前功皆歸於虛地若再發者則又自發日計數一百日少愈一周年快愈若十年二十年調養則必得高壽

4 凡少陽人間有鼻血少許或口鼻間痰涎中有血雖細微皆吐血之屬也又口中暗有冷涎逆上者雖不嘔吐亦嘔吐之屬也少年有此證者多致夭折以其等閒任置故也此二證必在重病險病之列不可不預防服藥永除病根然後可保無虞

5 中風受病太重故治法不可期必吐血受病猶輕故治法可以期必中風吐血調養爲主服藥次之嘔吐以下腹痛食滯痞滿服藥調養則其病易愈

6 中風嘔吐宜用獨活地黃湯吐血宜用十二味地黃湯

7 浮腫爲病急治則生不急治則危用藥早則容易愈也用藥不早則孟浪死也此病外勢平緩似不速死故人必易之此病實是急證四五日内必治之疾謾不可以十日論之也浮腫初發當用木通大安湯或荊防地黃湯加木通日再服則六七日内浮腫必解浮腫解後百日内必用荊防地黃湯加木通二三錢每日一二貼用之以清小便以防再發再發難治浮腫初解飮食尤宜忍飢而小食若如平人大食則必不免再發大畏小便赤也小便清則浮腫解小便赤則浮腫結

8 少陽人中消者腹脹則必成鼓脹鼓脹不治少陽人鼓脹病如少陰人藏結病

* Part Ⅲ-3 General Remarks on the Lesser Yang Person

皆經歷五六七八月或周年而竟死蓋少陰人藏結表陽溫氣雖在幾絶裡陰溫氣猶恃完壯少陽人鼓脹裡陽清氣雖在幾絶表陰清氣猶恃完壯故皆經歷久遠而死也

9 少陽人傷寒喘促宜先用靈砂一分溫水調下因煎荊防瓜蔞等藥用之則必無煎藥時刻遲滯救病

10 靈砂藥力急迫可以一再用而不可屢用蓋救急之藥敏於救急而已藥必湯服然後充滿腸胃能爲補陰補陽

11 痢疾之比結胸則痢疾爲順證也而痢疾之謂重證者以其與浮腫相近也嘔吐之比腹痛則嘔吐爲逆證也而嘔吐之謂惡證者以其距中風不遠也

12 少陽人痢疾宜用黃連清腸湯

13 少陽人瘧疾有間兩日發者卽勞瘧也可以緩治不可急治此證瘧不發日用獨活地黃湯二貼朝暮服瘧發日預煎荊防敗毒散二貼待惡寒發作時二貼連服一月之內以獨活地黃湯四十貼荊防敗毒散二十貼爲準的則其瘧必無不退之理

14 少陽人內發咽喉外腫項頰者謂之纏喉風二三日內殺人最急又上唇人中穴瘇謂之唇瘇凡人中左右逼近處一指許發瘇雖微如粟粒亦危證也此二證始發而輕者當用凉膈散火湯陽毒白虎湯重者當用水銀熏鼻方一炷熏鼻而項頰汗出則愈若倉卒無熏鼻藥則輕粉末一分五厘乳香沒藥甘遂末各五分和匀糊丸一服盡

15 少陽人小兒食多飢瘦宜用蘆會肥兒丸忍冬藤地骨皮湯

16 嘗見少陽人肩上有毒瘇火熬香油灌瘡肌肉焦爛而不知其熱有醫教以牛角片置火炭上燒而熏之煙入瘡口毒汁自流其瘇立愈

17 嘗見少陽人七十老人發腦疽有醫教以河豚卵作末傅之其疽立愈河豚卵至毒彘犬食之則立死掛於林木間烏鵲不敢食

18 嘗治少陽人蛇頭瘡河豚卵作末少許點膏藥上傅之而一日一次易以新末傅藥五六日病效而新肉急生而有妬肉因以磨刀砥末傅之妬肉立消而疾愈又用之於連珠痰多日傅之者必效用之於爲炭火所傷與狗咬蟲咬無不得效

19 嘗治少陽人六十老人中風一臂不遂病用輕粉五厘其病輒加少陽人二十歲少年一脚微不仁痺風用輕粉甘遂龍虎丹二三次用之得效

20 嘗治少陽人咽喉水醬不入大便不通三日病至危境用甘遂天一丸卽效

21 嘗治少陽人七十老人大便四五日不通或六七日不通飮食如常兩脚膝寒無力用輕粉甘遂龍虎丹大便卽通後數日大便又秘則又用屢次用之竟以大便一日一度爲準而病愈此老竟得八十壽

22 嘗見少陽人當門二齒齦縫血出頃刻間數碗將至危境有醫教以火熬香油以新綿點油乘熱灼齒縫仍爲血止

23 嘗見少陽人一人每日一次梳頭數月後得口眼喎斜病其後又見少陽人日梳得喎斜病者凡三人蓋日梳少陽人禁忌也嘗見太陰人八十老人日梳者老人自言曰日梳極好我之日梳已爲四十年云

3-1

張仲景傷寒論中少陽人病經驗設方藥十方*

1 白虎湯石膏五錢知母二錢甘草七分粳米半合

2 猪苓湯猪苓赤茯苓澤瀉滑石阿膠各一錢

3 五苓散澤瀉二錢五分赤茯苓猪苓白朮各一錢五分肉桂五分

4 小柴胡湯柴胡三錢黃芩二錢人蔘半夏各一錢五分甘草五分

5 大青龍湯石膏四錢麻黃三錢桂枝二錢杏仁一錢五分甘草一錢薑三片棗二枚

6 桂婢各半湯石膏二錢麻黃桂枝白芍藥各一錢甘草三分薑三片棗二枚

7 小陷胸湯半夏製五錢黃連二錢五分瓜蔞大者四分之一

8 大陷胸湯大黃三錢芒硝二錢甘遂末五分

9 十棗湯芫花微炒甘遂大戟炒等分爲末別取大棗十枚水一盞煎至半盞去棗調藥末强人一錢弱人半錢服大便利下水以粥補之

10 腎氣丸六味地黃湯加五味子一味

* Part III-3-1 Ten Prescriptions for the Lesser Yang Person's Disease from Zhang Zhongjing's 『*Shanghanlun*』

3-2

元明二代醫家著述中少陽人病經驗行用要藥九方*

1 凉膈散連翹二錢大黃芒硝甘草各一錢薄荷黃芩梔子各五分此方出於局方治積熱煩躁口舌生瘡目赤頭昏今考更定此方當去大黃甘草黃芩

2 黃連猪肚丸雄猪肚一箇黃連小麥炒各五兩天花粉白茯神各四兩麥門冬二兩右爲末入猪肚中封口安甑中蒸爛搗作丸梧子大此方出於危亦林得效方書中治强中證今考更定此方中麥門冬一味肺藥也肺與腎一升一降上下貫通腎藥五味中肺藥一味雖爲贅材亦自無妨不必苛論

3 六味地黃湯熟地黃四錢山藥山茱萸各二錢澤瀉牧丹皮白茯苓各一錢五分此方出於虞博醫學正傳書中治虛勞今考更定此方中山藥一味肺藥也

4 生熟地黃丸生乾地黃熟地黃玄參石膏各一兩糊丸梧子大空心茶清下五七十丸此方出於李梴醫學入門書中治眼昏

5 導赤散木通滑石黃柏赤茯苓生地黃山梔子甘草梢各一錢枳殼白朮各五分此方出於龔信萬病回春書中治尿如米泔色不過二服愈今考更定此方當去枳殼白朮甘草

6 荊防敗毒散羌活獨活柴胡前胡赤茯苓荊芥穗防風枳殼桔梗川芎人蔘甘草各一錢薄荷少許治傷寒時氣發熱頭痛項强肢體煩疼今考更定此方當去枳殼桔梗川芎人蔘甘草(此方出於某書疊出故省略下同)

7 肥兒丸胡黃連五錢使君子肉四錢五分人蔘黃連神麴麥芽山查肉各三錢五分白茯苓白朮甘草灸各三錢蘆薈煆二錢五分右爲末黃米糊和丸菉豆大米飮下二三十丸治小兒疳積今考更定此方當去人蔘白朮山查肉甘草而使君子一味未能經驗的知藥性故不敢輕論

8 消毒飮牛蒡子二錢荊芥穗一錢生甘草防風各五分治痘不快出及胸前稠密急用三四服快透解毒神效右三方出於龔信醫鑑書中今考更定此方當去甘草

---

* Part III-3-2 Nine Prescriptions for the Lesser Yang Person's Disease Mentioned in the Writings of Famous Doctors in the Yuan and Ming Dynasties

9 水銀熏鼻方黑鉛水銀各一錢朱砂乳香沒藥各五分血竭雄黃沈香各三分右爲末和勻捲作紙燃七條用香油點燈放床上令病人放兩脚包住上用單被通身蓋之口噤凉水頻換則不損口初日用三條後日每用一條熏鼻此方出於朱震亨丹溪心法書中治楊梅天疱瘡甚奇論曰水銀破積熱淸頭目制陽回陰於下焦爲少陽抑陽扶陰藥中無敵之藥而秪可用之於當日救急之用不可用之於連日補陰之用者以其拔山扛鼎之力一擧而直搗大敵之巢穴再擧則敵已解散反有倒戈之患故也纏喉風必用之藥少陽人一脚不遂兩脚不遂者輕粉末五厘或一分連三日服無論病之差不差必不過三日服又不過日服五厘或一分謹風冷愼禁忌一臂不遂半身不遂口眼喎斜不可用用之必危急病可以急治緩病不可以急治輕粉劫藥不可銳意用之以望速效緩病緩愈然後可謂眞愈緩病速效則終必更病難治有連三日用之者有間一二三日連服連三次用之者嘗見少陽人咽喉病眼鼻病脚痺病用水銀連三四日或熏鼻或內服病愈者病愈後一月之內必不可內處冷外觸風尤不可任意洗手洗面更着新衣梳頭也犯此禁者必死又不可冷室冷室則觸冷而猝死又不可燠室燠室則煩熱開牖觸風而亦猝死此皆目擊者也一人病愈十餘日更着新衣而猝死一人病愈二十日後梳頭而猝死一人咽喉病熏鼻初日二條翌日一條當夜燠室觸風而猝死時俗服水銀者忌鹽醬者以醬中有豆豉能解水銀毒故也然毒藥害毒容或無妨則不必苛忌塩醬

3-3

新定少陽人病應用要藥十七方*

1 荊防敗毒散羌活獨活柴胡前胡荊芥防風赤茯苓生地黃地骨皮車前子各一錢右方治頭痛寒熱往來者宜用

2 荊防導赤散生地黃三錢木通二錢玄蔘瓜蔞仁各一錢五分前胡羌活獨活荊芥防風各一錢右方治頭痛胸膈煩熱者宜用

3 荊防瀉白散生地黃三錢茯苓澤瀉各二錢石膏知母羌活獨活荊芥防風各一錢右方治頭痛膀胱㷡躁者宜用

4 猪苓車前子湯茯苓澤瀉各二錢猪苓車前子各一錢五分知母石膏羌活獨活荊芥防風各一錢右方治頭腹痛有泄瀉者宜用

5 滑石苦參湯茯苓澤瀉滑石苦參各二錢川黃連黃柏羌活獨活荊芥防風各一錢右方治腹痛無泄瀉者宜用

6 獨活地黃湯熟地黃四錢山茱萸二錢茯苓澤瀉各一錢五分牧丹皮防風獨活各一錢右方治食滯痞滿者宜用

7 荊防地黃湯熟地黃山茱萸茯苓澤瀉各二錢車前子羌活獨活荊芥防風各一錢咳嗽加前胡血證加玄參牧丹皮偏頭痛加黃連牛蒡子食滯痞滿者加牧丹皮有火者加石膏頭痛煩熱與血證者用生地黃加石膏者去山茱萸荊芥防風羌活獨活俱是補陰藥荊防大清胸膈散風羌獨大補膀胱眞陰無論頭腹痛痞滿泄瀉凡虛弱者數百貼用之無不必效屢試屢驗

8 十二味地黃湯熟地黃四錢山茱萸二錢白茯苓澤瀉各一錢五分牧丹皮地骨皮玄蔘枸杞子覆盆子車前子荊芥防風各一錢

9 地黃白虎湯石膏五錢或一兩生地黃四錢知母二錢防風獨活各一錢

10 陽毒白虎湯石膏五錢或一兩生地黃四錢知母二錢荊芥防風牛蒡子各一錢右方治陽毒發斑便秘者宜用

---

* Part Ⅲ-3-3 Seventeen Newly Created Prescriptions for the Lesser Yang Person's Disease

11 凉膈散火湯生地黃忍冬藤連翹各二錢山梔子薄荷知母石膏防風荊芥各一錢右方治上消者宜用

12 忍冬藤地骨皮湯忍冬藤四錢山茱萸地骨皮各二錢川黃連黃柏玄蔘苦參生地黃知母山梔子枸杞子覆盆子荊芥防風金銀花各一錢右方治中消者宜用

13 熟地黃苦參湯熟地黃四錢山茱萸二錢白茯苓澤瀉各一錢五分知母黃柏苦參各一錢右方治下消者宜用

14 木通大安湯木通生地黃各五錢赤茯苓二錢澤瀉車前子川黃連羌活防風荊芥各一錢右方治浮腫者宜用險病始終用藥當至百餘貼黃連澤瀉爲貴材則貧者或去連澤

15 黃連清腸湯生地黃四錢木通茯苓澤瀉各二錢猪苓車前子川黃連羌活防風各一錢右方治痢疾者宜用去木通二錢加荊芥一錢痲疾者宜用

16 朱砂益元散滑石二錢澤瀉一錢甘遂五分朱砂一分右爲末溫水或井華水調服夏月滌暑宜用

17 甘遂天一丸甘遂末一錢輕粉末一分和勻糊丸分作十丸朱砂爲衣作丸乾久則堅硬難和每用時以紙二三疊包炮以杵搗碎作麤末三四五片口含末因飮井華水和下候三四辰刻內不下利則再用二丸下利三度爲適中六度爲快過預煎米飮下利二三度因進米飮否則氣陷而難堪耐治結胸水入還吐甘遂一錢輕粉五分分作十丸則名曰輕粉甘遂龍虎丹輕粉甘遂各等分作十丸則名曰輕粉甘遂雌雄丹輕粉一錢乳香沒藥甘遂各五分分作三十丸則名曰乳香沒藥輕粉丸輕粉發汗甘遂下水輕粉藥力一分則快足五厘則無不及甘遂藥力一分五厘則快足七八厘則無不及輕粉甘遂自是毒藥俱不可輕易過一分用之斟酌輕重病欲頭腦滌火則輕粉爲君病欲胸膈下水則甘遂爲君右少陽人藥諸種不可炮炙炒煨用

1

太陰人胃脘受寒表寒病論*

1 張仲景曰太陽傷寒頭痛發熱身疼腰痛骨節皆痛惡寒無汗而喘麻黃湯主之註曰傷寒頭痛身疼腰痛以至牽連百骨節俱痛者此太陽傷寒榮血不利故也

2 論曰此卽太陰人傷寒背顀表病輕證也此證麻黃湯非不當用而桂枝甘草皆爲蠹材此證當用麻黃發表湯

3 張仲景曰傷寒四五日而厥者必發熱厥深者熱亦深厥微者熱亦微傷寒厥四日熱反三日復厥五日厥多熱少其病爲進傷寒發熱四日厥反三日厥少熱多其病當自愈

4 論曰此謂之厥者但惡寒不發熱之謂也非手足厥逆之謂也太陰人傷寒表證寒厥四五日後發熱者重證也此證發熱其汗必自髮際而始通於額上又數日後發熱而眉稜通汗又數日後發熱而顴上通汗又數日後發熱而脣頤通汗又數日後發熱而胸臆通汗也而額上之汗數次而後達於眉稜眉稜之汗數次而後達於顴上顴上之汗數次而後達於脣頤脣頤之汗不過一次而直達於胸臆矣此證首尾幾近二十日凡寒厥六七次而後病解也此證俗謂之長感病凡太陰人病先額上眉稜有汗而一汗病不解屢汗病解者名曰長感病

5 太陰人病寒厥六七日而不發熱不汗出則死也寒厥二三日而發熱汗出則輕證也寒厥四五日而發熱得微汗於額上者此之謂長感病其病爲重證也此證原委勞心焦思之餘胃脘衰弱而表局虛薄不勝寒而外被寒邪所圍正邪相爭之形勢客勝主弱譬如一團孤軍困在垓心幾於全軍覆沒之境先鋒一隊倖而跳出決圍一面僅得開路後軍全隊尙在垓心將又屢次力戰然後方爲出來則爻象正是凜凜之勢也額上通汗者卽先鋒一隊決圍跳出之象也眉稜通汗者卽前軍全隊決圍全面氣勢勇敢之象也顴上通汗者中軍半隊緩緩出圍之象也此病汗出眉稜則快免危也汗出顴上則必無危也

---

* Part Ⅳ-1 Discourse on the Greater Yin Person's Exterior Cold Disease Induced from the Epigastrium Affected by Cold

6 太陰人汗無論額上眉稜上顴上汗出如黍粒發熱稍久而還入者正强邪弱快汗也汗出如微粒或淋漓無粒乍時而還入者正弱邪强非快汗也

7 太陰人背部後面自腦以下有汗而面部髮際以下不汗者匈證也全面皆有汗而耳門左右不汗者死證也大凡太陰人汗始自耳後高骨面部髮際大通於胸臆間而病解也髮際之汗始免死也額上之汗僅免危也眉稜之汗快免危也顴上之汗生路寬闊也脣頤之汗病已解也胸臆之汗病大解也嘗見此證額上汗欲作眉稜汗者寒厥之勢不甚猛也顴上汗欲作脣頤汗者寒厥之勢甚猛至於寒戰叩齒完若動風而其汗直達兩腋張仲景所云厥深者熱亦深厥微者熱亦微蓋謂此也此證寒厥之勢多日者病重之勢也寒厥之勢猛峻者非病重之勢也

8 此證京畿道人謂之長感病咸鏡道人謂之四十日痛或謂之無汗乾病時俗所用荊防敗毒散藿香正氣散補中益氣湯個個誤治惟熊膽雖或盲人直門然又連用他藥病勢更變古人所云病不能殺人藥能殺人者不亦信乎百病加減之勢以凡眼目觀之固難推測而此證又有甚焉此證之汗在眉稜顴上時雖不服藥亦自愈矣而病人招醫妄投誤藥則顴上之汗還爲額上之汗而外證寒厥之勢則稍減矣於是焉醫師自以爲信藥效病人亦自以爲得藥效又數日誤藥則額上之汗又不通而死矣此證當以汗之進退占病之輕重不可以寒之寬猛占病之輕重張仲景曰其病當自愈云者豈非珍重無妄之論乎然長感病無疫氣者待其自愈則好也而瘟病疫氣重者若明知證藥無疑則不可尋常置之待其勿藥自愈恐生奇證

9 論曰太陰人病寒厥四日而無汗者重證也寒厥五日而無汗者險證也當用熊膽散或寒多熱少湯加蠐螬五七九箇大便滑者必用乾栗薏苡仁等屬大便燥者必用葛根大黃等屬若額上眉稜上有汗則待其自愈而病解後用藥調理否則恐生後病

10 嘗治太陰人胃脘寒證瘟病有一太陰人素有怔忡無汗氣短結咳矣忽焉又添出一證泄瀉數十日不止卽表病之重者也用太陰調胃湯加樗根皮一錢日再服十日泄瀉方止連用三十日每日流汗滿面素證亦減而忽其家五六人一時瘟疫此人緣於救病數日不服藥矣此人又染瘟病瘟證粥食無味全不入口仍以太陰調胃湯加升麻黃芩各一錢連用十日汗流滿面疫氣少減而有二日大便不通之證仍用葛根承氣湯五日而五日內粥食大倍疫氣大減而病解又用太陰調胃湯加升麻黃芩四十日調理疫氣旣減素病亦完

11 結咳者勉强發咳痰欲出不出而或出曰結咳少陰人結咳謂之胸結咳太陰人結咳謂之頷結咳

12 大凡瘟疫先察其人素病如何則表裏虛實可知已素病寒者得瘟病則亦寒證也素病熱者得瘟病則亦熱證也素病輕者得瘟病則重證也素病重者得瘟病則險證也

13 有一太陰人素病咽嗌乾燥而面色青白表寒或泄蓋咽嗌乾燥者肝熱也面色青白表寒或泄者胃脘寒也此病表裏俱病素病之太重者也此人得瘟病其證自始發日至于病解二十日大便初滑或泄中滑末乾每日二三四次無日不通初用寒多熱少湯病解後用調理肺元湯四十日調理僅僅獲生

14 此病始發大便或滑或泄而六日內有額汗眉稜汗顴汗飲食起居有時如常六日後始用藥七日全體面部髮際以下至于脣頤汗流滿面淋漓洽足而汗後面色帶青有語訥證八日九日語訥耳聾而脣汗還爲顴汗顴汗還爲眉稜汗汗出微粒乍出乍入而只有額汗呼吸短喘矣至于十日夜額汗還入而語訥耳聾尤甚痰涎壅喉口不能喀病人自以手指探口拭之而出十一日呼吸

短喘尤甚至于十二日忽然食粥二碗斯時若論其藥則熊膽散或者可也而熊膽闕材自念此人今夜必死矣當日初昏呼吸暫時少定十三日鷄鳴時髮際有汗十四日十五日連三日食粥二三碗額汗眉稜汗顴汗次次發出面色脫青十六日臆汗始通稍能喀痰語訥亦愈至于二十日臆汗數次大通遂能起立房中諸證皆安而耳聾證則自如也病解後用藥調理四十日耳聾目迷自祛

2

太陰人肝受熱裏熱病論*

1 朱肱曰陽毒面赤斑斑如錦紋咽喉痛唾膿血宜葛根解肌湯黑奴丸陽毒及壞傷寒醫所不治精魄已竭心下尚煖斡開其口灌黑奴丸藥下咽卽活

2 李梴曰微惡寒發熱宜葛根解肌湯目疼鼻乾潮汗閉澁滿渴狂譫宜調胃承氣湯熱在表則目疼不眠宜解肌湯熱入裏則狂譫宜調胃承氣湯

3 龔信曰陽明病目疼鼻乾不得臥宜葛根解肌湯

4 三陽病深變爲陽毒面赤眼紅身發斑黃或下利黃赤六脈洪大宜黑奴丸

5 論曰右諸證當用葛根解肌湯黑奴丸

6 靈樞曰尺膚熱深脈盛燥者病瘟也

7 王叔和曰瘟病脈陰陽俱盛病熱之極浮之而滑沈之散澁

8 脈法曰瘟病二三日體熱腹滿頭痛食飮如故脈直而疾八日死瘟病四五日頭痛腹滿而吐脈來細而强十二日死八九日頭身不痛目不赤色不變而反利脈來澁按之不足擧時大心下堅十七日死

9 龔信曰瘟病穰穰大熱脈細小者死瘟病下利痛甚者死

10 萬曆丙戌余寓大梁瘟疫大作士民多斃其證增寒壯熱頭面項頰赤腫咽喉腫痛昏憒余發一秘方名二聖救苦丸大黃四兩猪牙皂角二兩麵糊和丸菉豆大五七十丸一服卽汗一汗卽愈稟壯者百發百中皂角開關竅發其表大黃瀉諸火通其裏

11 感四時不正之氣使人痰涎壅盛煩熱頭疼身痛增寒壯熱項强睛疼或飮食如常起居依舊甚至聲啞或赤眼口瘡大小腮腫喉痺咳嗽稠粘噴嚏

12 論曰右諸證增寒壯熱燥澁者當用皂角大黃湯葛根承氣湯頭面項頰赤腫者當用皂角大黃湯葛根承氣湯體熱腹滿自利者熱勝則裏證也當用葛根解肌湯寒勝則表證而太重證也當用太陰調胃湯加升麻黃芩

* Part Ⅳ-2 Discourse on the Greater Yin Person's Interior Febrile Disease Induced from the Liver Affected by Heat

13 嘗治太陰人肝熱熱證瘟病有一太陰人素病數年來眼病時作時止矣此人得瘟病自始發日用熱多寒少湯三四五日大便或滑或泄至六日有大便一日不通之證仍用葛根承氣湯連三日粥食大倍又用三日疫氣大減病解後復用熱多寒少湯大便燥澁則加大黃一錢滑泄太多則去大黃如此調理二十日其人完健此病始發嘔逆嘔吐昏憒不省重痛矣末境反爲輕證十二日而病解

14 一太陰人十歲兒得裏熱瘟病粥食全不入口藥亦不入口壯熱穰穰有時飮冷水至于十一日則大便不通已四日矣恇怯譫語曰有百蟲滿室又有鼠入懷云奔遑匍匐驚呼啼泣有時熱極生風兩手厥冷兩膝伸而不屈急用葛根承氣湯不憚啼泣强灌口中卽日粥食大倍疫氣大解倖而得生此病始發四五日飮食起居如常無異平人矣末境反爲重證十七日而病解

15 內經曰諸澁枯涸皺揭皆屬於燥

16 論曰太陰人面色青白者多無燥證面色黃赤黑者多有燥證蓋肝熱肺燥而然也嘗治太陰人燥熱證手指焦黑癍瘡病自左手中指焦黑無力二年內一指黑血焦凝過掌心而掌背浮腫以刀斷指矣又一年內癍瘡遍滿全體大者如大錢小者如小錢得病已爲三年而以壯年人手力不能役勞一半刻足力不能日行步三十里以熱多寒少湯用藁本二錢加大黃一錢二十八貼用之大便始滑不過一二日又秘燥又用二十貼大便不甚滑泄而面部癍瘡少差手力足力稍快有效矣又用二十貼其病快差

17 靈樞曰二陽結謂之消飮一溲二死不治註曰二陽結謂胃及大腸熱結也

18 扁鵲難經曰消渴脈當得緊實而數反得沈濇而微者死

19 張仲景曰消渴病小便反多如飮水一斗小便亦一斗腎氣丸主之

20 論曰此病非少陽人消渴也卽太陰人燥熱也此證不當用腎氣丸當用熱多寒少湯加藁本大黃

21 嘗治太陰人年五十近衰者燥熱病引飮小便多大便秘者用熱多寒少湯藁本二錢加大黃一錢二十貼得效矣後一月餘用他醫藥五貼此人更病復用熱多寒少湯加藁本大黃五六十貼用藥時間其病僅僅支撑後終不免死又嘗治太陰人年少者燥熱病用此方三百貼得支撑一周年此病亦不免死此人得病一周年或間用他醫方未知緣何故也蓋燥熱至於飮一溲二而病劇則難治凡太陰人大便秘燥小便覺多而引飮者不可不早治豫防

22 此病非必不治之病也此少年得病用藥一周年後方死蓋此病原委侈樂無厭慾火外馳肝熱大盛肺燥太枯之故也若此少年安心滌慾一百日而用藥則焉有不治之理乎蓋自始病日至于終死日慾火無日不馳故也諺曰先祖德澤雖或不得一一個報而恭敬德澤必無一一不受報凡無論某病人恭敬其心蕩滌慾火安靜善心一百日則其病無不愈二百日則其人無不完恭敬德澤之個個受報百事皆然而疾病尤甚

23 危亦林曰陰血耗竭耳聾目暗脚弱腰痛宜用黑元丹

24 凡男子方當壯年而眞氣猶怯此乃稟賦素弱非虛而然滋益之方群品稍衆藥力細微難見功效但固天元一氣使水升火降則五臟自和百病不生宜用拱辰丹

25 論曰此證當用黑元與拱辰丹當歸山茱萸皆爲蠹材藥力未全欲收全力宜用拱辰黑元丹鹿茸大補湯

26 太陰人證有食後痞滿腿脚無力病宜用拱辰黑元丹鹿茸大補湯太陰調胃湯調胃升清湯

27 太陰人證有泄瀉病表寒證泄瀉當用太陰調胃湯表熱證泄瀉當用葛根蘿蔔子湯

28 太陰人證有咳嗽病宜用太陰調胃湯鹿茸大補湯拱辰黑元丹

29 太陰人證有哮喘病重證也當用麻黃定喘湯

30 太陰人證有胸腹痛病危險證也當用麻黃定痛湯

31 太陰人小兒有泄瀉十餘次無度者必發慢驚風宜用補肺元湯豫備慢風

32 太陰人有腹脹浮腫病當用乾栗蠐螬湯此病極危險證而十生九死之病也雖用藥病愈三年内不再發然後方可論生侈樂禁嗜慾三年内宜恭敬心身調養愼攝必在其人矣凡太陰人病若待浮腫已發而治之則十病九死也此病不可以病論之而以死論之可也然則如之何其可也凡太陰人勞心焦思屢謀不成者或有久泄久痢或痳病小便不利食後痞滿腿脚無力病皆浮腫之漸已爲重險病而此時以浮腫論而蕩滌慾火恭敬其心用藥治之可也

33 太陰人證有夢泄病一月内三四發者虛勞重證也大便秘一日則宜用熱多寒少湯加大黃一錢大便每日不秘則加龍骨減大黃或用拱辰黑元丹鹿茸大補湯此病出於謀慮太多思想無窮

34 太陰人證有卒中風病胸臆格格有窒塞聲而目瞪者必用瓜蔕散手足拘攣眼合者當用牛黃清心丸素面色黃赤黑者多有目瞪者素面色青白者多有眼合者面色青白而眼合者手足拘攣則其病急危也不必待拘攣但見眼合而素面色青白者必急用清心丸古方清心丸每每神效目瞪者亦急發而稍緩死眼合者急發急死然目瞪者亦不可以緩論而急治之

35 牛黃清心丸非家家必有之物宜用遠志石菖蒲末各一錢灌口因以皂角末三分吹鼻此證手足拘攣而項直則危也傍人以兩手執病人兩手腕左右撓動兩肩或執病人足腕屈伸兩脚太陰人中風撓動病人肩脚好也少陽人中風大忌撓動病人手足又不可抱人起坐少陰人中風傍人抱病人起坐則可也而不可搖動兩肩可以徐徐按摩手足

36 中毒吐瀉宜用麝香

2-1

張仲景傷寒論中太陰人病經驗設方藥四方*

1 麻黃湯麻黃三錢桂枝二錢甘草六分杏仁十枚薑三片棗二枚

2 桂麻各半湯麻黃一錢五分白芍藥桂枝杏仁各一錢甘草七分薑三片棗二枚

3 調胃承氣湯大黃四錢芒硝二錢甘草一錢

4 大柴胡湯柴胡四錢黃芩白芍藥各二錢五分大黃二錢枳實一錢五分治少陽轉屬陽明身熱不惡寒反惡熱大便硬小便赤譫語腹脹潮熱

* Part Ⅳ-2-1 Four Prescriptions for the Greater Yin Person's Disease from Zhang Zhonjing's 『*Shanghanlun*』

2-2

唐宋明三代醫家著述中太陰人經驗行用要藥九方*

1 石菖蒲遠志散石菖蒲遠志爲細末每服一錢酒飮任下日三令人耳目聰明此方出於孫思邈千金方書中

2 調中湯大黃一錢五分黃芩桔梗葛根白朮白芍藥赤茯苓藁本甘草各一錢治夏發燥疫口乾咽塞今考更定此方當去白朮芍藥茯苓甘草

3 黑奴丸麻黃大黃各二兩黃芩釜底煤芒硝竈突墨樑上塵小麥奴各一兩右爲末蜜丸彈子大每一丸新汲水和服須臾振寒汗出而解陽毒及壞傷寒醫所不治精魄已竭心下尙煖斡開其口灌藥下咽卽活右二方出於朱肱活人書中今考更定此方當去芒硝

4 生脈散麥門冬二錢人蔘五味子各一錢夏月代熟水飮之令人氣力湧出今考更定此方當去人蔘

5 樗根皮丸樗根白皮爲末酒糊和丸治夢遺此藥性凉而燥不可單服右二方出於李梴醫學入門書中

6 二聖救苦丸大黃四兩猪牙皂角二兩麵糊和丸菉豆大五七十丸一服卽汗一汗卽愈此方出於龔信萬病回春書中治天行瘟疫

7 葛根解肌湯葛根升麻黃芩桔梗白芷柴胡白芍藥羌活石膏各一錢甘草五分治陽明病目疼鼻乾不得臥今考更定此方當去柴胡芍藥羌活石膏甘草

8 牛黃淸心丸山藥七錢甘草炒五錢人蔘蒲黃神麴竝炒各二錢五分犀角二錢大豆黃卷炒肉桂阿膠炒各一錢七分白芍藥麥門冬黃芩當歸白朮防風朱砂水飛各一錢五分柴胡桔梗杏仁白茯茯川芎各一錢三分牛黃一錢二分羚羊角龍腦麝香各一錢雄黃八分白蘞乾薑炮各七分金箔一百四十箔内四十箔爲衣大棗二十枚蒸取肉硏爲膏右爲末棗膏入煉蜜和匀每一兩作十丸金箔爲衣每取一丸溫水和下治卒中風不省人事痰涎壅塞精神昏

* Part Ⅳ-2-2 Nine Prescriptions for the Greater Yin Person's Disease Mentioned in the Writings of Famous Doctors in the Tang, Song and Ming Dynasties

憒言語蹇澁口眼喎斜手足不遂等證右二方出於龔信醫鑑書中今考更定此方當去白朮人蔘甘草神麴肉桂阿膠芎藥當歸川芎乾薑大棗淸蜜柴胡茯苓雄黃朱砂

9 麻黃定喘湯麻黃三錢杏仁一錢五分黃芩半夏桑白皮蘇子款冬花甘草各一錢白果去殼碎炒二十一箇黃色歌曰諸病原來有藥方惟愁齁喘難當病人遇此仙丹藥服後方知定喘湯此方出於龔信萬病回春書中治哮喘神方今考更定此方當去半夏蘇子甘草

2-3

新定太陰人病應用要藥二十四方*

1 太陰調胃湯薏苡仁乾栗各三錢蘿葍子二錢五味子麥門冬石菖蒲桔梗麻黃各一錢

2 葛根解肌湯葛根三錢黃芩藁本各一錢五分桔梗升麻白芷各一錢

3 調胃升淸湯薏苡仁乾栗各三錢蘿葍子一錢五分麻黃桔梗麥門冬五味子石菖蒲遠志天門冬酸棗仁龍眼肉各一錢

4 淸心蓮子湯蓮子肉山藥各二錢天門冬麥門冬遠志石菖蒲酸棗仁龍眼肉柏子仁黃芩蘿葍子各一錢甘菊花三分

5 麻黃定喘湯麻黃三錢杏仁一錢五分黃芩蘿葍子桑白皮桔梗麥門冬款冬花各一錢白果炒黃色二一箇

6 麻黃定痛湯薏苡仁三錢麻黃蘿葍子各二錢杏仁石菖蒲桔梗麥門冬五味子使君子龍眼肉柏子仁各一錢乾栗七箇

7 熱多寒少湯葛根四錢黃芩藁本各二錢蘿葍子桔梗升麻白芷各一錢

8 寒多熱少湯薏苡仁三錢蘿葍子二錢麥門冬桔梗黃芩杏仁麻黃各一錢乾栗七箇

9 葛根承氣湯葛根四錢黃芩大黃各二錢桔梗升麻白芷各一錢本方加大黃二錢則名曰葛根大承氣湯減大黃一錢則名曰葛根小承氣湯

10 調理肺元湯麥門冬桔梗薏苡仁各二錢黃芩麻黃蘿葍子各一錢

11 麻黃發表湯桔梗三錢麻黃一錢五分麥門冬黃芩杏仁各一錢

12 補肺元湯麥門冬三錢桔梗二錢五味子一錢加山藥薏苡仁蘿葍子各一錢則尤妙

13 鹿茸大補湯鹿茸二三四錢麥門冬薏苡仁各一錢五分山藥天門冬五味子

---

* Part Ⅳ-2-3 Twenty Four Important Newly Formulated Prescriptions for the Greater Yin Person's Disease

杏仁麻黃各一錢虛弱人表症寒證多者宜用

14 拱辰黑元丹鹿茸四五六兩山藥天門冬各四兩蠐螬一二兩麝香五錢煮烏梅肉爲膏和丸梧子大溫湯下五七十丸或燒酒下虛弱人裏症多者宜用

15 皂角大黃湯升麻葛根各三錢大黃皂角各一錢用之者不可過三四貼升麻三錢大黃皂角同局藥力峻猛故也

16 葛根浮萍湯葛根三錢蘿葍子黃芩各二錢紫背浮萍大黃各一錢蠐螬十箇治浮腫裏症熱多者宜用

17 乾栗蠐螬湯乾栗百箇蠐螬十箇湯服或灸食黃栗蠐螬十箇作末別用黃栗湯水調下治浮腫表症寒多者宜用

18 乾栗樗根皮湯乾栗一兩樗根白皮三四五錢治痢疾或湯服或丸服而丸服者或單用樗根白皮五錢

19 瓜蔕散瓜蔕炒黃爲末三五分溫水調下或乾瓜蔕一錢急煎湯用治卒中風臆膈格格有窒塞聲及目瞪者必可用此藥此病此證可用他病他證必不可用胸腹痛寒咳喘尤忌用雖滯食物不可用此藥而用他藥面色青白而素有寒證表虛者卒中風則當用熊膽散牛黃清心元石菖蒲遠志散而不可用瓜蔕散

20 熊膽散熊膽三五分溫水調下

21 麝香散麝香三五分溫水調下或溫酒調下只擧三五分則四分在其中

22 石菖蒲遠志散遠志石菖蒲各一錢猪牙皂角並末三分溫水調下或遠志菖蒲末溫水調下皂角末吹鼻

23 麥門冬遠志散麥門冬三錢遠志石菖蒲各一錢五味子五分

24 牛黃清心元山藥七錢蒲黃炒二錢五分犀角二錢大豆黃卷炒一錢七分麥門冬黃芩各一錢五分桔梗杏仁各一錢三分牛黃一錢二分羚羊角龍腦麝香各一錢白蘞七分金箔七十箔內二十箔爲衣烏梅二十枚蒸取肉研爲膏右爲末烏梅膏和匀每一兩作二十丸金箔爲衣每取一丸溫水和下右太陰人藥諸種杏仁去雙仁去皮尖麥門冬遠志去心白果黃栗去殼大黃或酒蒸或生用鹿茸皂角酥炙酸棗仁杏仁白果炒用

1

太陽人外感腰脊病論*

1 內經曰尺脈緩澁謂之解㑊釋曰尺爲陰部肝腎主之緩爲熱中澁爲亡血故謂之解㑊解㑊者寒不寒熱不熱弱不弱壯不壯獰不可名謂之解㑊也

2 靈樞曰髓傷則消爍䯒痠體解㑊然不去矣不去謂不能行去也

3 論曰此證卽太陽人腰脊病太重證也必戒深哀遠嗔怒修清定然後其病可愈此證當用五加皮壯脊湯

4 解㑊者上體完健而下體解㑊然脚力不能行去也而其脚自無痲痺腫痛之證脚力亦不甚弱此所以弱不弱壯不壯寒不寒熱不熱而其病爲腰脊病也有解㑊證者必無大惡寒發熱身體疼痛之證也太陽人若有大惡寒發熱身體疼痛之證則腰脊表氣充實也其病易治其人亦完健

---

* Part V-1 Discourse on the Greater Yang Person's Lumbar Vertebrae Disease Induced by Exopathogen

2

太陽人內觸小腸病論*

1 朱震亨曰噎膈反胃之病血液俱耗胃脘乾枯其枯在上近咽則水飮可行食物難入入亦不多名之曰噎其枯在下近胃則食雖可入難盡入胃良久復出名之曰膈亦曰反胃大便秘少若羊屎然名雖不同病出一體又曰上焦噎膈食下則胃脘當心而痛須臾吐出食出痛乃止中焦噎膈食物可下難盡入胃良久復出下焦噎膈朝食暮吐暮食朝吐氣血俱虛者口中多出沫但見沫多出者必死大便如羊屎者難治不淡飮食者難治

2 張鷄峯曰噎當是神思間病惟內觀自養可以治之

3 龔信醫鑑曰反胃也膈也噎也受病皆同噎膈之證不屬虛不屬實不屬冷不屬熱乃神氣中一點病耳

4 論曰此證卽太陽人小腸病太重證也必遠嗔怒斷厚味然後其病可愈此證當用獼猴藤植腸湯

5 食物自外入而有所妨碍曰噎自內受而有所拒格曰膈朝食暮吐暮食朝吐曰反胃然朝食而暮吐暮食而朝吐者非全食皆吐也有所妨碍而拒格於胃之上口者經宿而自吐也則反胃亦噎膈也蓋噎膈者胃脘之噎膈也反胃者胃口之噎膈也同是一證也有噎膈證者必無腹痛腸鳴泄瀉痢疾之證也太陽人若有腹痛腸鳴泄瀉痢疾之證則小腸裏氣充實也其病易治其人亦完健

6 解㑊噎膈俱是重證而重證之中有輕重之等級焉解㑊而無噎膈則解㑊之輕證也噎膈而無解㑊則噎膈之輕證也若解㑊兼噎膈噎膈兼解㑊則其爲重險之證不可勝言而重險中又有輕重也太陽人解㑊噎膈不至死境之前起居飮食如常人必易之視以例病故入於危境而莫可挽回也余稟賦太陽人嘗得此病六七年嘔吐涎沫數十年攝身倖而免夭錄此以爲太陽人有病者戒若論治法一言蔽曰遠嗔怒而已矣

7 太陽人意强而操弱意强則胃脘之氣上達而呼散者太過而越也操弱則小

* Part V-2 Discourse on the Greater Yang Person's Small Intestine Disease Induced by Endopathogen

腸之氣中執而吸聚者不支而餒也所以其病爲噎膈反胃也

8 問朱震亨論噎膈反胃曰血液俱耗胃脘乾枯食物難入其說如何曰水穀納於胃而脾衛之出於大腸而腎衛之脾腎者出納水穀之府庫而迭爲補瀉者也氣液呼於胃脘而肺衛之吸於小腸而肝衛之肺肝者呼吸氣液之門戶而迭爲進退者也是故少陽人大腸出水穀陰寒之氣不足則胃中納水穀陽熱之氣必盛也太陽人小腸吸氣液陰凉之氣不足則胃脘呼氣液陽溫之氣必盛也胃脘陽溫之氣太盛則胃脘血液乾枯其勢固然也然非但乾枯而然也上呼之氣太過而中吸之氣太不支故食物不吸入而還呼出也

9 或曰朱震亨所論噎膈反胃者安知非少陰少陽太陰人病而吾子必名目曰太陽人病內經所論解㑊者安知非少陰少陽太陰人病而吾子必名目曰太陽人病莫非牽强附會耶願問其說曰少陽人有嘔吐則必有大熱也少陰人有嘔吐則必有大寒也太陰人有嘔吐則必病愈也今此噎膈反胃不寒不熱非實非虛則此非太陽人病而何也解㑊者上體完健而下體解㑊然胻瘧不能行去之謂也少陰少陽太陰人有此證則他證疊出而亦必無寒不寒熱不熱弱不弱壯不壯之理矣

10 或曰吾子論太陽人解㑊病治法曰戒深哀遠嗔怒修淸定論噎膈病治法曰遠嗔怒斷厚味意者太陽人解㑊病重於噎膈病而哀心所傷者重於怒心所傷乎曰否太陽人噎膈病太重於解㑊病而怒心所傷者太重於哀心所傷也太陽人哀心深着則傷表氣怒心暴發則傷裏氣故解㑊表證以戒哀遠怒兼言之也曰然則少陽人怒性傷口膀胱氣哀情傷腎大腸氣少陰人樂性傷目膂氣喜情傷脾胃氣太陰人喜性傷耳腦顀氣樂情傷肺胃脘氣乎曰然

11 太陽人大便一則宜滑也二則宜體大而多也小便一則宜多也二則宜數也面色宜白不宜黑肌肉宜瘦不宜肥鳩尾下不宜有塊塊小則病輕而其塊易消塊大則病重而其塊難消

2-1

本草所載太陽人病經驗要藥單方十種及李梴龔信經驗要藥單方二種*

1 本草曰五加皮治兩脚疼痺骨節攣急痿躄小兒三歲不能行服此便行走松節療脚軟弱木瓜止嘔逆煮汁飲之最佳葡萄根止嘔噦濃煎取汁細細飲之佳獼猴桃治熱壅反胃取汁服之藤汁至滑主胃閉吐逆取汁服之甚佳蘆根治乾嘔噎及五噎煩悶蘆根五兩水煎頓服一升不過三升卽差蚌蛤治反胃吐食鯽魚治反胃蓴和鯽魚作羹食之主反胃食不下止嘔蕎麥實腸胃益氣力

2 李梴曰杵頭糠主噎食不下咽喉塞細糠一兩白粥清調服

3 龔信曰螃蛤治反胃

---

* Part V-2-1 Ten Recommended Herbs for the Greater Yang Person's Disease (Mentioned in the "Materia Medica") Based on My Experiences, and Two Herbs Based on the Experiences of Li Chan and Gong Xin

2-2

新定太陽人病應用設方藥二力*

1 五加皮壯脊湯五加皮四錢木瓜青松節各二錢葡萄根蘆根櫻桃肉各一錢蕎麥米半匙青松節闕材則以好松葉代之右方治表證

2 獼猴藤植腸湯獼猴桃四錢木瓜葡萄根各二錢蘆根櫻桃肉五加皮松花各一錢杵頭糠半匙獼猴桃闕材則以藤代之右方治裏證凡菜果之屬淸平疏淡之藥皆爲肝藥蛤屬亦補肝論曰藥驗不廣者病驗不廣故也太陽人數從古稀少故古方書中所載證藥亦稀少也今此五加皮壯脊湯獼猴藤植腸湯立方草草雖欠不博而若使太陽人有病者因是二方詳究其理而又變通置方則何患乎無好藥哉

* Part V-2-2 Two Newly Formulated Prescriptions Applicable to the Greater Yang Person's Disease

1

廣濟說*

1 初一歲至十六歲曰幼十七歲至三十二歲曰少三十三歲至四十八歲曰壯四十九歲至六十四歲曰老

2 凡人幼年好聞見而能愛敬如春生之芽少年好勇猛而能騰捷如夏長之苗壯年好交結而能修飭如秋斂之實老年好計策而能秘密如冬藏之根

3 幼年好文字者幼年之豪傑也少年敬長老者少年之豪傑也壯年能汎愛者壯年之豪傑也老年保可人者老年之豪傑也有好才能而又有十分快足於好心術者眞豪傑也有好才能而終不十分快足於好心術者才能而已

4 幼年七八歲前聞見未及而喜怒哀樂膠着則成病也慈母宜保護之也少年二十四五歲前勇猛未及而喜怒哀樂膠着則成病也智父能兄宜保護之也壯年三十八九歲前則賢弟良朋可以助之也老年五十六七歲前則孝子孝孫可以扶之也

5 善人之家善人必聚惡人之家惡人必聚善人多聚則善人之臟氣活動惡人多聚則惡人之心氣强旺酒色財權之家惡人多聚故其家孝男孝婦受病

6 好權之家朋黨比周敗其家者朋黨也好貨之家子孫驕愚敗其家者子孫也

7 人家凡事不成疾病連綿善惡相持其家將敗之地惟明哲之慈父孝子處之有術也

8 嬌奢減壽懶怠減壽偏急減壽貪慾減壽爲人嬌奢必耽侈色爲人懶怠必嗜酒食爲人偏急必爭權勢爲人貪慾必殉貨財

9 簡約得壽勤幹得壽警戒得壽聞見得壽爲人簡約必遠侈色爲人勤幹必潔酒食爲人警戒必避權勢爲人聞見必淸貨財

10 居處荒凉色之故也行身闒茸酒之故也用心煩亂權之故也事務錯亂貨之故也

* Part Ⅵ-1 Discourse on General Health Maintenance

11 若敬淑女色得中道若愛良朋酒得明德若尚賢人權得正術若保窮民貨得全功

12 酒色財權自古所戒謂之四堵墻而比之牢獄非但一身壽夭一家禍福之所繫也天下治亂亦在於此若使一天下酒色財權無乖戾之氣則庶幾近於堯舜周召南世矣

13 凡人簡約而勤幹警戒而聞見四材圓全者自然上壽簡約勤幹而警戒或聞見警戒而勤幹三材全者次壽嬌奢而勤幹警戒而貪慾或簡約而懶怠偏急而聞見二材全者恭敬則壽怠慢則夭

14 凡人恭敬則必壽怠慢則必夭勤幹則必壽虛貪則必夭飢者之腸急於得食則腸氣蕩矣貧者之骨急於得財則骨力竭矣飢而安飢則腸氣有守貧而安貧則骨力有立是故飲食以能忍飢而不貪飽爲恭敬衣服以能耐寒而不貪溫爲恭敬筋力以能勤勞而不貪安逸爲恭敬財物以能謹實而不貪苟得爲恭敬

15 山谷之人沒聞見而禍夭市井之人沒簡約而禍夭農畝之人沒勤幹而禍夭讀書之人沒警戒而禍夭

16 山谷之人宜有聞見有聞見則福壽市井之人宜有簡約有簡約則福壽鄉野之人宜有勤幹有勤幹則福壽士林之人宜有警戒有警戒則福壽

17 山谷之人若有聞見非但福壽也此人卽山谷之傑也市井之人若有簡約非但福壽也此人卽市井之傑也鄉野之人若有勤幹非但福壽也此人卽鄉野之傑也士林之人若有警戒非但福壽也此人卽士林之傑也

18 或曰農夫元來力作最是勤幹者也而何謂沒勤幹士人元來讀書最是警戒者也而何謂沒警戒耶曰以百畝之不治爲己憂者農夫之任也農夫而比之士人則眞是懶怠者也士人頗讀書故心恒妄矜農夫目不識字故心恒佩銘士人而擬之農夫則眞不警戒者也若農夫勤於識字士人習於力作則才性調密臟氣堅固

19 嬌奢者之心藐視閭閻生活輕易天下室家眼界驕豪全昧產業之艱難甚劣財力之方略每爲女色所陷終身不悔

20 懶怠者之心極其麤猛不欲積工之寸累每有虛大之甕算蓋其心甚憚勤幹故欲逃其身於酒國以姑避勤幹之計也凡懶怠者無不縱酒但見縱者則必知其爲懶怠人心麤猛也

21 酒色之殺人者人皆曰酒毒枯腸色勞竭精云此知其一未知其二也縱酒者厭勤其身憂患如山惑色者深愛其女憂患如刀萬端心曲與酒毒色勞幷力攻之而殺人也

22 狂童必愛淫女淫女亦愛狂童愚夫必愛妬婦妬婦必愛愚夫以物理觀之則淫女斷合狂童之配也愚夫亦宜妬婦之匹也蓋淫女妬婦可以爲惡人賤人之配匹也不可爲君子貴人之配匹也七去惡中淫去妬去爲首惡而世俗不知妬字之義但以憎疾衆妾爲言貴人之繼嗣最重則婦人必不可憎疾貴人之有妾而亂家之本未嘗不在於衆妾則婦人之憎疾衆妾之邪媚者猶爲婦人之賢德也何所當於妬字之義乎詩云桃之夭夭其葉蓁蓁之子于歸宜其家人宜其家人者好賢樂善而宜於家人之謂也不宜其家人者妬賢嫉能而不宜於家人之謂也凡人家疾病連綿死亡相隨子孫愚蚩資產零落者莫非愚夫妬婦妬賢嫉能之所做出也

23 天下之惡莫多於妬賢嫉能天下之善莫大於好賢樂善不妬賢嫉能而爲惡

則惡必不多也不好賢樂善而爲善則善必不大也歷稽往牒天下之受病都出於妬賢嫉能天下之救病都出於好賢樂善故曰妬賢嫉能天下之多病也好賢樂善天下之大藥也

2

四象人辨證論*

1 太少陰陽人以今時目見一縣萬人數大略論之則太陰人五千人也少陽人三千人也少陰人二千人也太陽人數絶少一縣中或三四人十餘人而已

2 太陽人體形氣像腦傾之起勢盛壯而腰圍之立勢孤弱少陽人體形氣像胸襟之包勢盛壯而膀胱之坐勢孤弱太陰人體形氣像腰圍之立勢盛壯而腦傾之起勢孤弱少陰人體形氣像膀胱之坐勢盛壯而胸襟之包勢孤弱

3 太陽人性質長於疏通而材幹能於交遇少陽人性質長於剛武而材幹能於事務太陰人性質長於成就而材幹能於居處少陰人性質長於端重而材幹能於黨與

4 太陽人體形元不難辨而人數稀罕故最爲難辨也其體形腦傾之起勢强旺性質疏通又有果斷其病噎膈反胃解㑊證亦自易辨而病未至重險之前別無大證完若無病壯健人也少陰人老人亦有噎證不可誤作太陽人治

5 太陽女體形壯實而肝小脇窄子宮不足故不能生産以六畜玩理而太陽牝牛馬體形壯實而亦不生産者其理可推

6 少陽人體形上盛下虛胸實足輕剽銳好勇而人數亦多四象人中最爲易辨

7 少陽人或有短小靜雅外形恰似少陰人者觀其病勢寒熱仔細執證不可誤作少陰人治

8 太陰少陰人體形或略相彷彿難辨疑似而觀其病證則必無不辨太陰人虛汗則完實也少陰人虛汗則大病也太陰人陽剛堅密則大病也少陰人陽剛堅密則完實也太陰人有胸膈怔忡證也少陰人有手足悗亂證也太陰人有目眥上引證又有目睛內疼證也少陰人則無此證也少陰人平時呼吸平均而間有一太息呼吸也太陰人則無此太息呼吸也太陰人瘧疾惡寒中能飮冷水少陰人瘧疾惡寒中不飮冷水太陰人脈長而緊少陰人脈緩而弱太陰人肌肉堅實少陰人肌肉浮軟太陰人容貌詞氣起居有儀而修整正大少陰

* Part Ⅵ-2 Discourse on Identifying the Four Constitutions

人容貌詞氣體任自然而簡易小巧

9 少陰人體形矮短而亦多有長大者或有八九尺長大者太陰人體形長大而亦或有六尺矮短者

10 太陰人恒有怯心怯心寧靜則居之安資之深而造於道也怯心益多則放心桎梏而物化之也若怯心至於怕心則大病作而怔忡也怔忡者太陰人病之重證也

11 少陽人恒有懼心懼心寧靜則居之安資之深而造於道也懼心益多則放心桎梏而物化之也若懼心至於恐心則大病作而健忘也健忘者少陽人病之險證也

12 少陰人恒有不安定之心不安定之心寧靜則脾氣卽活也太陽人恒有急迫之心急迫之心寧靜則肝血卽和也

13 少陰人有咽喉證其病太重而爲緩病也不可等閒任置當用蔘桂八物湯或用獐肝金蛇酒

14 太陽人有八九日大便不通證其病非殆證也不必疑惑而亦不可無藥當用獼猴藤五加皮湯

15 太陽人小便旺多則完實而無病太陰人汗液通暢則完實而無病少陽人大便善通則完實而無病少陰人飮食善化則完實而無病

16 太陽人噎膈則胃脘之上焦散豁如風太陰人痢病則小腸之中焦窄塞如霧少陽人大便不通則胸膈必如烈火少陰人泄瀉不止則臍下必如冰冷明知其人而又明知其證則應用之藥必無可疑

17 人物形容仔細商量再三推移如有迷惑則參互病證明見無疑然後可以用藥最不可輕忽而一貼藥誤投重病險證一貼藥必殺人

18 華佗曰養生之術每欲小勞但莫大疲有一老人曰人可日再食而不四五食也又不可旣食後添食如此則必無不壽

19 余足之曰太陰人察於外而恒寧靜怯心少陽人察於內而恒寧靜懼心太陽人退一步而恒寧靜急迫之心少陰人進一步而恒寧靜不安定之心如此則必無不壽

20 又曰太陽人恒戒怒心哀心少陽人恒戒哀心怒心太陰人恒戒樂心喜心少陰人恒戒喜心樂心如此則必無不壽

21 大舜自耕稼陶漁無非取諸人以爲善夫子曰三人行必有我師以此觀之則天下衆人之才能聖人必博學審問而兼之故大而化也太少陰陽人識見才局各有所長文筆射御歌舞揖讓以至於博弈小技細鎖動作凡百做造面面不同皆異其妙儘乎衆人才能之浩多於造化中也

22 靈樞書中有太少陰陽五行人論而略得外形未得臟理蓋太少陰陽人早有古昔之見而未盡精究也

3

跋文*

此書自癸巳七月十三日始作晝思夜度無頃刻休息至于翌年甲午四月十三日少陰少陽人論則略得詳備太陰太陽人論則僅成簡約蓋經驗未遍而精力已憊故也記曰開而不達則思若太陰太陽人思而得之則亦何損乎簡約哉

萬室之邑一人陶則器不足也百家之村一人醫則活人不足也必廣明醫學家家知醫人人知病然後可以壽世保元

光緖甲午四月十三日咸興李濟馬畢書于漢南山中

甲午畢書後乙未ˉ並阝至于庚子因本改抄自醫源論至太陰人諸論各有增删而其餘諸論未有增删故　依新舊本刊行

* Part Ⅵ-3 Epilogue

Notes

Part I-1 Discourse on Nate and Order

1) King Yao (堯)

Formally, in Chinese mythology, a legendary emperor of the golden age (c. 24th century B.C.) of antiquity, exalted by Confucius as an inspiration and perennial model of virtue and righteousness, and always mentioned with King Shun (舜王), his successor, to whom Yao gave his two daughters in marriage. Legends recount that after 70 years of Yao's rule, the sun and moon were as resplendent as jewels, the five planets shone like strung pearls, phoenixes nested in the palace courtyards, crystal springs flowed from the hills, pearl grass covered the countryside, rice crops were plentiful, two unicorns (omens of prosperity) appeared in the capital at Pingyang (平陽), and the wondrous calendar bean made its appearance, producing a pod a day for half a month before the 15 pods withered one by one on successive days. Two remarkable events marked Yao's reign: a rampaging flood was controlled by Da Yu (大禹); and Hou I (后羿), the Lord Archer, saved the world from destruction by shooting down nine of the ten suns burning up the earth. Like Fuhsi (伏犧), Shennong (神農), and Huangdi (黃帝) before him, Yao had special temples dedicated in his honour. He is said to have offered sacrifices and to have practiced divination. In choosing a successor, Yao bypassed his own less worthy son in favors of Shun and served as counselor to the new emperor.

2) King Shun (舜)

In Chinese mythology, a legendary emperor (c. 23rd century B.C.) of the golden age of antiquity, singled out by Confucius as a model of integrity and resplendent virtue. His name is invariably associated with that of Yao, his legendary predecessor. Though Shun's father repeatedly tried to murder him, the boy's filial piety never faltered. Because Heaven and Earth knew of his virtue, birds came to assist in weeding his paddies, and animals appeared from nowhere to drag the plow. Yao bypassed his own son in choosing Shun as the most worthy to rule. He likewise gave Shun his two daughters, Ohuang (娥皇) and Nuying (女英), in marriage. Shun offered sacrifice to the Six Honoured Ones (whose identity is uncertain) and the springs of earth. He is credited with standardizing weights and measures, regulating waterways, and organizing the kingdom into 12 provinces. During his reign, marvelous phenomena occurred in the heavens and on earth.

3) King Chieh (桀)

The last king of the legendary Xia (夏) dynasty in ancient China. He is a typical despot who forms a striking contrast to King Yao and King Shun. The state of the Xia dynasty under his rule had already been so weakened that many feudal lords broke their relations with him. He was killed while trying to escape. The stories and dates attributed to him are unreliable, since they vary considerably in the Chinese and Western sources.

4) King Chou (紂)

Also called Ti Hsin (帝辛), last sovereign of the Shang (商), or Yin (殷) dynasty, who according to legend lost his empire because of his extreme debauchery. To please his concubine, Tachi, it is said that he built a lake of wine around which naked men and women were forced to chase one another. His cruelty was such that the nearby forests were littered with corpses. Moreover, he provoked the resentment of the people by levying taxes to build, over the course of seven years, the elaborate Deer Tower Palace (鹿臺). It was supposed to have been 600 feet high and a half mile in circumference, with doors and chambers constructed of precious stones. When King Wu, the founder of the succeeding Zhou (周) dynasty (1111 - 255 B.C.), overthrew the Shang, Chou set fire to his palace and committed suicide by leaping into the flames.

5) Confucius (孔子)

Original name Kung Chiu (孔丘), China's most famous teacher, philosopher, and political theorist whose ideas have influenced the civilizations of eastern Asia. A brief account of the life and works of Confucius follows. Although little reliable information exists on Confucius' ancestry and early life, his family was probably of the impoverished nobility. He was orphaned at an early age and grew up poor. He was largely self-educated, but apparently became the most learned man of his day. Learning, however, was not his greatest interest. Confucius was deeply disturbed by the political and social conditions of his times. Unable to obtain an official position in which he might affect his ideas of reform, he spent the greater part of his life educating a small group of disciples. Confucius was not a religious leader in the ordinary sense, for his teachings were essentially social ethics. Though his interest in books was secondary to his passion for reform, many ancient classics were attributed to his authorship and editorship. These books, interpreted in Confucian terms, were the basic curriculum of Chinese education for more than 2,000 years, and explain why Confucius must be counted among the most influential men of all time.

6) King Wen (文)

Father of King Wu, the founder of the Zhou dynasty and one of the sage rulers regarded by Confucian historians as a model king. Wen was a ruler of Zhou, one of the semi-barbaric states on the western frontier of China, a long-time battleground between the civilized Chinese and nomadic invaders. By 1144 B.C., he had begun to threaten the Shang dynasty and was captured and imprisoned by King Chou, the last Shang ruler. After King Wen returned to Chou, he spent the rest of his life remonstrating against the cruelty and corruption of his age. Upon his death, his son and successor, King Wu (武), destroyed the Shang and founded the Zhou dynasty.

7) King Wu (武)

The founder and the first ruler of the Zhou dynasty. Wu was respected by later Confucians as a wise king. He succeeded his father, the famous King Wen, as head of the semi-barbaric state of Zhou, located on the western border of China. Wu continued his father's work and formed a coalition with eight other border states, which defeated the last other evil border states and also defeated the evil ruler of the Shang. After establishing the Zhou dynasty, Wu, assisted by his brother, known as the Duke of Zhou (周公), consolidated his rule by establishing a feudalistic form of government, which parceled out territory to relatives and vassals willing to acknowledge Zhou sovereignty.

8) Cao Cao (曹操)

One of the greatest generals at the end of the Han (漢) dynasty. He was the adopted son of the chief eunuch of the imperial court, and wielded much influence in the last years of the Han. Cao rose to prominence as a general when he suppressed the Yellow Turban (黃巾賊) Rebellion, which threatened the last years of Han rule. The dynasty, however, was greatly weakened by the rebellion, and in the ensuing chaos, the country was divided among the major generals into three parts. Cao occupied the strategic northern section around the emperor's capital prerogatives. Cao's large armies and his skillful maneuvering have long been notorious in

Chinese history. He was described by Confucian historians and in popular legends as the archetypal shrewd, bold and unscrupulous villain. He was portrayed in this role in the great 14th century historical novel, 『*Sanguo Yanyi*』 (三國演義: "Story of the Three Kingdoms"), and since then he has been one of the most popular figures of Chinese legend and folklore, with various evil magic powers ascribed to him. Modern historians tend to view Cao as a skillful general and pragmatic politician. After Cao's death, his son Cao Pi (曹丕) usurped the Han throne and proclaimed the Wei (魏) dynasty.

9) Emperor of Chin (秦始皇)

Shih Huangdi (始皇帝), creator of the first unified Chinese empire (259~210 B.C.) and emperor of the Chin (秦) dynasty. He was born while his father was being held hostage in the state of Chao (趙). His mother was a former concubine of the rich merchant Lu Puwei (呂不韋). By 221 B.C., with the help of espionage, extensive bribery, and the ruthlessly effective leadership of gifted generals, he had marked his final triumph: For the first time, China was united, under the supreme rule of the Chin. With unbounded confidence, he claimed that his dynasty would last "10,000 generations." However, it collapsed only four years after his death. It seems certain that Shih Huangdi had an imposing personality and showed an unbending will in pursuing his aim of uniting and strengthening the empire. His despotic rule and the draconian punishments he meted out were dictated largely by his legalistic (法家) ideas. With few exceptions, the traditional historiography of Imperial China has regarded Shih Huangdi as the villain par excellence, inhuman, uncultivated, and superstitious.

10) 『*Shijing*』 (詩經)

"Classics of Poetry", the first anthology of Chinese poetry. It was compiled by the ancient sage Confucius (551~479 B.C.) and cited by him as a model of literary expression; for, despite its numerous themes, the subject matter was always "expressive of pleasure without being licentious and of grief without being hurtfully expressive." The book, one of the Five Classics (五經), contains 305 poems (and six poem titles) classified either as popular songs or ballads, courtly songs, or eulogies.

Part I-2 Discourse on the Four Principles

1) Mencius (孟子)

(371~239 B.C., ancient state of Tsou (趨), China), early Chinese philosopher whose development of orthodox Confucianism earned him the title "The Second Sage (亞聖)." Chief among his basic tenets was an emphasis on the obligation of rulers to provide for the common people. Mencius' book,『*Mengzi*』(孟子)records his doings and sayings and contains statements on the innate goodness of human nature, a topic heatedly debated by Confucianists up to modern times. The philosophical ideas of Mencius might be regarded as an amplification of the teachings of Confucius. Confucius taught the concept of Ren (仁), love or humanity, as the basic virtue of mankind. Mencius made the original goodness of human nature the keynote to his system. While Mencius has always been regarded as a major philosopher, special importance was attributed to him and his work by the Neo-Confucianists of the Song dynasty (AD 960~1279). For the last 1,000 years, Mencius has been revered among the Chinese people as the co-founder of Confucianism, second only to Confucius himself.

2) Yu (禹): King Yu

Yu the Great, in Chinese mythology, the Tamer of the Flood, one of China's saviour-heroes and reputed founder of China's oldest dynasty, the Xia. King Yu, after years of strenuous labors, dredged outlets to the sea with the aid of dragons, thus making the world suitable for human habitation.

Part I-5 Discourse on the Origin of Eastern Medicine

1)『*Shujing*』(書經)

The "Classic of Document", also called the『*Shangshu*』(商書: "Official History"), one of the Five Classics of Chinese antiquity. The『*Shujing*』consists of fifty eight chapters. The first five chapters purport to preserve the sayings and to recall the deeds of such illustrious emperors as Yao and Shun. Chapters six to nine are devoted to the Xia dynasty (c. 2205~1766 B.C.), the historicity of which has not been definitively established. The next 17 chapters deal with the Shang dynasty and its collapse in 1122 B.C.. The final 32 chapters cover the Western Zhou dynasty that ruled China until 771 B.C..

2) Shennong (神農)

The second of ancient China's mythical emperors, said to have been born in the 28th century B.C., with the head of a bull and the body of a man. By inventing the cart and plow, taming the ox, yoking the horse, and teaching his people to clear the land with fire, Shennong is said to have established a stable agricultural societyin China. His catalog of 365 species of medicinal plants became the basis of later herbological studies. Marvelous tales of his youth relate that he spoke after three days, walked within a week, and could plow a field at the age of three.

3) Huangdi (黃帝)

The third of ancient China's mythological emperors, a cultural hero and patron saint of Taoism. Huangdi is reputed to have been born in 2,704 B.C., and begun his rule as emperor in 2,697 B.C.. His legendary reign is credited with the introduction of wooden houses, carts, boats, the bow and arrow, and writing. Huangdi himself is credited with defeating "barbarians" in a great battle somewhere in what is now Shansi. The victory won him the leadership of tribes throughout the Huang He (黃河: Yellow River) plain. Some traditions also credit him with the introduction of governmental institutions and the use of coined money. His wife was reputed to have discovered sericulture (silk production) and to have taught women how to breed silkworms and weave fabrics of silk. Huangdi is held up in some ancient sources as a paragon of wisdom whose reign was a golden age. He is said to have dreamed of an ideal kingdom whose tranquil inhabitants lived in harmonious accord with natural law and possessed virtues remarkably like those espoused by early Taoism. Upon waking from his dream, Huangdi sought to inculcate these virtues in his own kingdom and to ensure order and prosperity among the inhabitants. Upon his death, he was said to have become an immortal.

4) 『*Bencao*』 (本草)

The "Herbal", 『*Shennong Bencaojing*』 (神農本草經), the earliest book on Materia Medica, and believed to have been a product of the first century B.C., with its authorship attributed to the ancient emperor "the Divine Peasant" Shennong. There are 365 kinds of drugs listed. The drugs are divided into three classes: superior, common and inferior.

5) 『*Suwen*』 (素問)

The "*Plain Questions*", also called the 『*Huangdi Neijing Suwen*』 (黃帝內經素問),

originally consisting of nine volumes, with 81 articles. After the Wei and Jin dynasties, there were only eight volumes extant. In the Tang dynasty, while making notes and commentaries on the book, Wang Bing (王冰) divided it into 24 volumes and supplemented some of the lost articles. In the Northern Song dynasty, Lin Yi (林億) and other scholars, read proofs and made notes on it again. All later extant editions were based on the Northern Song version. The book includes a variety of subjects, such as human anatomy, physiology, etiology, pathology, diagnosis, pattern identification, treatment, disease prevention, health preservation, relations between man and nature, the application of yin-yang and five phases in medicine, the theory of promoting the flow of qi, etc. The book has been prized by physicians of all generations.

6) Zhang Zhongjing (張仲景)

(150?~219? A.D.), Also called Zhang Ji (張機), and is considered one of the most influential figures in the history of Chinese medicine. He was the first to advocate the methods of analysing and differentiating pathological conditions in accordance with the six stages and the eight principal syndromes/patterns. He stressed the principle of treating diseases according to the method of differentiating symptoms and signs. He is also ascribed the authorship of several medical books on various topics, the most important of which, now extant, are the『*Shanghan Zabinglun*』(傷寒雜病論: "Treatise on Cold-induced and Miscellaneous Diseases") and『*Jinkui Yaolue Fanglun*』(金匱要略方論: "Synopsis of Prescriptions of the Golden Chamber").

7) Zhu Gong (朱肱)

A famous physician in the Song dynasty. He studied Zhang Zhongjing's theory for many years, and wrote the『*Shanghan Baiwen*』(傷寒百聞, 1108), which is in the form of 100 questions and answers. In 1114 (A.D.), he wrote the『*Huorenshu*』(活人書), which is a 22volume rewrite of the『*Shanghan Baiwen*』. In this book, he analyzed Zhang Zhongjing's *liujing* (六經) through the theory of the six meridians.

8)『*Huorenshu*』(活人書)

The "*Book for Saving Lives*", also called the『*Nanyang Huorenshu*』(南陽活人書),『*Leizheng Huorenshu*』(類證活人書), written in 22 volumes by Zhu Gong (朱肱) in 1108 A.D.. He divided the volumes into four parts and introduced the febrile diseases and miscellaneous diseases separately. The『*Huorenshu*』was influential to the early commentaries pertaining to Zhang Zhongjing's theory.

9) Li Gao (李杲)

(1180~1251 A.D.) Also called Li Mingzhi (李明之) or Li Dongyuan (李東垣), a disciple of Zhang Yuansu (張元素), who held that diseases, apart from external changes, were mainly caused by the "internal injury" of the spleen and stomach (i.e., intemperance in drinking and eating or overwork), and advocated the regulation of the spleen and stomach and nourishing the original qi. He is considered the founder of the school of strengthening the spleen and stomach. His masterpiece was the 『*Piweilun*』(脾胃論: "Treatise on the Spleen and Stomach").

10) Wang Haogu (王好古)

Also called Wang Jinzhi (王進之), or Wang Haizang (王海藏). A distinguished physician in the 13th century, whose chief contribution was his plea in support of using tonics and stimulants for infectious diseases in the later stage when the metabolic function is weakened, and the avoidance of purgatives. Five of his publications are still in existence, including the 『*Tangye Bencao*』(湯液本草: "Materia Medica of Decoction", 1289 A.D.).

11) Zhu Zhenheng (朱震亨)

(1282~1358 A.D.) A native of Danxi (丹溪), Jinhua County, Zhejiang Province, also known as the Master of Danxi, who took indulgence as the root of all troubles and exhorted the value of tonics for the purpose of supplementing the yin-deficiency. He advocated the theory that yang was always in excess while yin was often deficient, and thus belonged to the school of nourishing yin. He was the author of 『*Gezhi Yulun*』(格致餘論: "Inquiry into the Properties of Things", 1347 A.D.) and 『*Jufang Fahui*』(局方發揮: ":n Expounding on the Formularies of the Bureau of the People's Welfare Pharmacies").

12) Wei Yilin (危亦林)

(1277~1347 A.D.) Also called Wei Dazhai (危達齋) was thought to have been a bone physician famous for setting bones. Based on the experience and findings of his ancestors, not a few of whom were noted physicians, he compiled a large number of prescriptions in a book entitled 『*Shiyi Dexiaofang*』(世醫得效方: "Effective Formulas Tested by Generations of Physicians").

13) Li Chan (李梴)

Also called Li Jianzhai (李健齋). A physician in the 16th century who summarized the prescriptions used at that period in medical practice and divided them into 18 different categories. Li was the author of the『*Yixue Rumen*』(醫學入門: "Introduction to Medicine", 1575 A.D.), and『*Xiyi Guige*』(習醫規格: "Rules for the Study of Medicine", 1575 A.D.).

14) Gong Xin (龔信)

A famous physician of the Ming dynasty and the author of the『*Yijianshu*』(醫鑑書), which was completed by his son, Gong Tingxian .

15) Heo Jun (許浚)

Heo Jun was born in 1546, and became the head physician during the reign of King Seonjo (宣祖) and Gwanghaegun (光海君) in the Joseon dynasty. Additionally, Heo Jun contributed several works to the literature of traditional Korean medicine. The most brilliant of them is the『*Dongui Bogam*』, which he finished compiling in 1610. His medical philosophy drew heavily from the『*Suwen*』,『*Lingshu*』and『*Nanjing*』. The theories of Zhang Zhongjing and the "Four Masters" of the Jin-Yuan dynasties were influential as well.

16)『*Dongui Bogam*』(東醫寶鑑)

The "*Treasure Mirror of Eastern Medicine*" was compiled by Heo Jun and was published in 1611 A.D. (Joseon dynasty) in 25 volumes. Heo Jun gathered and organized the traditional Chinese medical books, which had been published until the Ming dynasty. The『*Dongui Bogam*』consisted of five parts: Internal Medicine (內景篇), External Diseases (外形篇), Miscellaneous Diseases (雜病篇), Drugs and Decoctions (湯液篇), and Acupuncture and Moxibustion (鍼灸篇). The scope of this work is very broad and well organized. Eventually, it became one of the most important books in east Asian traditional medicine.

17)『*Tangye Bencao*』(湯液本草)

The "*Materia Medica of Decoction*", written by Wang Haogu (王好古) and published in 1298 A.D., lists 238 kinds of drugs, in which the flavor, taste, therapeutic properties as well as the mutual influence of mixing medicines are all described. This text is used in combination with the study of the Materia Medica.

18)『*Shiliao Bencao*』(食療本草)

The "*Dietetic Materia Medica*" is a monograph by the Tang dynasty's Meng

Xian (孟詵), recording herbs, which can be used as both food and drugs. The original has been lost, but its text can be found in the 『*Leizheng Bencao*』(類證本草: "Classified Materia Medica").

19) Meng Xian (孟詵)

(621~713 A.D.) A herbalist in the Tang dynasty and author of the 『*Shiliao Bencao*』. The original has been lost, but the text can be found in the 『*Leizheng Bencao*』.

20) Chen Zangqi (陳藏器)

An herbalist in the Tang dynasty, and author of the 『*Bencao Shiyi* 』(本草拾遺).

21) 『Bencao Shiyi』(本草拾遺)

The "*Supplement to Materia Medica*" was written in ten volumes by Chen Zangqi (陳藏器) in the Tang dynasty, and added medical substances not included in the 『*Xinxiu Bencao*』(新修本草: "Newly Compiled Materia Medica").

22) Fang Anshang (龐安常)

Also called Fang Anshi, a noted physician known for having written several medical works, among which the most widely read was a detailed and comprehensive treatise on various kinds of fevers under the title of 『*Shanghan Zhongbinglun*』(傷寒總病論: "General Treatise on Cold-induced Disease", 1100 A.D.).

23) 『*Rihuazi Bencao*』(日華子本草)

Written in 20 volumes by Rihuazi (日華子). The original copy is lost, but parts of its contents are found in the 『*Zhenglei Bencao*』(證類本草).

24) 『*Suse Bowon*』(壽世保元)

The "*Longevity and Life Preservation*", written by Lee Je-ma and published in 1894. Its full name is 『*Dongui Suse Bowon*』(東醫壽世保元: "Longevity and Life Preservation in Eastern Medicine"), and is the text upon which Sasang Constitutional Medicine is based.

25) 『*Shanghanlun*』(傷寒論)

The "Treatise on Cold-induced Diseases", a new edition of Zhang Zhongjing's "Treatise on Cold-induced and Miscellaneous Diseases", rearranged by Wang Shuhe (王叔和) in the Jin dynasty. In this work, acute febrile diseases are analyzed and differentiated in accordance with the theory of the six stages. The book is regarded as one of the most influential works in the traditional practice of Chinese medicine.

26) Qibo (岐伯)

A famous mythical physician in the reign of Huangdi, the Yellow Emperor (2698~2589 B.C.), who was asked by the Emperor to taste various kinds of herbs and to study medicine and pharmacy. The first and greatest medical work in China, the 『*Huangdi Neijing*』, consists of questions and answers between Huangdi and Qibo and other officials on problems of medicine and pharmacy.

27) 『*Lingshu*』 (靈樞)

The "*Miraculous Pivot*" or "*Divine Axis*", one of the two parts of the *Huangdi Neijing*, also called *Huangdi Neijing Lingshujing*(黃帝內經靈樞經, "Miraculous Pivot of Huangdi' s Internal Classic"). The subjects of "*Miraculous Pivot*" are similar to those of *Suwen* ("Plain Questions") but the former has a more detailed description of meridians and needling, and is less concerned with the basic theories about the functions of the internal organs and the vital substances. In introducing basic theories and clinical practice, the two books supplement each other. This book, like 『*Suwen*』, has been prized by physicians of all generations.

Part II-1 Discourse on the Lesser Yin Person's Exterior Febrile Disease Induced From the Kidney Affected by Heat

1) 『*Dexiaofang*』 (得效方)

The 『*Effective Formulas*』, also called the 『*Shiyi Dexiaofang*』 (世醫得效方: "Effective Formulas Tested by Physicians for Generations"), compiled by Wei Yilin (危亦林) in 1345 A.D., is based on the author' s family experiences as physicians for five successive generations, and in which the contents are prescriptions for children' s disease, internal medicine, ophthalmology, oral disease, dentistry, bone-setting, war wounds, ulcers and carbuncles.

2) 『*Yijian*』 (醫鑑)

The "*Mirror of Medicine*", also called the 『*Yijianshu*』 (醫鑑書): a comprehensive medical work by Gong Xin and Gong Tingxian; it was later supplemented by Wang Kentang (王肯堂). It deals with the theories from the time of 『*Neijing*』 and

『*Nanjing*』 to the Jin-Yuan (金元) dynasties' schools. It covers the methods of using acupuncture and moxibustion, and lists many prescriptions.

3) 『*Benshifang*』 (本事方)

The "*Effective Prescriptions*", also called the 『*Leizheng Puji Benshifang*』 (類證普濟本事方: "Classified Effective Prescriptions for Universal Relief"), is a work of ten volumes written by Xu Shuwei (許叔微) in the Southern Song (南宋) dynasty and published in the middle of the 12th century. This text mainly deals with common diseases related to internal medicine, listing 23 kinds of treatment with more than 300 prescriptions. At the end of each prescription, the authors' proven cases are described.

4) Xu Shuwei (許叔微)

(1079~1154 A.D.) A famous physician in the Song dynasty and a close follower of Zhang Zhongjing. Xu prepared graphic illustrations of thirty six varieties of pulse based on Zhang Zhongjing's work, and propounded the theory of using drugs in relation to the intensity of the disease. Xu was the author of several medical works, among which 『*Leizheng Puji Benshifang*』 in ten volumes has been one of his most widely read.

5) 『*Haizangshu*』 (海藏書)

Haizang is Wang Haogu's other name. See Wang Haogu.

6) 『*Yixue Gangmu*』 (醫學綱目)

The "*Compendium of Medicine*", a comprehensive medical work by Lou Ying (樓英) in forty volumes. He gathered many traditional medicine treatises and descriptions to support his opinions. The scope of this work is very broad. It is well organized and the explanations to the descriptions are precise.

7) 『*Minglilun*』 (明理論)

The "*Expounding on the Treatise*" (1156) written by Cheng Wuji (成無己) in the Jin (金) dynasty, is a concise reference book for beginners studying the 『*Shanghanlun*』, in which the ideas related to the compatibility of ingredients are stressed.

8) 『*Danxi Xinfa*』 (丹溪心法)

The "*Danxi's Experiential Therapy*" was written by Zhu Zhenheng (朱震亨) in the Yuan (元) dynasty, but rearranged and edited by his disciples. In 1481 A.D., the book was reedited with supplements and corrections by Cheng Chong (程充), who added six treatises on medical theories and 100 articles dealing with various diseases, most of which are concerned with internal medicine. The author' s theory that "Yang is ever excessive and yin is ever deficient" is reflected throughout the book.

9) 『*Yixue Rumen*』(醫學入門)
The "*Introduction to Medicine*", a comprehensive medical work written by Li Chan in 1575. The book covers basic medical theories, explanatory diagrams of meridians, internal organs, diagnosis, acupuncture and moxibustion, herbal drugs, infection due to both exogenic and endogenic pathogens, internal medicine, gynecology, pediatrics, surgery, etc.

Part II-2 Discourse on the Lesser Yin Person's Interior Cold Disease Induced from the Stomach Affected by Cold

1) 『*Dongyuanshu*』(東垣書)
A collection of 10 articles from various physicians including Li Gao published in 1529.

2) Cheng Wuji (成無己)
(1066~1155 A.D.) He is known for his assiduous study of Zhang Zhongjing's "Treatise on Cold-induced and Miscellaneous Diseases" and for writing several books on its comment. His 『*Zhujie Shanghanlun* (註解傷寒論: "Commentary on the Treatise on Cold-induced Diseases", 1142 A.D.)』 is considered the earliest of its kind in Chinese medical literature.

3) 『*Maijing*』(脈經)
The "Classic of Pulse", written by Wang Shuhe (王叔和) in the third century, generally acknowledged as the standard work on the subject and the earliest comprehensive work dealing with pulse diagnosis now extant.

4) Wang Shuhe (王叔和)
(About 210~285 A.D.) Also called Wang Xi, versed in pulse taking, commissioner of the Imperial Academy of Medicine, and author of the 『Maijing』, the first comprehensive book on pulse diagnosis now extant in China. He perfected and systemized the art of pulse taking, yet emphasized the use of all four methods of

diagnosis, visual inspection, audio-olfactive investigation, interrogation, and palpation and pulse diagnosis. He rearranged Zhang Zhongjing's 『*Shanghan Zabinglun*』, which contributed much towards the preservation of that important medical classic.

Part II-3-2 Thirteen Prescriptions and Six Other Prescriptions Containing Semen Crotonis for the Lesser Yin Person's Disease Mentioned in the Writings of Famous Doctors in the Song, Yuan and Ming Dynasties

1) 『*Wanbing Huichun*』(萬病回春)

The "Recovery from All Ailments", a comprehensive medical work consisting of eight volumes by Gong Tingxian, published in 1587. The book describes in detail numerous diseases and patterns. It explains treatments and prescriptions in detail. This work was a great influence on later practitioners.

2) 『*Jufang*』(局方)

The "Formularies of the Burean of People Welfare Pharmacies", 『*Taiping Huimin Heji Jufang*』(太平惠民和劑局方), or simply 『*Heji Jufang*』(和劑局方), compiled by Chen Shiwen (陳師文) and others, in 1151 A.D.. It is a ten volume work dividing 788 oft-used and effective prescriptions into fourteen categories.

Part III-1 Discourse on the Lesser Yang Person's Exterior Cold Disease Induced from the Spleen Affected by Cold

1) Du Ren (杜任)

He is cited in the 『*Yixue Gangmu*』(醫學綱目), but he has not been identified.

2) 『*Shanghan Shiquanlun*』(傷寒十卷論)

The "Ten Pieces of Advice on Exogenous Febrile Disease", written by Li Zijian.

3) Li Zijian (李子建)

A famous physician in the Song dynasty, and author of the 『*Shanghan Shiquanlun*』. Little is known about him except that he studied Zhang Zhongjing (張仲景)'s works and concluded that febrile diseases were not as dangerous to people as mediocre doctors who gave out erroneous prescriptions.

4) Zhu Danxi (朱丹溪)

Danxi is Zhu Zhenheng's other name. See Zhu Zhenheng.

Part Ⅲ-2 Discourse on the Lesser Yang Person's Interior Febrile Disease Induced from the Stomach Affected by Heat

1) 『*Dongui Uibang Yuchui*』(東醫醫方類聚)

The "Classified Collection of Eastern Medical Prescriptions". King Sejong (世宗) of the Joseon dynasty ordered his officers to gather all the traditional medical books and to compile a comprehensive medical work for the sake of medical practice improvement. It comprises 266 volumes.

2) Sun Simiao (孫思邈)

(581~682 A.D.) A prominent physician of the Tang dynasty and author of the 『*Qianjin Yaofang*』(千金要方: "Essential Prescriptions Worth a Thousand Gold Pieces", 652 A.D.) and 『*Qianjin Yifang*』(千金翼方: "Supplement to Prescriptions Worth a Thousand Gold Pieces", 682 A.D.), which are considered a collection of the medical achievements before the 7th century.

3) 『*Qianjinfang*』(千金方)

The "Essential Prescriptions Worth a Thousand Gold Pieces", also called the 『*Beiji Qianjin Yaofang*』(備急千金要方: "Essential Prescriptions Worth a Thousand Gold Pieces for Emergencies") or 『*Qianjin Yaofang*』, compiled by Sun Simiao (孫思邈) at the end of the seventh century in thirty volumes. This text gives a general introduction, deals with the prescriptions of various clinical branches, diet, pulse taking, acupuncture, etc.

4) 『*Ijing*』(易經)

The "Classic of Changes", an ancient Chinese text that is one of the Five Classics of Confucianism. The uniqueness of 『*Ijing*』 is in its presentation of 64 symbolic hexagrams that, if properly understood and interpreted, are said to contain profound meanings applicable to daily life. Throughout the ages, the 『*Ijing*』 enthusiasts have claimed that the book is a means of understanding, and even controlling, future events.

Part Ⅲ-3-2 Nine Prescriptions for the Lesser Yang Person's Disease Mentioned in the Writings of Famous Doctors in the Yuan and Ming Dynasties

1) 『*Yixue Zhengzhuan*』(醫學正傳)

The "Orthodox Medical Record" (1515), a comprehensive medical work by Yu Tuan (虞博) in eight volumes. With reference to many schools' theories, he stated his own experiences in medicine. He criticised the method of using incantation and *yunqi* (運氣: the theory of five circuits and six qi) in estimating the pathological period, symptoms and treatment.

2) Yu Tuan (虞博)

Yu Tuan (1438~1517) is also called Yu Tianmin (虞天民). He collected over thirty important medical works and edited his own 『*Yixue Zhengzhuan*』.

Part Ⅳ-2 Discourse on the Greater Yin Person's Interior Febrile Disease Induced from the Liver Affected by Heat

1) 『*Neijing*』(內經)

The 『*Huangdi Neijing*』, the oldest and greatest medical classic extant in China, with its authorship ascribed to the ancient Emperor Huangdi (2698~2589 B.C.). The work was actually a product of various unknown authors from the Warring States Period (475~221 B.C.) to the Late Han dynasty (25~220 A.D.). The book consists of two parts: the 『*Suwen*』(素問: "Plain Questions"), and 『*Lingshu*』(靈樞: "Miraculous Pivot" or "Divine Axis", also known as the "Canon of Acupuncture").

2) Bianque (扁鵲)

(circa 500 B.C.) Also known as Qin Yueren (秦越人), the earliest noted physician who was famous for his medical knowledge and well versed in diagnosis and treatment, especially pulse taking and acupuncture. He was ascribed the authorship of some medical works such as the 『*Bianque Neijing*』(扁鵲內經: "The Internal Classic of Bianque") and 『*Bianque Waijing*』(扁鵲外經: "The External Classic of Bianque"), all of which have been lost.

3) 『*Nanjing*』(難經)

The "Classic of Difficult Issues", a book that appeared in the first or second century

B.C. with its authorship unknown, though it is often ascribed to Qin Yueren (秦越人). It deals with fundamental medical theories and expounds the 『*Neijing*』's main points in the form of questions and answers. The points of acupuncture and moxibustion, the method of needling, the physiological and pathological conditions related to the meridians and collaterals, and the method of feeling the pulse are all discussed.

Part V-2 Discourse on the Greater Yang Person's Small Intestine Disease Induced by Endopathogen

1) Zhang Jihfeng (張鷄峰)
His history is not well documented. His theory was recorded in the 『*Danxi Xinfa*』 (丹溪心法) and quoted in the 『*Dongui Bogam*』.

Part VI-3 Epilogue

1) 『*Liji*』 (禮記)
The "Record of Rites", one of the Five Classics of Chinese Confucian literature, the original text of which is said to have been compiled by the ancient sage Confucius himself. In general, the 『*Liji*』 underscores the moral principles in such subjects as royal regulations, rites, ritual objects and sacrifices, education, music, the behaviors of scholars, and the doctrine of the mean. In 1190, Zhu Xi, a Neo-Confucian philosopher, took two chapters from the 『*Liji*』, gave them separate titles, and published them together with two other Confucian texts under the name 『*Sishu*』 (四書: "Four Books"). This collection is generally used to introduce Chinese students to Confucian literature.

Selected Bibliography

Classical Sources

(Chinese-Language)

Chen Shiwen et al. (陳師文等). *Formularies of the Bureau of People's Welfare Pharmacies* (Taiping Huimin Heji Jufang 太平惠民和劑局方). Beijing: People's Health Press, 1959. First appeared 1241.

Cheng Wuji (成無己). *Expounding on the Treatise* (*Minglilun* 明理論). Shanghai: Shanghai People's Health Press, 1957. First appeared 1156.

Classic of Difficult Issues with Annotations (*Nanjing Jiaoshi* 難經校釋), Edited by Nanjing Traditional Chinese Medical Collage. Beijing: People's Health Press, 1979.

Gong Tingxian (龔廷賢). *Recovery from All Ailments* (*Wanbing Huichun* 萬病回春). Shanghai: Shanghai Jinzhang Book Press, 1955. First appeared 1587.

Gong Xin (龔信). *Mirror of Medicine* (*Yijian* 醫鑑). Nanjing: Jiangxi Science and Technology Press, 1990. First appeared 1576.

Heo Jun et al. (許浚 等). *Treasure Mirror of Eastern Medicine* (*Dongui Bogam* 東醫寶鑑). Beijing: People's Health Press, 1982. First appeared 1611.

Kim Ye-mong et al.(金禮蒙 等). *Classified Collection of Eastern Medical Prescriptions* (*Dongui Uibang Yuchui* 東醫醫方類聚). Seoul: Geumyoung Press, 1977. First appeared 1445.

Li Chan (李梴). *Introduction to Medicine* (*Yixue Rumen* 醫學入門). Shanghai: Shanghai Jinzhang Book Press, 1941. First appeared 1575.

Li Gao (李杲). *Book of Dongyuan* (*Dongyuanshu* 東垣書). Shanghai: Shanghai Shougu Book Store, 1929. First appeared 1529.

Liu Wansu (劉完素). *Profound Ideas and Etiology Based on Plain Question* (*Suwen Xuanji Yuanbingshi* 素問玄機原病式). Beijing: People's Health Press, 1983. First appeared 1186.

Lou Ying (樓英). *Compendium of Medicine* (*Yixue Gangmu* 醫學綱目). Beijing: People's Health Press, 1987. First appeared 1565.

Meng Xian (孟詵). *Dietetic Materia Medica* (*Shiliao Bencao* 食療本草). Beijing: People's Health Press, 1984. First appeared 704.

Shennong's Materia Medica (*Shennong Bencaojing* 神農本草經). Beijing: People' s Health Press, 1963.

Sun Si-miao (孫思邈). *Prescription Worth a Thousand Gold Pieces* (*Qianjinfang* 千金方). Taipei: Nanjing Traditional Chinese Medical Research Bureau, 1965. First appeared 652 A.D.

Wang Haogu (王好古). *Materia Medica of Decoction* (*Tangye Bencao* 湯液本草). Beijing: People' s Health Press, 1987. First appeared 1289.

Wang Shu-he (王叔和). *Classic of Pulse* (*Maijing* 脈經). Hong Kong: Taiping Book Publishers, 1961. First appeared 280 A.D.

Wei Yilin (危亦林). *Effective Formulas Tested by Physicians for Generations* (*Shiyi Dexiaofang* 世醫得效方). Shanghai: Shanghai Science and Technology Press, 1964. First appeared 1337.

Xu Shu-wei (許叔微). *Effective Prescriptions for Universal Relief* (*Puji Benshifang* 普濟本事方). Shanghai: Shanghai Science and Technology Press, 1978. First appeared 1132.

Yellow Emperor's Canon of Internal Medicine: Miraculous Pivot with Annotations (*Huangdi Neijing Lingshu Jiaoshi* 黃帝內經靈樞校釋). Edited by Hebei Medical College. Beijing: :eople' s Health Press, 1982.

Yellow Emperor's Canon of Internal Medicine:Plain Questions with Annotations (*Huangdi Neijing Suwen Jiaoshi* 黃帝內經素問校釋). Edited by Shandong Traditional Chinese Medical Collage and Hebei Medical College. Beijing: People' s Health Press, 1982.

Yu Tuan (虞博). *Orthodox Medical Record* (*Yixue Zhengzhuan* 醫學正傳). Beijing: People' s Health Press, 1965. First appeared 1515.

Zhu Gong (朱肱). *Book for Saving Life* (*Huorenshu* 活人書). Beijing: People' s Health Press, 1993. First appeared 1107.

Zhu Zhenheng (朱震亨). *Danxi's Experiential Therapy* (*Danxi Xinfa* 丹溪心法). Shanghai: Shanghai Science and Technology Press, 1959. First appeared 1601.

(English-Language)

Legge, James. *Book of Changes* (周易), The Chinese-English Bilingual Series of Chinese Classics. Zhangsha, China: Hunan Publishing House, 1992.

Legge, James. *The Four Books* (四書), The Chinese-English Bilingual Series of Chinese Classics. Zhangsha, China: Hunan Publishing House, 1992.

Luo Xiwen (羅希文), trans. and comp. *Treatise on Cold-induced Diseases* (傷寒論) *with*

500 Cases. Beijing, China: New World Press, 1993.

Xu Yuanchong (許淵沖). *Book of Poetry* (詩經), The Chinese-English Bilingual Series of Chinese Classics. Zhangsha, China: Hunan Publishing House, 1992.

Contemporary Sources

(Korean-Language)

Choi Seung-hoon (崔昇勳). *Pathology of Yellow Emperor's Canon of Internal Medicine* (內經病理學). Seoul: Tongnamu Press, 1993.

Lee Eul-ho (李乙浩) and Hong Soon-yong(洪淳用). *The Principle of Sasang Constitutional Medicine* (四象醫學原論). Seoul: Soomoon Press, 1973.

(Chinese-Language)

Joseon Medicine (朝醫學) as a series of Encyclopedia of Chinese Medicine. Shanghai: Shanghai Science and Technology Press, 1992.

Joseon Medicine (朝醫學). Edited and printed by the Institute of Traditional Medicine in Yanbian Joseon Racial Autonomous Region. Yanbian, 1985.

(English-Language)

Beith, Ilza. *The Yellow Emperor's Classic of Internal Medicine*. Berkeley and Los Angeles, California: University of California Press, 1972.

Chan Wingtsit (陳筝捷), trans. and comp. *A Source Book in Chinese Philosophy*. Princeton, N.J.: Princeton University Press, Princeton Paperbacks, 1963.

Fung Yulan (馮友蘭). *A History of Chinese Philosophy*. vol. I. Translated by Derk Bodde. Princeton, N.J.: Princeton University Press, 1953.

Ou Ming et al. (歐明 等). *Chinese-English Manual of Common-Used Prescriptions in Traditional Chinese Medicine*. Hong Kong: Joint Publishing Co., 1989.

Wiseman, Nigel et al. *Fundamentals of Chinese Medicine*. Taipei, Taiwan: Southern Materials Center, Inc., 1986.

World Health Organization, Western Pacific Regional Office. *WHO International Standard Terminologies on Traditional Medicine in the Western Pacific Region*. Manila, Philippines, 2007.

Xie Zhufan et al. (謝竹藩 等). *Classified Dictionary of Traditional Chinese Medicine*. Beijing, China: New World Press, 1994.

Index

General Terms

E

M

N

O

R

S

Prescription

C

D

E

F

G

H

J

K

L

M

N

P

Q

R

S

T

V

W

X

Y

Z

Drugs

A

B

C

Persons

Books